OXFORD MEDICAL PUBLICATIONS

Operative Surgery

Operative Surgery

Second edition

Edited by

Greg R. McLatchie
Professor of Sports Medicine and Surgical Sciences,
University of Sunderland, UK

David J. Leaper
Emeritus Professor of Surgery,
University of Newcastle upon Tyne, UK

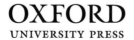

OXFORD
UNIVERSITY PRESS

Great Clarendon Street, Oxford OX2 6DP

Oxford University Press is a department of the University of Oxford.
It furthers the University's objective of excellence in research, scholarship,
and education by publishing worldwide in

Oxford New York

Auckland Cape Town Dar es Salaam Hong Kong Karachi
Kuala Lumpur Madrid Melbourne Mexico City Nairobi
New Delhi Shanghai Taipei Toronto

With offices in

Argentina Austria Brazil Chile Czech Republic France Greece
Guatemala Hungary Italy Japan Poland Portugal Singapore
South Korea Switzerland Thailand Turkey Ukraine Vietnam

Oxford is a registered trade mark of Oxford University Press
in the UK and in certain other countries

Published in the United States
by Oxford University Press Inc., New York

British Library Cataloguing in Publication Data
Data available

Library of Congress Cataloging in Publication Data
Data available

Typeset by Newgen Imaging Systems (P) Ltd., Chennai, India
Printed in Italy
on acid-free paper by Legoprint S.p.A.

ISBN 0–19–851056–X (flexicover: alk.paper)   978–0–19–851056–7 (flexicover: alk.paper)

10 9 8 7 6 5 4 3 2 1

Preface to first edition

This book is a practical guide for the surgeon or surgical trainee about to perform or assist at an operation. The procedures described are those commonly carried out in general, urological, and orthopaedic surgical practice with an introduction on perioperative management and anaesthetics. These should also prove of interest to operating department nurses, assistants, and students of medicine. Indications for and complications of procedures are given but more extensive descriptions of these can be found in surgical text books to which the reader should refer.

We emphasize that the book is not for the first-time operator nor does it embrace the philosophy of 'see one, do one, teach one'. Anyone aspiring to be a surgeon must acquire the basic skills of safe knot-tying and familiarity with surgical instruments. Only by witnessing, assisting at, and then performing many procedures within the structure of a formal surgical training course can the trainee develop the skill, judgement, and the ability to select patients correctly—the recipe for safe surgery.

GRM
Hartlepool
DJL
Stockton on Tees
1996

Preface to second edition

The text and increased numbers of contributors reflect the changes that have occurred in General Surgery over the past ten years. It is unlikely that in the future we will encounter General Surgical Units. They will be replaced by specialised departments catering for specific areas of surgical expertise. These changes will also fashion future editions of this text in that almost every chapter will become a handbook in itself and the training of surgeons become significantly changed.

GRM
DL
North Tees and Hartlepool NHS Trust
April 2006

Dedications

For Ross, Cameron, Ailidh, Claire, Calum, Charles, Alice, Stephen, Rebecca, and Amy

Acknowledgements

We are grateful to all who have helped us to produce this book, in particular the staff of Oxford University Press. We thank Luca Di Franco for some of the illustrations and Paul Rodgers who took photographs. Staff on the Surgical Wards at the University Hospital of Hartlepool; Debbie Blackwood, Dean Trainer, Nicola Jones and Elizabeth Redden, deserve special mention, as does Anneli Thornton who prepared the manuscript.

Contributors

Mr A. K. Agarwal
Consultant Surgeon,
North Tees & Hartlepool
NHS Trust

Mr S. Aspinall
Specialist Registrar,
Northern Deanery

Professor B. S. Avery
Consultant Oral &
Maxillofacial Surgeon,
James Cook University Hospital,
Middlesbrough

Mr R. Carter
Lister Department of
Pancreatico-biliary surgery,
Glasgow Royal Infirmary

Mr A. E. Clason
Consultant Vascular Surgeon,
James Cook University Hospital,
Middlesbrough

Mr F. Di Franco
Specialist Registrar,
Northern Deanery

A. J. Dickenson
Consultant Maxillofacial Surgeon

Mr. S. Dresner
Consultant Surgeon,
James Cook University Hospital,
Middlesbrough

Mr H. El-Khalifa
Associate Specialist,
North Tees & Hartlepool
NHS Trust

Mr M. El-Sheikh
Consultant Surgeon,
Nottingham City Hospital
NHS Trust

Mr T. Friesem
Consultant Spinal Surgeon,
North Tees & Hartlepool
NHS Trust

Mr A. Gilliam
Specialist Registrar,
Northern Deanery

Mr C. Harding
Consultant Urologist,
North Tees & Hartlepool
NHS Trust

Mr L. Horgan
Consultant Surgeon,
Upper GI and Laproscopic
Surgical Unit,
North Tyneside General
Hospital

Professor C. W. Imrie
Lister Department of
Pancreatico-biliary Surgery,
Glasgow Royal Infirmary

Dr P. Kalia
Consultant Anaesthetist,
North Tees & Hartlepool
NHS Trust

Mr V. J. Kurup
Consultant Surgeon,
North Tees & Hartlepool
NHS Trust

Mr Q. King
Consultant Urologist,
North Tees & Hartlepool
NHS Trust

Professor David J. Leaper
Emeritus Professor of Surgery,
North Tees & Hartlepool
NHS Trust

Mr P. A. Lear
Consultant Vascular and
Transplant Surgeon,
North Bristol NHS Trust

Professor T. Lennard
School of Surgical and
Reproductive Sciences,
Newcastle upon Tyne

Professor G. R. McLatchie
Consultant Surgeon,
North Tees & Hartlepool
NHS Trust

Dr D. Monkhouse
Specialist Registrar,
Anaesthetics,
Northern Deanery

A. N. Morritt
Consultant Cardiothoracic
Surgeon,
James Cook University Hospital,
Middlesbrough

Mr G. O'Dair
Specialist Registrar
Northern Deanery

Mr P. Raine
Royal Hospital for Sick Children,
Glasgow

Mr S. Rawat
Upper GI and Laparoscopic
Surgical Unit,
North Tyneside General Hospital

Mr C. M. S. Royston
Department of General Surgery,
Hull Royal Infirmary

Mr J. Shenfine
Specialist Registrar

Mr D. Southward
Consultant in Accident &
Emergency,
North Tees & Hartlepool
NHS Trust

Mr Y. K. S. Visnarath
Consultant Surgeon,
James Cook University
Hospital,
Middlesbrough

Mr G. Walker
Specialist Registrar in Paediatric
Surgery,
Glasgow

Contents

Symbols and abbreviations

>	greater than
<	less than
↑	increased
↓	decreased
±	and/or
≥	greater than or equal to
A&E	accident and emergency
ABC	airway, breathing, circulation
ABPI	Association of the British Pharmaceutical Industry
ACE	angiotensin-converting enzyme
ACTH	adrenocorticotropic hormone
AGNB	aerobic Gram-negative bacilli
AJCC	American Joint Committee on Cancer
APE	abdomino-perineal excision
APLS	antiphospholipid antibody syndrome
APTTR	activated partial thromboplastin time ratio
ARDS	acute respiratory distress syndrome
ASIS	American Society for Information Science or anterior superior iliac spine
ATLS	advanced trauma life support
BKA	below knee amputation
BMI	body mass index
Bpm	beats per minute
BXO	balanitis xerotica obliterans
CBD	chronic beryllium disease
CCF	congestive cardiac failure
CCU	Coronary Care Unit
CDH	congenital diaphragmatic hernia
CJD	Creutzfeld–Jakob disease
CMV	cytomegalovirus
CNS	central nervous system or coagulase negative staphylococcus
COH	congenital diaphragmatic hernia
CRF	chronic renal failure

CSF	cerebrospinal fluid
CT	computed tomography
CVP	central venous pressure
CXR	chest X-ray
DGF	delayed graft function
DJ	duodenal-jejunal
DPL	diagnostic peritoneal lavage
DVT	deep vein thrombosis
EBV	Epstein–Barr virus
ECG	electrocardiogram
EHL	extensor hallucis longus
EMLA	entectic mixture of local anaesthetic
ENT	ear, nose, throat
ERCP	endoscopic retrograde cholangio-pancreatography
ESWL	extracorporeal shockwave lithotripsy
EUA	examination under anaesthetic
EUS	endoscopic ultrasound
FBC	full blood count
FEV_1	forced expiratory volume (in 1 second)
FHL	familial erythrophagocytic lymphohistiocytosis or flexor hallucis longus
FNAC	fine needle aspiration cytology
FVC	forced expiratory vital capacity
GERD	gastrooesophageal reflux disease
GJ	gastro-jejunal
GKI	glucose/potassium/insulin
GOJ	gastro-oesophageal junction
GOS	Great Ormond Street
H&P	history and physical examination
HDU	high dependency unit
Hib	*Haemophilus influenza* type b
HIV	human immunodeficiency virus
HLA	human leucocyte antigen
HRT	hormone replacement therapy
HSV	herpes simplex virus
ICU	intensive care unit
IL-1	interleukin 1
IM	intramuscular

IMA	inferior mesenteric artery
IMV	inferior mesenteric vein
INR	international normalized ratio
IPF	initial poor function
IPMT	intraductal papillary mucinous tumour
ITU	intensive therapy unit
IVC	inferior vena cava
JVP	jugular vein catheterization
kPa	kilo Pascals
LES	lower esophageal sphincter
LFT	liver function tests
LIF	left iliac fossa
LMU	lower, middle, upper
LMWH	low molecular weight heparin
LOS	lower oesophageal sphincter
LSV	long saphenous vein
LUS	laproscopic ultrasonography
MAO-A	monoamine oxidase A
MI	myocardial infarction
MIBG	meta iodo benzyl guanidine
MIBI	myocardial perfusion imaging
MIDN	minimally invasive donor nephrectomy
MITS	minimally invasive thoracoscopic splanchnicectomy
MOA	monoamine oxidase inhibitors
MRCP	magnetic resonance cholangio-pancreatography
MRI	magnetic resonance imaging
MRSA	methicillin-resistant *Staphylococcus aureus*
NG	naso-gastric
NHB	non-heart beating
OA	oesophageal atresia
OGD	oesophagogastroduodenoscopy
OTE	otitis media with effusion
PAC	pulmonary artery catheterization
PAIs	plasminogen activator inhibitor
PAK	pancreas after kidney
PALS	paediatric advanced life support
PCA	patient-controlled analgesia

PCNL	percutaneous nephrolithotomy
PE	pulmonary embolism
PEEP	positive end expiratory pressure
per anum	though the anus
PNF	primary non-function
PONV	postoperative nausea and vomiting
PPPD	pylorus preserving pancreatico-duodenectomy
PSARP	posterior sagittal anorectoplasty
PT	prothrombin time
PTA	pancreas transplantation alone
PTFE	polytetrafluoroethylene
PTH	parathormone
PTLD	post-transplant lymphoproliferative disease
PTT	partial thromboplastin time
PUJ	pelviureteric junction
PVC	polyvinylchloride
RA	right atrium
RCC	renal cell carcinoma
RI	resistance index
RIF	right iliac fossa
RIND	reversible ischaemic neurological deficit
RSTL	relaxed skin tension line
rTPA	recombinant tissue plasminogen activator
SAGB	Swedish adjustable gastric band
SEPS	subfascial endoscopic perforator surgery
SFA	superficial femoral artery
SMA	superior mesenteric artery
SMV	superior mesenteric vein
SPK	simultaneous pancreas-kidney
SSRIs	selective serotonin reuptake inhibitors
SSSI	superficial surgical site infection
SVC	superior vena cava
TAPP	transabdominal preperitoneal
TB	tuberculosis
TBSA	total body surface area
TCC	transitional cell carcinoma
TED	thromboembolic deterrent

TEP	totally extraperitoneal
TNF	tumour necrosis factor
TOF	tetralogy of Fallot
TOR	target of rapamycin
tPA	tissue plasminogen activator
TRAM	tranverse rectus abdominis myocutaneous
TURBT	transurethral resection of bladder tumour
TURP	transurethral resection of prostate
U	units
ULTRA	Unrelated Live Transplant Regulatory Authority
UTI	urinary tract infection
UVPPP	uvulopalatopharyngoplasty
VATS	video assisted thoracic surgery
VT	ventricular tachycardia
YAG	yttrium aluminum garnet

Perioperative anaesthetic care and practical procedures

P. Kalia and D. Monkhouse

Preoperative evaluation

Assessment of the patient before elective inpatient, day case, or emergency surgery is mandatory. Unnecessary cancellations are thereby avoided. Lack of preoperative assessment increases the risks associated with anaesthetics and surgery. The main goals of the preoperative visit are to:

- Establish rapport with the patient besides allaying apprehensions and anxieties.
- Assess fitness for anaesthesia and surgery by detailed history, physical examination, and laboratory investigations.
- Control of medical conditions before elective surgery.
- Plan the anaesthetic technique.
- Discuss options with the patient (general versus local anaesthesia).
- Prescribe premedication and drugs that need to be continued or stopped.
- Plan postoperative care, including pain relief, HDU, or ICU care.
- Obtain informed consent.

Airway assessment
Factors leading to difficult intubation should be identified. Assessment of the airway is the most important part of preoperative assessment, as failure to maintain the airway can result in life-threatening hypoxia. Any past history of a difficult intubation should be documented. Obesity, short neck, limited neck movement, decreased mouth opening, prominent upper incisors, micrognathia, congenital abnormalities (cystic hygroma, Pierre Robin, and Treacher Collins syndrome), and facial trauma can lead to difficult intubation. A thyromental distance of less than 6.5cm can be indicative of a difficult intubation.

Respiratory system
Patients with pre-existing lung disease (such as chronic obstructive airway disease or asthma) and poor lung function have a higher incidence of postoperative pulmonary complications. Upper respiratory tract infection should be treated before elective surgery. Asthmatic patients have increased airway reactivity and can develop acute bronchospasm during laryngoscopy or intubation. Local or regional anaesthesia may be a safer option.

Cardiovascular system
A detailed history should be taken regarding dyspnoea, angina, palpitations, orthopnoea and paroxysmal nocturnal dyspnoea. The patient's functional capacity should be determined as this correlates well with maximum oxygen uptake on treadmill testing and can be prognostically significant. Physical examination should include assessment of heart rate and rhythm with measurement of blood pressure and JVP. The chest should be auscultated to detect murmurs or additional heart sounds.

Myocardial infarction (MI) and congestive cardiac failure (CCF)

A history of recent MI or CCF places the patient in a high-risk category. This necessitates full investigation and treatment prior to elective surgery. The incidence of reinfarction following surgery has been reported to range from 0–37% depending on the timing of surgery relative to MI. Surgery performed 3–6 months after MI is associated with a reinfarction rate of 15%. Mortality from postoperative infarction is in the order of 40–60%. Consequently, *elective* surgery should be deferred until 6 months after a MI.

Patients with symptomatic coronary artery disease should be investigated preoperatively to stratify risk. Exercise stress testing and angiography may be of value in deciding whether the patient will benefit from coronary revascularisation prior to elective general surgery. The duration and type of surgery is also important. Vascular surgery carries a higher risk of perioperative MI (10.9%) than abdominal surgery (4.3%).

Hypertension

Affected patients should be assessed for adequacy of control and involvement of target organs (heart and kidney). Patients with uncontrolled hypertension exhibit wide fluctuations of blood pressure intraoperatively because of increased reactivity of blood vessels to sympathetic stimulation. Wide swings of blood pressure can precipitate myocardial ischaemia or stroke.

Valvular and congenital heart disease

Patients with either valvular pathology or congenital heart disease present a major anaesthetic challenge. The exact nature of the cardiac problems should be known preoperatively and the condition optimised. Concurrent problems such as chest infection and cardiac failure should be treated aggressively. These patients are at risk of acquiring infective endocarditis and prophylactic antibiotic administration is mandatory.

Diabetes mellitus

Diabetic control should be assessed. Random blood glucose levels are of limited value. Glycosylated haemoglobin levels are preferable. Patients should be assessed for complications of diabetes such as hypertension, ischaemic heart disease, renal disease, infection and autonomic and peripheral neuropathy. Preoperative assessment should be geared towards optimising perioperative blood glucose control and minimising complications associated with the coexisting pathologies.

Renal system

There is a broad clinical spectrum of disease from mild renal dysfunction to end-stage renal failure. Patients with preoperative renal dysfunction are more likely to develop postoperative renal failure, particularly after aortic or cardiac surgery.

Anaemia, hypertension, ischaemic heart disease and diabetes may complicate the picture. Care should be exercised when administering drugs requiring renal metabolism or excretion. This has a major impact upon the choice of anaesthetic agents and provision of postoperative analgesia. Meticulous attention to fluid and electrolyte balance is essential.

Hepatic system

Patients with liver dysfunction represent a high-risk group for anaesthesia. They must be fully assessed and optimised prior to theatre. Preoperative clinical assessment should be geared towards detecting jaundice, ascites and signs of decompensated liver disease. All medication administered should take into account altered drug handling. Correction of coagulopathy may be required. Deranged electrolytes and acid–base balance are common findings. Deeply jaundiced patients may require preoperative hydration and mannitol to reduce the risk of postoperative renal failure.

Haemopoetic system

Anaemia should be treated preoperatively before elective surgery as oxygen carrying capacity is decreased. Haemoglobin values of 10g/dL are acceptable as decreased blood viscosity improves blood flow with a consequent increase in oxygen delivery to the tissues. In patients with chronic anaemia, haemoglobin values of 8g/dL are satisfactory as there is an increase in 2,3 diphosphoglycerate which causes a right shift in the oxygen dissociation curve promoting release of oxygen at tissue level.

Patients of certain ethnic origin or with a family history of haemoglobinopathy should have haemoglobin estimation and electrophoresis performed. If scheduled for emergency surgery, a Sickledex test should be used for screening and followed by electrophoresis if positive to distinguish between sickle cell disease and trait.

Pregnancy

Elective surgery is best delayed until the second trimester of pregnancy because of potentially detrimental effects on the fetus during organogenesis. In addition, conditions requiring abdominal surgery are associated with an increased risk of premature labour or miscarriage.

From 16 weeks onwards there is an increased risk of acid aspiration during anaesthesia. Hypotension can occur due to aortocaval compression if the patient is placed in supine position.

Social history

Smoking decreases the oxygen carrying capacity, increases irritability of airway and decreases ciliary function. Ideally smoking should be stopped 4–6 weeks prior to surgery. Cessation of smoking 24 hours before surgery increases oxygen carrying capacity as carbon monoxide is rapidly eliminated.

Chronic alcoholics require increased doses of anaesthetics drugs due to enzyme induction.

Substance abuse may present problems in the form of difficult venous access, high risk of hepatitis and HIV, resistance to intravenous anaesthetic agents, opiate analgesia and acute withdrawal states.

Family history

There are several genetically inherited diseases that influence anaesthetic management, notably malignant hyperthermia, suxemethonium apnoea, porphyria, and myotonic dystrophy. A detailed family history should be taken preoperatively to allow conduct of a safe, appropriate anaesthetic technique.

Laboratory investigations

Most fit patients (ASA 1) undergoing minor surgery do not need any investigations.
- Haemoglobin should be checked in female patients of reproductive age group and clinically anaemic patients.
- Full blood count, urea and electrolytes should be checked in patients with cardiac, respiratory, or renal disease and in patients on digoxin, diuretics, and ACE inhibitors.
- Patients with a history of liver disease or heavy alcohol consumption should have liver function tests performed.
- A coagulation screen should be checked on all patients with impaired liver function, coagulopathies and those treated with anticoagulants.
- Chest X-ray and ECG should be performed in patients with a history of respiratory or cardiac disease respectively.
- Patients with symptomatic pulmonary disease should be subjected to spirometry and blood gas analysis. Obstructive lung disease can be differentiated from restrictive lung disease by measuring the FEV_1/FVC ratio.

Preoperative medication—continue or stop?

It is important to review the prescribed medications. The surgical team and ward staff must be aware of which medications to continue and which to stop in the preoperative period. Lack of knowledge can lead to dangerous consequences.

Medications to be continued

- **Cardiovascular medication** such as calcium channel blockers, β blockers, nitrates, and antiarrhythmic agents should be continued as sudden withdrawal can precipitate hypertension, ischaemia, and myocardial infarction.
- **Bronchodilators** should be continued as withdrawal can precipitate bronchospasm.
- **Antiepileptic** treatment should be continued.
- **Steroid** intake can cause adrenal suppression. History of steroid intake (prednisolone 10mg or more) within the last three months requires hydrocortisone supplementation perioperatively.
- **Aspirin** inhibits platelet function and is the mainstay of secondary prevention in patients with history of myocardial infarction or stroke. It should be continued unless major bleeding is expected (cardiac or prostate surgery) or minor bleeding is best avoided (retinal or intra cranial surgery). The risk of bleeding should be weighed against the risk of precipitating a thromboembolic event.

Medications to be stopped

- **Anticoagulants** Warfarin should be stopped at least four days before surgery as these patients are at increased risk of bleeding. The effect of warfarin can be reversed with vitamin K (or fresh frozen plasma in an emergency). An International Normalised Ratio (INR) of 1.5–2 is acceptable. In patients with a high risk of thromboembolism, a continuous intravenous infusion of unfractionated heparin should be commenced at 1000 U/hour and the rate adjusted to keep APTTR between 1.5–2.5. This should be stopped 6 hours before surgery, recommenced 12 hours post surgery and continued until warfarin is reinstituted and INR >2.0. For patients with a low risk of thrombo-embolism, the use of subcutaneous low molecular weight heparin is recommended until warfarin therapy can be restarted and INR >2.0.
- **Anticoagulants and central neuraxial block (spinal and epidural)** These techniques should be avoided in patients with a coagulopathy or those on warfarin therapy. In patients requiring DVT prophylaxis, a spinal or epidural can be performed six hours after subcutaneous injection of unfractionated heparin and 12 hours after low molecular weight heparin. Aspirin is not a contraindication to use these blocks.

- **ACE inhibitors and angiotensin II receptor antagonists** may be associated with severe hypotension on induction or during maintenance of anaesthesia. These drugs are usually stopped 24 hours prior to surgery.
- **Oral hypoglycaemic agents** like chlorpropamide and metformin should be stopped 48 hours before surgery. Long-acting agents should be substituted by short-acting drugs like gliclazide. For minor surgery, it is acceptable to omit the morning dose of oral hypoglycaemic agent. However, a GKI infusion is required for those undergoing major surgery and patients with poor preoperative glycaemic control.
- **Contraceptive pill and anaesthesia** Synthetic oestrogens increase the risk of thromboembolism by increasing the activity of clotting factors. Oestrogen-only and the combined pill should be stopped four weeks before elective surgery; other forms of contraception should be offered. Heparin should be given if emergency surgery is contemplated. The progestogen-only pill and HRT do not need to be discontinued.
- **Monoamine oxidase inhibitors** should be discontinued two weeks before elective surgery. They can precipitate a fatal reaction if used concurrently with indirectly acting vasopressors (ephedrine) or pethidine. The reaction occurs as a consequence of excessive levels of monoamines and inhibition of hepatic enzymes. Non-selective MAO inhibitors (phenelzine, and tranylcypromine) can be replaced with meclobemide, a short acting selective inhibitor of MAO-A. Meclobemide can be stopped 12 hours before surgery.
- **Selective serotonin reuptake inhibitors (SSRIs)** lack anticholinergic effects and are frequently used as alternative to tricyclic antidepressants. Fluoxetine and paroxetine increase serotonergic transmission. When concurrent serotonergic medications such as pethidine, tramadol, and pentazocine are used, a fatal serotonin syndrome can occur (hypertension, fever, hyperreflexia, and coma).

Intraoperative complications

Most intraoperative problems are foreseeable and preventable. They are minimised by a thorough preoperative assessment of the patient, meticulous checking of anaesthetic equipment and use of appropriate anaesthetic and surgical techniques by suitably skilled personnel. Intraoperative problems occur in 9% of all patients undergoing surgery.

The risks of intraoperative complications can be related to:

Patient factors
- Extremes of age
- Morbid obesity
- Nature of underlying disease process
- Co-existing morbidity.

Surgical factors
- Complexity, timing, and duration of operation
- Urgency of procedure
- Experience of surgeon.

Anaesthetic factors
- Adequacy of preoperative preparation
- Lack of appropriate monitoring
- Urgency of anaesthesia
- Experience of anaesthetist.

Should an adverse event occur, it is imperative that it is promptly recognised and effectively managed to minimise the risk to the patient.

Cardiovascular problems

Hypotension during surgery may be defined as a fall in systolic blood pressure in excess of 25% of the patient's preoperative value. This may result in inadequate tissue perfusion, ischaemia, and ultimately organ dysfunction.

The causes of hypotension are usually multifactorial and are often confounded by hypovolaemia due to inadequate preoperative fluid replacement or excess intraoperative loss.

Immediate management involves confirmation of the blood pressure reading, delivery of a high concentration of oxygen, and implementation of measures to restore cardiac output (fluid bolus, head down tilt, reduction in concentration of anaesthetic agents or administration of vasopressor agents). In most instances, these measures are adequate to restore BP. If hypotension persists despite these measures, causes such as pneumothorax, myocardial ischaemia, embolism, and anaphylaxis should be considered. Subsequent management should be directed towards correcting the underlying problem.

Hypertension during surgery may be defined as an increase in systolic pressure in excess of 25% of the patient's preoperative value. This results in increased myocardial workload and hence oxygen demand. If myocardial oxygen supply is inadequate to meet demand, then ischaemia ensues. Hypertension also results in increased risk of cerebrovascular events.

The use of perioperative beta-blockade may circumvent this problem. Immediate management should involve a systematic search for the underlying cause. If hypertension persists, the alternative options include increasing the depth of anaesthesia and/or analgesia and administration of alpha-blockers, beta-blockers or vasodilators.

Bradycardia may be defined as a heart rate of <60bpm. It is commonly seen during anaesthesia, particularly in young healthy adults or where opioids are used as part of the anaesthetic. Surgical procedures which increase vagal tone may also produce bradycardia, for example, cervical dilatation, anal stretch, traction on extraocular muscles, and peritoneal traction.

   Treatment is reserved for clinically significant bradycardias where there is a reduction in cardiac output or where escape beats are seen on the ECG. Treatment options include anticholinergics such as glycopyrrolate and atropine. For refractory bradycardia with haemodynamic compromise, it may be necessary to use either an isoprenaline infusion or a temporary transvenous cardiac pacing wire.

Causes of intraoperative hypotension

Decreased preload

• Hypovolaemia	Dehydration/inadequate replacement
	Haemorrhage
	Gastrointestinal losses
	Insensible or third space losses
• Obstructed venous return	Embolism (thrombus, gas, fat, air)
	Aorto–caval compression
	Pericardial tamponade
• Increased intra-thoracic pressure	Positive pressure ventilation
	Pneumothorax

Decreased afterload

• Drugs	Induction agents
	Volatile agents
	Antihypertensives
	Histamine release
	Anaphylaxis/hypersensitivity reactions
• Anaesthetic technique	Spinal anaesthesia
	Epidural anaesthesia
• Sepsis	

Decreased contractility

• Drugs	Anaesthetic agents
	Beta-blockers
	Calcium antagonists
• Myocardial ischaemia	
• Acidosis	
• Arrhythmias	

Causes of intraoperative hypertension

Patient factors
- Pre-existing hypertension
- Raised intracranial pressure
- Pre-eclampsia
- Rebound hypertension (cessation of therapy)
- Phaeochromocytoma
- Thyroid storm

Surgical factors
- Prolonged tourniquet time
- Aortic-cross clamping
- Post-myocardial revascularisation
- Bladder distension

Anaesthetic factors
- Inadequate depth of anaesthesia
- Inadequate analgesia
- Hypoxaemia
- Hypercapnia
- Instrumentation of airway
- Hypothermia
- Malignant hyperthermia
- Hypervolaemia

Tachycardia may be defined as a heart rate of >100bpm. It can occur as a normal physiological response to sympathetic stimulation or as part of a pathological process such as sepsis, burns, hyperthyroidism or malignant hyperthermia. Increased sympathetic tone can be exacerbated by hypoxaemia, hypercapnia, hypotension, hypovolaemia and inadequate anaesthesia/analgesia. Treatment involves correction of the underlying cause. Pharmacological intervention may be required if persistent tachycardia produces myocardial ischaemia.

Arrhythmias occur frequently in the intraoperative period. They can be precipitated by the following:
- Hypoxaemia
- Hypercapnia
- Hypo/hyperkalaemia
- Myocardial ischaemia
- Surgical stimulation and light anaesthesia
- Deep inhalational anaesthesia, particularly halothane
- Central venous cannulation
- Mediastinal manipulation
- Chronotropic drugs, particularly epinephrine.

General management

- Correct the cause (hypoxia, hypercarbia, electrolyte imbalance, and acidosis).
- Inform the surgeon to stop the surgery as reflex bradycardia can occur during various procedures such as eye surgery, mesenteric traction, anal stretch, and laparoscopic procedures.
- Correct the hypotension.

Specific management

Aggressive management is required in the presence of haemodynamic instability. Specific treatment of various arrhythmias is described below.

Supraventricular arrhythmias

Atrial fibrillation. ECG shows loss of P waves with complete irregularity of the QRS complex. Because atrial contraction contributes up to 30% of the normal ventricular filling, the onset of AF often produces a marked fall in cardiac output.

Treatment

- Amiodarone to slow down the ventricular rate and chemically cardiovert.
- Digoxin to slow ventricular rate.
- Flecainide to restore sinus rhythm (but caution with LV dysfunction).
- Synchronised DC cardioversion in event of haemodynamic compromise.

Atrial flutter is seen in the intraoperative period as a paroxysmal arrhythmia precipitated by anaesthesia and surgery in a susceptible individual. ECG shows the classical 'saw-tooth' pattern of flutter waves.

Treatment

- Synchronised DC shock in an anaesthetised patient with any degree of cardiovascular compromise is the first-line treatment.
- Digoxin or amiodarone infusion would be an alternative.

Junctional/AV nodal tachycardias. ECG shows a narrow complex tachycardia with ventricular rate of 150–200/minute. A broad complex pattern may be seen if there is antegrade conduction down an accessory pathway.

Treatment

- Synchronised DC shock in a haemodynamically compromised patient.
- Carotid sinus massage or vagal manoeuvres may slow the rate to reveal the underlying rhythm.
- Adenosine slows atrioventricular conduction and is particularly useful for terminating the re-entry tachycardia of Wolff–Parkinson–White syndrome.
- Verapamil, beta-blockers or amiodarone may improve rate control or convert to sinus rhythm.

Ventricular arrhythmias

Ventricular tachycardia. The ECG shows a broad complex tachycardia with capture and fusion beats.

Treatment
- Synchronised DC shock is the first-line treatment of VT with cardiovascular compromise. Synchronisation is not required if the VT is very rapid or the patient is pulseless.
- Amiodarone is the first line pharmacological agent.

Ventricular fibrillation
There is chaotic ventricular contraction with no identifiable QRS complexes on ECG.

Treatment
This should be promptly managed with DC cardioversion according to the European Resuscitation Council guidelines.

Myocardial ischaemia occurs when myocardial oxygen demand exceeds supply. Oxygen supply to the myocardium is determined by coronary blood flow and oxygen content. Demand is determined by heart rate, contractility and wall tension. Tachycardia is the most important determinant of the supply/demand ratio because it causes a reduction in diastolic coronary filling, with a simultaneous increase in myocardial work. Patients most at risk perioperatively are those with a recent MI, poorly controlled angina, decompensated heart failure or severe valvular disease. Monitoring susceptible patients with a V5 ECG electrode and with continuous ST segment analysis will improve ischaemia detection rates. Intraoperative management should be geared towards ensuring adequate arterial oxygenation, maintaining normocapnia, normotension, and avoidance of tachycardia whilst ensuring adequate depth of anaesthesia and effective analgesia. The use of glyceryl trinitrate as a coronary vasodilator may be necessary if ischaemic changes persist.

Respiratory complications
Hypoxaemia can be defined as an arterial oxygen tension of <8kPa and causes specific to the intraoperative period are:

Equipment problems
- Oxygen supply failure
- Delivery of a hypoxic mixture
- Obstruction or leak in anaesthetic circuit
- Disconnection
- Ventilator failure
- Misplaced or obstructed endotracheal tube.

Patient factors
- Hypoventilation in a spontaneously breathing patient
- Increased airway resistance (bronchospasm, laryngospasm, anaphylaxis)
- Aspiration of gastric contents
- Atelectasis
- Pneumothorax
- Pulmonary oedema
- Embolus
- Low cardiac output state
- Increased oxygen demand (sepsis, malignant hyperthermia).

If hypoxaemia is detected, a systematic ABC approach should be adopted. Delivery of 100% oxygen (confirmed by oxygen analysis) is the first priority. Integrity of the breathing system should be confirmed by manual inflation of the lungs and checking for bilateral breath sounds and chest movement. The position and patency of the endotracheal tube should be confirmed. A search for clinical causes should then ensue with early exclusion of pneumothorax. Subsequent treatment is that of the underlying pathology.

Laryngospasm is a reflex, prolonged closure of the glottis by adduction of the vocal cords. It usually occurs in response to airway manipulation in the context of light anaesthesia. However, it may also occur in response to intense surgical stimulation such as incision and drainage of an abscess, peritoneal retraction, anal stretch or cervical dilatation. It occurs more commonly in smokers and those with recent upper respiratory tract infections because of increased airway reactivity. It may lead to complete or partial airway obstruction with resulting hypoxaemia and hypoventilation.

Management should include assessment of ABC followed by:
- Cessation of the provoking stimulus
- Administration of 100% oxygen
- Increase in depth of anaesthesia by intravenous route if necessary
- Laryngeal muscle relaxation with suxemethonium followed by ventilation with 100% and tracheal intubation if required.

Bronchospasm is an acute bronchoconstriction causing increased airway resistance, wheeze, and a prolonged expiratory phase of respiration. Susceptibility to bronchospasm during the intraoperative period is increased in smokers, asthmatics, and those with chronic obstructive pulmonary disease, a recent respiratory tract infection, or an atopic tendency.

Precipitating factors include:
- Surgical stimulation or airway manipulation during light anaesthesia
- Stimulation of the carina or bronchi by the tracheal tube
- Pharyngeal, laryngeal, or bronchial secretions or blood
- Aspiration of gastric contents
- Anaphylactic reactions
- Release of histamine
- Administration of beta-blockers.

Management aims are to maintain oxygenation, treat the underlying cause and reduce bronchoconstriction. 100% oxygen should be administered and the inspired concentration of volatile anaesthetic agent increased. The position and patency of the endotracheal tube should be checked. Bronchodilatation can be achieved by intravenous or nebulised salbutamol or by an intravenous infusion of aminophylline. Epinephrine is reserved for life-threatening emergencies.

Pneumothorax during the intraoperative period is rare but potentially life threatening. Patients with recent chest trauma, rib fractures, asthma, and chronic lung disease with bullae are most at risk. Iatrogenic causes include central venous cannulation, brachial plexus block, intercostal nerve block, tracheostomy, thoracic surgery, and barotrauma. Clinical signs include tachycardia, hypotension, hypoxaemia and high airway pressures. During anaesthesia, nitrous oxide can diffuse into air-filled spaces causing a pneumothorax to expand. Positive pressure ventilation also contributes to a rapid increase in size. If the pneumothorax is under tension, impaired venous return and cardiac output can precipitate cardiac arrest. Immediate management involves the ABC approach, cessation of nitrous oxide, delivery of 100% oxygen, and insertion of an intercostal drain. If the pneumothorax is under tension needle thoracocentesis should be performed prior to sitting an intercostal drain.

Embolism describes the entry of air/gas/thrombus/fat/amniotic fluid into the circulation usually via the venous route. This causes an obstruction to right ventricular outflow, reducing cardiac output and arterial blood pressure.

Risk factors for emboli include:
Anaesthetic factors
- Hypovolaemia
- Open central vascular access
- Pressurised infusions
- Prolonged use of a tourniquet
- Operation site higher than heart.

Surgical factors
- Multiple trauma
- Long bone surgery especially intramedullary nailing
- Hip and spinal surgery
- Laparoscopic procedures
- Neck surgery
- Vascular surgery
- Middle ear procedures.

Diagnosis is often difficult in the anaesthetised patient and relies upon a high degree of clinical suspicion in the context of tachycardia, hypoxaemia, and a fall in end-tidal carbon dioxide concentration. In the case of a large embolism, pulselessness and altered cardiac electrical activity may occur.

Management
- Follow the ABC approach.
- Maintain the airway, with 100% oxygen.
- Support the circulation with volume expansion and inotropes, to maintain the mean arterial pressure.
- In the event of gas/air embolism, subsequent management is aimed specifically at preventing further entry into the circulation. This may involve flooding the operative site with saline and covering it with wet gauze, compressing the major drainage vessels, lowering the operation site below the level of the heart or decompressing any gas-pressurised cavity.
- Gas can be aspirated from the right heart if a central venous catheter is in situ. Siting a central line for aspiration of gas is usually impractical, time consuming and not recommended.

Aspiration of gastric contents is a potential problem in all anaesthetised or unconscious patients as upper airway reflexes are depressed and lower oesophageal sphincter tone decreased.

Factors predisposing to aspiration include:
- Full stomach
- Known gastro-oesophageal reflux or hiatus hernia
- Raised intragastric pressure (gastrointestinal obstruction, pregnancy, laparoscopic surgery)
- Recent trauma
- Pain
- Opioid analgesia
- Diabetes mellitus
- Topically anaesthetised airway

Management of intraoperative aspiration should be aimed at minimising further regurgitation with clearance of gastric aspirate and subsequent airway protection. The patient should be placed in a left lateral head-down position, cricoid pressure applied and the trachea intubated. Gastric aspirate should be cleared by suctioning prior to initiation of positive pressure ventilation. Bronchoscopy ± bronchial lavage may be necessary to clear any remaining debris. If hypoxaemia ensues, ventilation with application of PEEP and delivery of high inspired oxygen concentrations may be required. Chest X-ray and blood gas analysis are mandatory. Respiratory support may need to be continued in ICU.

Adverse drug reactions

Anaphylaxis is an IgE mediated hypersensitivity reaction to an antigen which results in mast cell and basophil degranulation with release of histamine and serotonin. The incidence of anaphylaxis in anaesthetic practice is in the order of 1:10 000. It is more common in females and in patients with a history of allergy. 90% of reactions occur immediately after induction of anaesthesia.

Precipitating drugs include:
- Muscle relaxants, particularly suxemethonium
- Intravenous induction agents, most commonly thiopentone
- Opioid analgesics
- Local anaesthetics
- Colloid solutions
- Antibiotics especially penicillins
- Radio contrast media
- Latex.

Clinical features may vary from mild cutaneous manifestations such as urticaria and erythema to cardiovascular collapse and cardiac arrest.

Management
- Stop administration of offending drug.
- Maintain the airway and administer 100% oxygen.

- Administer intravenous epinephrine (0.5–1.0 ml 1:10 000) if the patient is haemodynamically compromised. If the intramuscular route is used, 0.5–1.0 ml of 1:1000 epinephrine should be given initially and repeated every 10 minutes until improvement is established. Epinephrine produces peripheral vasoconstriction, increased cardiac output, bronchodilatation and stabilisation of mast cells.
- Expand the intravascular volume with colloids or crystalloids.
- Administration of corticosteroids, antihistamines and bronchodilators (if required) is the second line treatment.
- Correct severe acidosis with sodium bicarbonate and continue epinephrine by infusion.
- Take a blood sample 1 hour after the start of the reaction and a further sample at 24 hours for tryptase estimation.
- Refer the patient for intradermal skin prick tests to identify the causative agent.
- Advise the patient to carry some form of hazard alert and a yellow card should be submitted to the Committee on Safety of Medicines.

Malignant hyperthermia is a rare genetic disorder with autosomal dominant inheritance characterised by a marked increase in skeletal muscle metabolism. Contact with a trigger agent can precipitate abnormal calcium release from the sarcoplasmic reticulum which leads to sustained muscle contraction. This produces a hypermetabolic state with increased carbon dioxide production, hyperthermia, metabolic acidosis, muscle breakdown, and hyperkalaemia. All inhalational anaesthetic agents and suxemethonium can trigger this response in a susceptible individual.

Management involves:
- Discontinuation of potential trigger agents
- Use of a vapour-free anaesthetic machine and circuit
- Administration of dantrolene 1mg/kg
- Supportive treatment
  - Hyperventilation with 100% oxygen
  - Correction of acidosis and hyperkalaemia
  - Active cooling
  - Treatment of any arrhythmias
  - Diuretic therapy to prevent renal damage by myoglobin
  - Invasive monitoring on ICU.

Mortality is in the order of 5%.

All suspected cases and their first degree relatives should be referred to a specialist centre for screening. This usually involves subjecting them to a muscle biopsy specimen for contracture testing.

Postoperative complications

Various complications can occur in the postoperative period because of the dysfunction of different systems, including respiratory, cardiac, central nervous, gastrointestinal, hepatic, and renal. The patient should be nursed on a tipping trolley, with 1:1 monitoring by trained recovery personnel until the patient is fully conscious. This section describes the diagnosis and management of common problems encountered in the postoperative period.

Hypoxia

Fall in the arterial oxygen tension results in tissue hypoxia and can be diagnosed by pulse oximetry. Immediate steps should be taken to improve the oxygenation before clinical signs of hypoxia (peripheral or central cyanosis) appear. Causes include airway obstruction due to decreased pharyngeal muscle tone and falling back of the tongue, residual effects of opioids, anaesthetic agents or muscle relaxants, ventilation perfusion mismatch, basal atelectasis, lung collapse and pneumothorax. Pulse oximetry is unreliable in the states of hypoperfusion, shock, and extreme vasoconstriction.

Management
- Ensure that the airway is patent.
- Correct airway obstruction by simple manoeuvres, such as head tilt, chin lift, or jaw thrust.
- Rule out the presence of foreign body (secretions, blood, or a fallen tooth) causing the airway obstruction.
- Administer 10 litres/minute of oxygen with a facemask.
- Introduce the Guedal's pharyngeal airway if the patient can tolerate and if the normal manoeuvres fail to remove the airway obstruction.
- Patients who are not breathing or are hypoventilating should be ventilated with bag and mask.

Nausea and vomiting

Predisposing factors
- Patient factors—female patients, past history of PONV, presence of blood in stomach, presence of nasogastric tube.
- Surgical factors—laparoscopic, middle ear, and abdominal surgery.
- Pharmacological factors—opioids, nitrous oxide, inhalational agents.
- Physiological factors—hypotension, hypoxia.

Management
- Prophylactic administration of antiemetic is indicated in high risk patients with one or more predisposing factors. Cyclizine 50mg or ondansetron 4mg can be injected intravenously.
- In case of PONV treat hypotension as it can cause PONV.
- Cyclizine should be used as the first line of treatment, failing which ondansetron can be given intravenously.

Hypotension

Causes
- Hypovolaemia
- Spinal or epidural anaesthesia

- Dysrhythmias
- Sepsis
- Myocardial infarction and left ventricular failure.

Management
- Administer oxygen 10 litres/minute by face mask.
- Ensure that blood volume status is optimized.
- Administer ephedrine 3–6mg intravenously.
- Treat the dysrhythmia.
- Restrict fluid administration in patients with LVF and MI. Start appropriate medical management.
- Transfer the patients with sepsis or cardiogenic problems to HDU or CCU for subsequent management.

Hypertension

Inadequate analgesia is the commonest cause of hypertension in the postoperative period. Antihypertensive medication should only be administered once adequate pain relief is provided to the patient.

Sore throat

Use of laryngeal mask airway, laryngoscopy, and intubation are all associated with high incidence if sore throat. Patients recover from this complication within 24–48 hours.

Practical procedures

Various practical procedures are required in patients requiring critical care and anaesthesia for various surgical operations. Universal precautions should be taken against cross-infection, while performing these procedures, where contact with blood or body fluids is likely.

Vascular access	Airway access
- Peripheral venous cannulation	- Oropharyngeal and nasopharyngeal airway insertion
- Arterial cannulation	- Laryngeal mask airway insertion
- Central venous cannulation	- Orotracheal intubation
- Pulmonary artery catheterisation	- Cricothyroidotomy
	- Percutaneous tracheostomy

Peripheral venous cannulation

Choose appropriate size of cannula depending upon the age of the patient: 24 gauge cannula in neonates, 22 gauge in small children, and 18 and 14 gauge in adults. The size of the cannula also depends on the rate of administration of the fluid. In small children topical anaesthesia with EMLA or Ametop cream should be applied, whereas in adult patients a small bleb can be raised by an intradermal injection of 1% lignocaine to alleviate the pain of venepuncture. Peripheral venous cannulation assembly consists of a cannula, mounted on the needle, an injection port, and a flash chamber (Fig. 1.1).

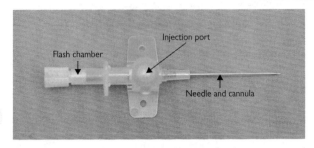

Fig. 1.1 Cannula for peripheral venous cannulation

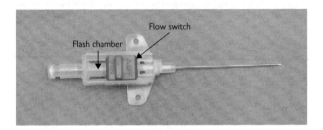

Fig. 1.2 Cannula with flow switch

- Clean the skin with an alcoholic antiseptic solution or swab.
- Insert the cannula after stretching the skin in the non-dominant arm.
- Puncture the skin at 15° angle and advance until blood is seen in the flash chamber.
- Make the cannula nearly parallel to the skin.
- Advance a little bit further so that both the tip of the needle and the cannula are in the lumen of the vein.
- Hold the needle and thread the cannula into the vein.
- Press the skin above tip of the cannula while withdrawing the needle, so that there is no spill over of blood and occlude the proximal end of the cannula with a bung.
- Discard the sharp in a disposable bin-box.

Arterial cannulation

Arterial cannulation is undertaken to monitor continuous blood pressure in critically ill patients and those requiring major surgery. A cannula can also be used where the repeated blood sample is required for arterial blood gas analysis. The most frequent site of arterial cannulation is the radial artery, although the femoral, brachial, and dorsalis pedis artery can also be cannulated. Allen's test should be performed to assess the adequacy of collateral circulation. The patient is asked to clench the fist very tightly while the radial and the ulnar arteries are compressed tightly to exsanguinate the palm. The patient is asked to open the fist and pressure on the ulnar artery is released. Collateral flow via the radial artery is adequate if the blanched palm of the hand becomes pink in less than six seconds.

Technique
The arm should be rested on a side support and a small, rolled sheet placed underneath the back of the wrist and the hand dorsiflexed. Clean the site with antiseptic solution. The site of puncture should be infiltrated with 1% lignocaine, using a 24 gauge needle. Usually a 20 gauge Teflon or polyethylene cannula with a flow switch (Fig. 1.2) is inserted at an angle of 30° to the skin, while palpating the radial artery, proximal to the point of insertion. As soon as the blood is seen in the flash chamber, the angle should be lowered to 15° and the assembly is pushed a little further so that both the needle and cannula are in the lumen of the artery. At this stage, the needle should be held firmly between the thumb and the index finger, while pushing the cannula into the artery. Withdraw the needle while pressing the tip of the cannula to avoid spilling of the blood and press the flow switch on after the needle is completely out. Complications include infection, thrombosis, and ischaemia.

Central venous cannulation
Central venous pressure (CVP) can be monitored by placing the tip of the cannula in intrathoracic portion of the superior or inferior vena cava. CVP reflects the filling pressure of the right side of the heart. CVP monitoring is done commonly to monitor the volume status and to enable accurate fluid therapy in hypovolaemic patients, without causing overload.

Routes of central venous cannulation
- Antecubital vein in cubital fossa
- External jugular vein
- Internal jugular vein
- Subclavian vein
- Femoral vein.

The right internal jugular vein is cannulated most commonly because of its straight course, ease of insertion and reduced incidence of certain complications, such as pneumothorax, as compared with the subclavian route.

- The patient should be positioned in Trendelenberg position with the head turned to the opposite side.
- A multiple lumen catheter is inserted into the internal jugular vein using Seldinger's technique. The catheter kit (Fig. 1.3) consists of a needle, J wire, dilator sheath, and multilumen catheter.
- A needle connected with a saline filled syringe is inserted at 30° to the skin at the apex of the triangle formed by the sternal and clavicular heads of sternocleidomastoid and clavicle, using aseptic technique.
- Advance the needle caudal and laterally towards the ipsilateral nipple until venous blood is aspirated. Never advance the needle more than 2.5cm.
- The syringe is disconnected and J tipped wire inserted through the needle.

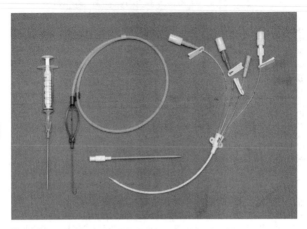

Fig. 1.3 Central venous catheter kit

- A CVP catheter is passed over the wire, after dilatation of puncture site, and wire is removed.
- A chest X-ray should be done to check the placement and to rule out pneumothorax.
- Central venous pressure can be measured by connecting the catheter to a pressure transducer or a saline filled manometer calibrated to midaxillary line as the reference point.

Complications
Immediate
- Carotid artery puncture
- Dysrhythmias
- Pneumothorax
- Air embolism
- Malpositioning.
Delayed
- Thrombosis
- Sepsis.

Pulmonary artery catheterisation (PAC)
This procedure is performed to measure pulmonary capillary wedge pressure which approximates the left atrial pressure in the presence of normal pulmonary vascular resistance. PAC can be used to monitor cardiac output, mixed venous oxygen saturation, systemic and pulmonary vascular resistance. The balloon tipped, 110cm long catheter (Fig. 1.4) is introduced through the introducer sheath placed in the internal jugular vein using Seldinger's technique (refer to CVP cannulation). The distal lumen is connected to a pressure transducer through a saline filled column. The balloon is inflated with 1.5ml of air after tip of catheter is in

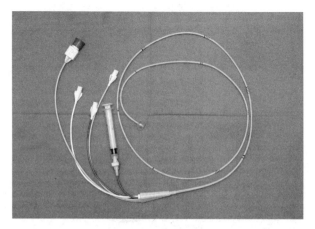

Fig. 1.4 Balloon tipped catheter

right atrium. The catheter is advanced and location of the tip of the catheter is guided by the pressure waveforms (Fig. 1.5). The catheter should not be advanced once the wedge trace is obtained. Deflation of the balloon should result in a pulmonary arterial trace.

Complications
Immediate
- Arterial puncture
- Haematoma
- Pneumothorax
- Dysrhythmias
- Air embolism
- Knotting
- Malpositioning

Delayed
- Infection
- Thrombosis
- Pulmonary haemorrhage, infarction.

Indications
- ARDS
- Severe sepsis
- Titration of inotropes in patients with poor cardiac function
- Major trauma and operations associated with major fluid shifts.

Oropharyngeal airway insertion

Guedal's airway should be inserted in patients with airway obstruction if simple manoeuvres like chin lift and jaw thrust fail. A conscious patient will not tolerate this airway.

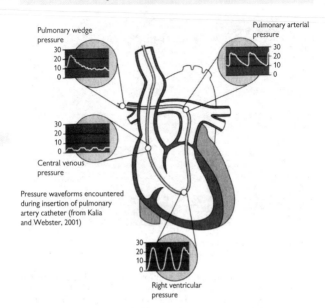

Fig. 1.5 Placement of pulmonary artery catheter showing related pressure valves

Technique
- Choose the appropriate size airway (Fig. 1.6) by placing the airway between tip of tragus and angle of mouth. A large airway can itself cause the obstruction whereas a smaller than ideal airway will not be able to remove the obstruction.
- Open the mouth, depress the tongue, and slide the airway posteriorly between tongue and hard palate, with concavity facing the front, until the flange is positioned and rests between lips and the teeth.
- In case of difficulty the airway can be inserted with concavity facing the hard palate. At the first point of resistance the airway should be rotated by 180° and pushed downwards gently till the flange rests between lips and teeth. Avoid this technique in small children as it can cause trauma to soft palate.

Nasopharyngeal airway insertion
Patients with intact pharyngeal reflexes tolerate nasopharyngeal airways better than oropharyngeal airways.

Technique
- Check the patency of nostrils and choose the nostril with greater patency.
- Lubricate the nasopharyngeal airway with jelly and insert in downward and posterior direction till the flange rests in front of the nostril.

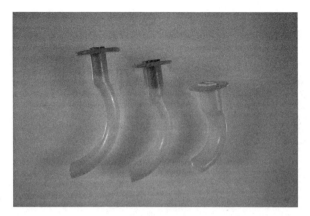

Fig. 1.6 Guedal's airways

Laryngeal mask airway (LMA)

It is introduced through the oral cavity after induction of anaesthesia. The laryngeal mask (Fig. 1.7) rests in front of the laryngeal inlet. It provides hands-free clear airway and obviates the need for tracheal intubation, thereby avoiding all the complications of intubation. It offers no protection from aspiration of gastric contents.

Indications
- Provision of a clear airway overcoming the need to hold a facemask.
- Avoidance of tracheal intubation in a spontaneously breathing patient.
- Airway maintenance in known or suspected cases of difficult intubation.
- Emergency management of failed intubation.
- Provision of a temporary airway during cardiopulmonary resuscitation.

The LMA does *not* protect against aspiration of gastric contents. In patients with a full stomach, delayed gastric emptying, gastro-oesophageal reflux, or a hiatus hernia, the use of a LMA is contraindicated.

Technique
- Adequate depth of anaesthesia/suppression of airway reflexes should be established.
- Extend the patient's head and open mouth. It may be necessary to hold down the lower jaw.
- Introduce the LMA into the oro-pharynx using a gloved finger. It is gently advanced along the hard palate until the tip of the cuff reaches the posterior pharyngeal wall. Advance it distally into the laryngo-pharynx until the cuff sits posterior to the larynx.
- When correctly positioned, inflate the cuff and the LMA is connected to a breathing system and secured.
- Confirm correct placement by manual inflation of the lungs or by observation of movement of a reservoir bag in spontaneously breathing patients.

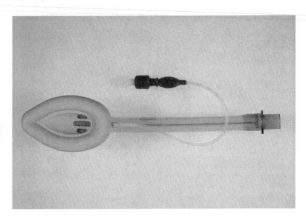

Fig. 1.7 Laryngeal mask airway

Orotracheal intubation

A definitive airway requires placement of a cuffed tube in the trachea. The tracheal tube (Fig. 1.8) is made of PVC and is radio-opaque. Most male patients require size 9 whereas female patients need size 8 tracheal tubes. Tracheal tube has a low pressure cuff designed to provide an airtight seal after inflation with air. Appropriate size and length of orotracheal tube in the children can be calculated by the formulae.

$$\text{Size} = \frac{\text{Age}}{4} + 4.5\text{mm} \qquad \text{Length} = \frac{\text{Age}}{2} + 12\text{cm}$$

Technique
- Check the laryngoscope and ensure that cuff of the tracheal tube is not leaking.
- Induce the conscious patient with an appropriate induction agent and muscle relaxant should be used to facilitate intubation.
- Position the patient in 'sniffing the morning air position' (flexion of neck by placing a 4 inch thick pillow under the occiput and extension at atlanto-occipital joint). Avoid manipulation of the neck in the patients with suspected cervical spine injury.
- Introduce the blade of the laryngoscope from right side of the mouth. Displace the tongue to the left by the flange of laryngoscope.
- Keep sliding the spatula of the blade on the tongue until the epiglottis is visualised.
- Tip of the blade should rest in the vallecula (junction of epiglottis and the base of tongue). Lift the laryngoscope in the direction of the handle.
- Identify the laryngeal inlet by the vocal cords and insert the tracheal tube gently into the trachea. Inflate the cuff of the tube with air, enough to prevent the audible leak of gases on positive pressure ventilation.
- Confirm the placement of the tube by auscultation and capnography.

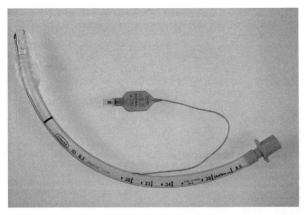

Fig. 1.8 Endotracheal tube

Indications for intubation
- Unconscious patient
- Risk of aspiration (patient with full stomach)
- Mechanical ventilation (apnoea, intrathoracic surgery)
- Operations with difficult airway access (ENT, prone position).

Complications of intubation
- Trauma to face, lips, tongue, and teeth
- Hypertensive response
- Arrhythmias.

Cricothyroidotomy

This procedure requires an opening in the cricothyroid membrane and the airway can be secured by placing the tube in the trachea through this opening. Cricothyroidotomy is a life-saving procedure in a patient with airway obstruction where airway access is impossible through the oropharyngeal or nasopharyngeal route. Cricothyroidotomy can be performed with the help of a needle or a proper tube can be introduced through the membrane using Seldinger's technique.

Technique
- Stabilise the cricothyroid membrane (extends between thyroid and cricoid cartilage) between thumb and index finger and puncture with a 12 or 14 needle connected with a saline filled syringe.
- Advance the needle at 45° angle until air is aspirated freely.
- Connect the needle to an oxygen source.
- Occlusion of the hole in the connecting tubing causes inflation of the chest and oxygenation of the patient. Inflate for one second and deflate for four seconds. Elimination of carbon dioxide is inadequate with this

technique and formal tracheostomy should be done within 45 minutes of this procedure to establish normal ventilation otherwise the patient will become hypercapnic.

- Seldinger's technique consists of the introduction of a J tipped wire through the needle once the tip of the needle is in the trachea. The needle is withdrawn and the dilator and cricothyroidotomy tube assembly is railroaded over the J wire. The dilator and J wire is withdrawn leaving the tube in the trachea.
- Confirm the placement of the tube by auscultation and capnography.

Complications
- Haematoma
- Aspiration
- Perforation of posterior wall of trachea
- Hoarseness
- Haemorrhage
- Subglottic stenosis
- Surgical emphysema
- False passage.

Tracheostomy (see Chapter 15)

Theatre procedures and prophylaxis

David J. Leaper

Theatre discipline

There are many time-honoured procedures in theatre which do not have an accepted evidence base. Nevertheless it would flaunt danger to disregard them, particularly as we currently enjoy the lowest figure of morbidity and mortality despite operating on a sicker and old cohort of patient. There are some downsides; the increase of emergent and resistant organisms such as *Cl. difficile* and MRSA serve as examples.

Theatre design and ventilation

- Modern operating theatres must be safe environments for patients and staff. Ideally they should have easy access to A&E, HDU, and ITU and general wards, with easily opened links to radiology and laboratories. High maintenance is required, not just for infection control, but for lighting, operating tables, anaesthetic machines, and other equipment.
- In general, operating theatre air is changed 20 times an hour using filters. The positive pressure (plenum) ceiling mounted, ventilation should ideally be of laminar flow to avoid turbulence. Ultraclean air, air changes up to 40 times per hour, and the use of exhaust suits in Charnley theatres is appropriate for orthopaedic operations when contamination can be disastrous. The evidence that such attention to ventilation is more effective than prophylactic antibiotics however is lacking. There must be satisfactory cleaning between lists and it is illogical to use designated orthopaedic theatre for dirty operations.
- Microbiological testing is undertaken regularly using a slit samplers. When there are outbrakes of resistant organisms, theatres may be need to be closed and sterilised, if they are the source, with infection control procedures to identify and treat carriers. Septic lesions on patients and staff should be reason to prevent their entry.
- Ceiling-mounted gases and vacuum facilities need similar maintenance and attention to infection control measures. It is impossible to connect the wrong gases to an anaesthetic machine. Most theatres have temperature and humidity control for both patient safety and staff comfort. Some theatres are fortunate enough to have some natural light but dignity and privacy must be ensured. It is appropriate to encourage as few personnel to be present in theatre and ensure as little movement as is practical.

Theatre clothing

- Vests, trousers and skirts are usually made of comfortable light cotton (ventiles) which can be used for a whole list of operations, unless they become soiled. It is inappropriate to use theatre clothing for trips to the ward or A&E, unless there is an emergency. On return, clothing should be changed; all hospitals see large amounts of linen disappear each year. Clogs or shoes are comfier than boots for many, but must be antistatic. Boots are appropriate for at risk operations, such as an HIV risk, or when there is gross contamination (when aprons should also have been anticipated).

- The use of caps and masks, in particular, is controversial. The control of hair is logical but both caps and masks afford protection to the staff from contamination. Masks and caps may be more important in prosthetic orthopaedic and vascular operations. Masks should not be handled and replaced—they are disposable, one per operation.
- Gowns and operating drapes can be cleaned, repaired and reautoclaved many times. They are less expensive than waterproof disposables (see HIV precautions) which can be justified in prosthetic surgery. The included cellulose is water-resistant but make gowns uncomfortable to wear in long operations.
- Aqueous antiseptics, chlorhexidine, triclosan, or povidone iodine (Betadine) are used for hand preparation prior to gowning up. Scrubbing the nails is only necessary for the first case on a list. Scrubbing the skin or repeat scrubbing risks contamination by deep skin organisms. After the first 4–5 minutes hand preparation (scrub-up), hand disinfection can be a simple hand washing between cases with antiseptic or a hand rub using an alcoholic preparation, unless there has been contamination. Alcoholic chlorhexidine and povidone iodine are used for patient skin preparation. Two applications should reduce resident flora by more than 95%. The use of incised drapes (adhesive polyurethane films), wound guards and drains has not been shown to reduce infection rates. If shaving is considered necessary it should be undertaken immediately prior to surgery or a depilatory cream can be used. Skin contamination is increased after shaving and may double the infection rate if shaving is undertaken >12–24 hours before surgery. The main reason for shaving is to facilitate removal of adhesive dressings.
- The use of heat for sterilisation is not particularly effective but steam under pressure (100–200kPa and 121–143°C) can kill all micro-organisms and spores and is very penetrative and therefore useful in sterilising materials and some instruments. Short cycle autoclaves are used in central sterile supply after cleaning and repairing equipment and linen.
- Disposable materials used in operation, for example, suture materials are sterilised by manufacturers in large (and expensive) gamma radiation units. Ethylene oxide is not used as it is explosive. Endoscopes and other delicate re-usable instruments need to be sterilised after cleaning by immersion in an antiseptic. Glutaraldehyde has been superseded by less toxic agents.

Patient care in operating theatre

Patients' consent must be taken by the operating surgeon or an experienced appropriate surrogate. It must be taken without coercion with a full explanation of the procedure intended, its benefits, and possible complications. Patients must have the opportunity to ask questions about the surgery and anaesthetic and discuss alternatives.

- The explanation of every complication presents difficulty but devastating complications, however rare, such as recurrent nerve damage during thyroid lobectomy, must be included.
- Each patient must be identified and an operating site or side marked before any premedication. Identity bracelets must match the notes, ID number, and what the patient says. Preoperative marking must use an indelible pen. Identification occurs on leaving the ward for surgery, at admission to the theatre and in the anaesthetic room. The surgeon should identify the patient and his/her marking before anaesthesia begins. The correct operation should be confirmed and that marking must be clear. Any doubt should mean the patient should be returned to the ward.
- Patients, and instruments, flow from 'clean to dirty' in a set pattern during the operating theatre stay. There are no new mistakes to make, we simply must try to avoid the time honoured ones. Once asleep or positioned on the operating table, it is the anaesthetist's responsibility, for example, to look after an arthritic cervical spine and the surgeon's responsibility to prevent damage to the lateral peroneal nerve in the Lloyds-Davies position, the ulnar nerve if arm boards are used and the brachial plexus if the arm is placed above the head. Pressure relieving aids must ensure bony prominences are protected from the risk of pressure sores. The patient must be secure, particularly if the table is tilted, and calves protected by the use of the heel pad.
- Hypothermia is common during long general anaesthetics, particularly when there is exposure. Hypothermia adds to postoperative complications, the risk of pressure sores, and wound infection. Core temperature, based on tympanic or oesophageal probes, can be maintained by the use of warmed IV fluids and either a forced warm-air blanket or warming mattress.
- Diathermy must be well maintained and should not be used if unfamiliar. It provides a high frequency alternating current of 400kHz which at the active electrode can produce heat up to 1000°C. In monopolar diathermy the indifferent plate must be checked with full contact to prevent burns. It is the surgeon's responsibility. Bipolar diathermy has both active and indifferent electrodes at the surgeon's fingertips and allows much more precision. Lasers need designated staff and must be operated with strict guidelines, including protective eye glasses and clear communication when being used.

Day case surgery

Day case surgery is by no means a recent concept but there is now strong evidence to show that 75% of elective surgery can be performed safely, according to the British Association of Day Surgery and the Audit Commission (the so-called 'basket' and 'trolley' of procedures). It may be extended into 24 hour facilities. This certainly fits with patient choice, allows seamless booking, and early return to work. For success it must be faultlessly driven by multidisciplinary and agreed protocols. Nurse assessment and discharge with pain relief and aftercare are shown to be highly effective. There is a culture change need to ask 'is there any reason not to do elective surgery as a day case?'

Apart from surgeon, nurse, and patient choice it is very cost effective and is ringfenced from invasion by medical admissions. Ideally the unit should be a stand alone, purpose built facility. All specialities in surgery can benefit and waiting lists can become controlled or ideally abolished and replaced with a diary system.

Evaluation of X-rays in surgery

- Imaging has become an indispensable adjunct to surgical procedures. They can be the road map to decision making and the approach and choice for an operation. Most hospital Trusts now have a weekly X-ray meeting at which decisions should be enabled preoperatively, as in cancer multidisciplinary meetings. Difficult imaging, particularly with real-time ultrasound, CT, and MRI can be interpreted together at these meetings. Radiologists are very friendly to surgeons and we need to be to them, particularly when CT is asked for at 2 a.m.! They can be approached for interpretation of emergency chest and abdominal X-rays but a personal touch is recommended! A chest X-ray can help you plan and consider postoperative care including physiotherapy but a radiologist can shown you that an erect plain abdominal X-ray may not help interpretation of intestinal obstruction. Always take their advice.

- Radiologists can bale out the need for emergency surgery and interventional radiology is a fulfilling career; as examples, the rise of endovascular aneurysmorrhaphy and guided aspiration of abdominal abscesses. Surgeons may take X-rays themselves in theatre, cholangiograms for example. To do this, it is imperative that the operator holds an irradiation protection certificate. Full radiation protection with gowns and exclusion of unnecessary staff must be complied with, including the cooperation of radiographers, radiologists, and planning of their time. Don't expect support at the last minute unless it is a true emergency. Planning should also make it clear to pregnant staff that they should avoid that operation on that particular day. It may be overlooked and then an operation has to be cancelled.

Prophylaxis of deep vein thrombosis

- Deep vein thrombosis (DVT) is an avoidable complication. Before prophylaxis 40–50% of patients undergoing total hip replacement for example would have a thrombosis in the soleal sinuses of the calf, or more proximal with a pulmonary embolus (PE) rate of 1–10%. Risk factors relate to hypercoagulability and the fibrinolytic system which depends on the balance of thrombin and antithrombin, tissue plasminogen activator (tPa) and plasminogen activator inhibitors (PAIs). Patients with genetic defects of protein C and S, and factor V Leiden defect for examples have the perioperative risk of hypercoagulability. The list of common clinical risk factors is shown in Table 2.1. In pregnancy it is always best to defer surgery and the stopping of HRT is logical. The effect of the pill, particularly low oestrogen types, is controversial. Common sense dictates cessation but not at the increased risk of pregnancy. Consult local agreed protocols.
- Diagnosis may be made clinically on classic signs but suspicion can be strengthened or confirmed by measuring D-dimers, contrast or isotope venography, duplex Doppler, or plethysmography. Local protocols usually apply.
- Prophylaxis includes early mobilization but in any level of risk thromboembolic deterrent (TED) stockings should be considered. In moderate to higher risk, intermittent calf compression or foot pumps should be used intraoperatively with prophylactic heparin in addition or in combination. Warfarin and aspirin probably have no role in prophylaxis.
- Low molecular weight heparin (LMWH) given once a day subcutaneously is now the prophylaxis of choice. It is associated with a minimum risk of bleeding and has replaced unfractionated calcium heparin. There is strong evidence based support for its use. For example tinzaparin can be given at 3500U daily subcutaneously, and in the case of DVT can be boosted as treatment until anticoagulation with warfarin is established.
- Local protocols must be consulted but Table 2.2 gives a template for DVT prophylaxis.

Table 2.1 Perioperative clinical risk factors for deep vein thrombosis

- Age (> 40 years, even more > 70 years)
- Obesity (BMI > 40)
- Immobilization (stroke or cardiac failure)
- Malignancy (pelvic)
- Pregnancy, the pill, HRT (oestrogen related)
- Sepsis and chronic inflammatory diseases
- Metabolic (diabetes, anaemia)
- Orthopaedic (THR and knee surgery)
- Previous thromboembolic disease

Table 2.2 Recommended DVT prophylaxis

	Clinical risk	Prophylaxis
Low	Minor surgery	Mobilization
	Major surgery age >40 years	Care in theatre
	Minor illness	TEDs
Moderate	Major surgery age >40 years	As low risk (TEDs)
	Major illness	Plus LMWH or
	Minor surgery with known risks	calf compression
High	Hip knee pelvic surgery	TEDs
	Major cancer resection	Plus LMWH
	Known hypercoagulability	Plus calf compression
	Previous DVT/PE	

Consider full dose IV heparin control in highest risk during withdrawal of warfarin and early postoperative period (discuss with haematologists).

Antibiotic prophylaxis

- The principles of antibiotic prophylaxis were laid down in the experiments of John Burke in the 1960s. If an appropriate antibiotic was given to an animal prior to an inoculation of *Staph. aureus* subsequent abscess formation was reduced. He described a decisive period when antibiotics protected against the development of infection whilst host defences were mounted in the four hours after the first incision. Since then many clinical trials have proven the worth of prohphylactic antibiotics to prevent wound infection (superficial surgical site infection—SSSI). They do not prevent wound or anastomotic failure but may reduce the risk of deep surgical site infections and intra-abdominal abscesses.

- Modern antibiotic prophylaxis gives empirical cover against the organisms expected at operation. Cover beyond 24 hours is not prophylaxis and should not exceed three doses (when it would be therapy). Wounds are classified into four categories (Table 2.3); prophylaxis is not appropriate for dirty wounds which need antibiotic therapy. Added risk factors are listed in Table 2.4.

- Local protocols ought to be adhered to otherwise there is a risk of antibiotic resistance. There may be rotating antibiotic policies in place and this should have been addressed by local clinical governance. Antibiotics are only an adjunct to surgical care and must be coupled to careful and gentle, meticulous surgery with perfect haemostasis. Theatre discipline must be obeyed, particularly in prosthetic surgery where strict asepsis is critical.

- In clean surgery without a prosthetic implant, antibiotic prophylaxis has not been proven to be effective. However, close surveillance of clean wound surgery into primary health care (where most infections occur or are detected) reveals a wound infection rate, albeit of minor nature, of up to 10%. Prophylaxis is effective in prosthetic surgery (where any surgical site infection is a disaster) and in clean-contaminated and contaminated wounds. Dirty surgery needs treatment for a minimum of 3–5 days. Suggested regimens are shown in Table 2.5, p43.

- In prosthetic surgery the major risk is from endogenous skin organisms (*Staph. aureus* and CNS), particularly those which are slime producers or when there is a biofilm production. There is a larger risk from resistant forms (Table 2.5). When a viscus is opened there is a risk from many other organisms, particularly the aerobic Gram-negative bacilli (AGNB) and anaerobes (mostly *Bacteroides* spp) which act in synergy.

- Patients who have rheumatic heart disease need prophylaxis for even minor procedures such as dental treatment and certainly invasive endoscopy (ERCP or urinary tract instrumentation). In endoscopic procedures a broad spectrum penicillin or second generation cephalosporin is recommended. Patients who have a splenectomy need pneumovax vaccination against pneumococcus with lifetime penicillin cover.

Table 2.3 Types and examples of surgical wounds

Clean	• No viscus opened • No inflammation • No breach in asepsis	• Varicose veins • Prosthetic, vascular, or orthopaedic surgery
Clean-contaminated	• Viscus opened • Minimal spillage	• Open cholecystectomy
Contaminated	• Viscus opened • Inflammatory disease • Significant spillage	• Elective colorectal surgery
Dirty	• Pus encountered • Perforation	• Faecal peritonitis (needs therapy)

Table 2.4 Risk factors for surgical infection

- Poor perfusion—(local ischaemia; shock of any cause)
- Malnutrition—(low albumin; obesity)
- Poor surgery—(haematoma; tension)
- Metabolic diseases—(diabetes, uraemia, jaundice)
- Immunosuppression—(steroids; cancer, chemo/radiotherapy)
- Perioperative care—(poor hygiene/hand washing, shaving.

Bowel preparation

- This must be considered for elective colorectal surgery, although many consider it unnecessary for right colon procedures. In obstruction intraoperative lavage may permit safe primary anastomoses. The Herculean attempts in the past to completely empty the bowel (5 days of enemas, magnesium sulphate, Epsom salts, mannitol, 10 litres of nasogastric saline) have been replaced by single sachets of cathartics such as Picolax. These should be given 12–24 hours before surgery but (i) respect the dignity of a patient who may be 'glued' to a toilet for 8 hours and (ii) remember obstruction may be induced, so carefully watch the patient for pain and abdominal distension and always ensure good hydration.
- Low residue diet for 5 days preoperatively may actually reduce patients fluid intake; this and attention to nutrition are equally important. Beware of the patient who has had a recent weight loss of 10–20%. The additional use of poorly absorbed antibiotics is controversial. Regard local protocols.
- Stoma siting must also be undertaken in the 24 hour preoperative period. Even in an anterior resection markings for an LIF end colostomy (following the unexpected need for a Hartmann's operation) or an RIF loop ileostomy (to dysfunction the distal anastomosis) should be considered.

Table 2.5 Suggested prophylactic regimens for operations at risk

Types of surgery	Organisms encountered	Prophylactic regimen suggested
• Vascular	• *Staphylococcus epidermidis* (or MRCNS) • *Staphylococcus aureus* (or MRSA) • Aerobic Gram-negative bacilli (AGNB)	• 3 doses flucloxacillin ± gentamicin, vanomycin or rifampicin if MRCNS/MRSA a risk
• Orthopaedic	• *Staphylococcus epidermidis/aureus*	• 1–3 doses wide-spectrum cephalosporin (with antistaphylococcal action) • Gentamicin beads
• Oesophagogastric	• Enterobacteriaceae • Enterococci (including anaerobic/viridans Streptococci)	• 1–3 doses second-generation cephalosporin and metronidazole in severe contamination
• Biliary	• Enterobacteriaceae (mainly *E. coli*) • Enterococci (including *Streptococcus faecalis*)	• 1 dose second-generation cephalosporin
• Small bowel	• Enterobacteriaceae • Anaerobes (mainly *Bacteroides*)	• 1–3 doses second-generation cephalosporin ± metronidazole
• Appendix/colorectal	• Enterobacteriaceae • Anaerobes (*Bacteriodes streptococci*)	• 3 doses second-generation cephalosporin (alternatively gentamicin) with metronidazole (oral, poorly absorbed antibiotics controversial)

All regimens are intravenous and should start preoperatively. In elective operations, antibiotics can be given at induction of anaesthesia. In emergency operations (or in contamination during elective surgery) antibiotics should be given at diagnosis and prolonged as therapy for 3–5 days if necessary.

HIV and AIDS precautions

- All medical and nursing staff are now expected to be immunised against hepatitis B. The current vaccination schedules use a genetically engineered antigen; three doses usually give good antibody levels with five year boosters. There is no vaccination yet against the non-B hepatitis viruses.

- Theatre precautions when operating on a patient who is, or who is at risk of being HIV positive, should always be preceded by the question, 'is this operation really necessary?' There will be local infection control guidelines.

- Theatre should be calm and contain as few personnel as possible with the operation probably at the end of a list with extra time allotted. Eye contact must be kept between the operating team with all instruments passed to and fro in a kidney dish. Glasses or a visor are needed by the whole team and as many disposables used (gowns, drapes, instruments etc.) as possible. Needle stick injuries can be minimised by double gloving and boots are more protective than clogs. Haemostasis should be meticulous with every effort made and anticipated to avoid spillage of body fluids.

- Surgeons who become HIV positive for any reason need professional advice on their limitations and modification of their presence in operative surgery.

Anatomy for surgeons

F. Di Franco and G. R. McLatchie

The female breast

Breasts are bilateral skin appendages that vary individually in size and shape.

Embryology

The breast arises from the mammary ridges that derive from the ectoderm.

Surface markings

The breast is contained within the superficial fascia. It rests on the pectoralis major extending:

- Superiorly to the 2nd rib.
- Inferiorly to 6th rib.
- Medially to the sternum.
- Laterally to mid axillary line.

The axillary tail is an extension of breast tissue into the axilla.

Structural features

The breast is composed of lobules. Within each lobule, glandular tissue is placed centrally whereas adipose tissue tends to be more laterally. The glands form a ductal system terminating in 15–20 lactiferous ducts radiating towards the nipple. Each lobe is separated by fibrous septa, a collagenous membrane that supports the glandular structure. The fibrous septa, along with the ligament of Cooper, form the suspensory mechanism of the breast by their attachment to the ribs and the skin.

Blood supply

Arterial

- Axillary artery via lateral thoracic and acromiothoracic branches.
- Internal mammary artery via its perforating branches.

Venous

- Venous plexus underneath the areola that drains towards the axillary vein.
- Veins draining towards the internal mammary vein.

Lymphatic drainage

- The lymphatics of the nipple drain along the surface of the breast underneath the skin.
- The lymphatics from the medial aspect of the breast drain towards the nodes of the internal mammary territory.
- Most of the lymphatics of the breast drain toward the axilla.

The majority of the lymph nodes are located in the territory of the axillary vein.

Nerve supply

It arises from the anterior and lateral branches of the 4th, 5th, and 6th thoracic nerves.

Practical hint

The status of the axillary lymph nodes is crucial in management of breast cancer because:

- It is a prognostic factor.
- It determines the need for adjuvant treatment.

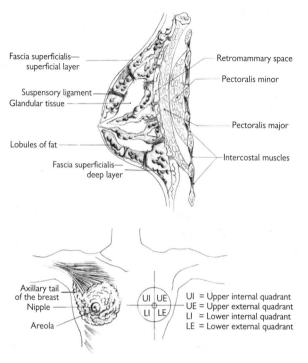

Fig. 3.1 The female breast

The endocrine system

The thyroid gland

This gland is highly vascular, enclosed in a fibrous capsule and bound by a sheath of pretracheal fascia to the larynx so it moves up and down during swallowing.

Structure

- Right and left lobes—pear-shaped, they lie at the sides of the larynx and trachea.
- An isthmus—connects the right and left lobe at the level of the second, third, and fourth tracheal rings.
- A pyramidal lobe—often projects upwards from the isthmus.

Relations

- **Superficial:** Sternothyroid, sternohyoid, omohyoid and their nerves from the ansa hypoglossi. These are overlapped below by the sterno-mastoid.
- **Medial:** Cricoid cartilage, thyroid cartilage, inferior constrictor above and recurrent laryngeal nerve.
- **Posterior:** Carotid sheath, inferior thyroid artery, prevertebral muscles.

Blood supply

- **Arterial**

Superior thyroid artery. This is the first branch of the external carotid. It passes to the upper pole under the infrahyoid muscles close to the external branch of the superior laryngeal nerve. Damage to the nerve leads to loss of timbre of the voice, which becomes monotone. The superior pedicle should therefore be tied close to its origin.

Inferior thyroid artery. It arises from the thyrocervical trunk, a branch of the subclavian artery. It ascends to the carotid sheath and enters the posterior part of the gland. The inferior pedicle should be tied well out to avoid recurrent laryngeal nerve damage.

- **Venous**

Superior thyroid vein emerges from the upper pole and drains into the internal jugular vein.

Middle thyroid vein from the lower part of the lateral border of the lobes crosses the common carotid and drains into the internal jugular vein.

Inferior thyroid vein from the isthmus or lower medial lobe passes along the front of the trachea to the left innominate vein.

Lymphatic drainage

To the middle and lower deep jugular, pretracheal, and mediastinal nodes.

Recurrent laryngeal nerve

Arises from the vagus and runs upwards in the tracheo-oesophageal groove behind or in front of the inferior thyroid arteries. It supplies all the intrinsic muscles of the larynx. Damage or division causes paralysis of the vocal cords on that side.

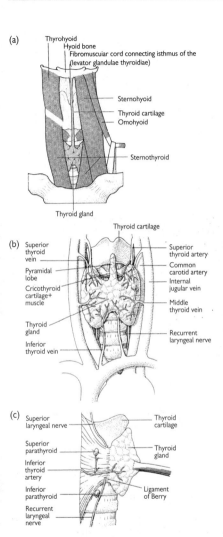

(a)
- Thyrohyoid
- Hyoid bone
- Fibromuscular cord connecting isthmus of the (levator glandulae thyroidiae)
- Sternohyoid
- Thyroid cartilage
- Omohyoid
- Sternothyroid
- Thyroid gland

(b)
- Superior thyroid vein
- Pyramidal lobe
- Cricothyroid cartilage + muscle
- Thyroid gland
- Inferior thyroid vein
- Thyroid cartilage
- Superior thyroid artery
- Common carotid artery
- Internal jugular vein
- Middle thyroid vein
- Recurrent laryngeal nerve

(c)
- Superior laryngeal nerve
- Superior parathyroid
- Inferior thyroid artery
- Inferior parathyroid
- Recurrent laryngeal nerve
- Thyroid cartilage
- Thyroid gland
- Ligament of Berry

Fig. 3.2. Structure of the thyroid gland. a) The infrahyoid muscles related to the thyroid. The sternohyoid muscle has been removed on the right-hand side. From *Textbook of Anatomy*, (ed. A. W. Rogers), 1992. Reproduced with permission from Churchill Livingstone

Parathyroid glands

These paired reddish-brown glands, each about the size of a small pea, lie behind the upper and lower aspects of the thyroid lobes. They are derived from the third (lower gland) and fourth pharyngeal (upper gland) pouches and lie within the pretracheal fascia often within the thyroid itself. Occasionally there may be more than four.
- Superior glands. Each is fairly constant in position, lying behind the upper third of the lobe inside the pretracheal fascia lateral to the trachea. Occasionally each may be more anterior and liable to injury during subtotal thyroidectomy.
- Inferior glands. Their position is more variable. They are usually found behind the lower part of each lobe either above or below the inferior thyroid artery as it enters the substance of the gland.

Unusual positions include retro-oesophageal, either in the neck or posterior mediastinum or the anterior mediastinum in relation to the thymus gland.

Adrenal glands

The right and left adrenal glands are intrabdominal. They lie above or medial to each kidney. Their total weight is 10g.

Structure
- Adrenal cortex
  - Zona glomerulosa, outer layer, produces aldosterone.
  - Zona fasciculata, middle layer, produces cortisol.
  - Zona reticularis, inner layer, produces sex hormones.
- Adrenal medulla.
  - Secretes catecholamines—adrenaline and noradrenaline

Relations
- Right adrenal gland
  - Anteriorly—bare area of the liver.
  - Posteriorly—diaphragm.
  - Medially—inferior vena cava.
  - Inferiorly—right kidney.
- Left adrenal gland
  - Anteriorly—splenic artery, pancreas and peritoneum of lesser sac.
  - Posteriorly—diaphragm (left crus).
  - Laterally—left kidney.

Blood supply
- Arterial
  - Superior adrenal arteries (from inferior phrenic artery on each side)
  - Middle adrenal arteries (from the aorta)
  - Inferior adrenal arteries (from the renal artery)
- Venous drainage
  - This is represented by a central vein
  - The right adrenal vein drains into the inferior vena cava
  - The left adrenal vein drains into the left renal vein

Practical hint
The right adrenal vein is very short. This may make surgery of the right adrenal more difficult.

The respiratory system

The trachea

The trachea is a fibroelastic organ composed by 15–20 U-shaped cartilaginous rings. It is approximately 11cm long. The trachea commences at the lower aspect of the cricoid cartilage and terminates at the level of the sternal angle where it bifurcates into the right and left main bronchi. The point where the trachea bifurcates is also known as carina.

Relations
- Anteriorly
  - Neck—isthmus of thyroid gland, inferior thyroid veins, sternohyoid, sternothyroid.
  - Thorax—brachiocephalic and left common carotid artery, left brachiocephalic vein.
- Posteriorly
  - Neck and thorax: oesophagus and recurrent laryngeal nerves.
- Laterally
  - Neck—lobes of thyroid gland, carotid sheath.
  - Thorax—on the right: vagus nerve, azygos vein and pleura—on the left: aortic arch, left common carotid artery, left subclavian artery, left recurrent laryngeal nerve, pleura.

Blood supply
It derives from the branches of the inferior thyroid arteries.

The bronchi

The bronchi arise at the bifurcation of the trachea. The right main bronchus is shorter and more vertical and has a greater diameter than the left one. It is 2.5cm long. Before entering the hilum of the lung, it divides into an upper lobe bronchus. After entering the hilum, it gives off a middle lobe and lower lobe bronchus. The 5cm long left bronchus divides into the bronchi to the upper and lower lobes just after entering the hilum of the lung. The bronchial tree reduces in diameter and length with each successive division.

The lungs

The lungs are paired organs. They are conical in shape.
- Each lung presents a:
  - Apex, extending above the first rib
  - Base, related to the diaphragm
  - Parietal surface, related to the rib cage
  - Mediastinal surface, related to the pericardium.
- The right lung has three lobes:
  - Superior (upper) lobe
  - Middle lobe
  - Inferior lobe.

The superior lobe is separated from the middle one by the horizontal fissure. The middle lobe is separated from the inferior one by the oblique fissure.

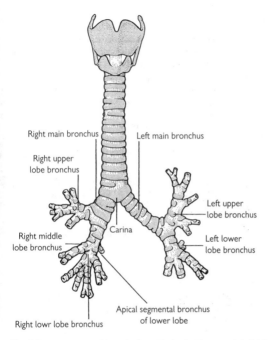

Fig. 3.3. The trachea and bronchi. From *Textbook of Anatomy*, (ed. A. W. Rogers), 1992. Reproduced with permission from Churchill Livingstone

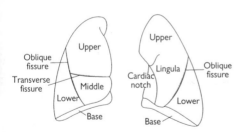

Fig. 3.4. The lungs and their lobes. From *Applied Basic Science for Basic Surgical Training*, (ed. A. T. Raftery), 2000. Reproduced with permission from Churchill Livingstone

The left lung has two lobes
- Superior lobe
- Inferior lobe.

The oblique fissure separates them. The deficiency of the superior lobe of the left lung is called cardiac notch. The lingula is the part of the left lung between the oblique fissure and the cardiac notch. It is the equivalent of the middle lobe of the right lung.

Bronchopulmonary segments

The lobar bronchi divide further to form the bronchopulmonary segments. There are ten segments per lung.

A bronchopulmonary segment is composed of :
- A tertiary bronchus
- The portion of lung it ventilates
- An artery
- A vein

There is no communication between segments. The bronchopulmonary segments represent the 'surgical units of the lung'. Their identification allows excising one segment without interfering with the adjacent ones.

Blood supply

The pulmonary trunk, which arises from the right ventricle, divides into the right and left pulmonary arteries.

The pleura

The lungs are invaginated by a serous membrane called pleura.
- *Visceral pleura*: this is the part of the membrane that lines the lungs.
- *Parietal pleura*: membrane that lines the mediastinum, diaphragm and inner aspect of the chest wall.

The parietal pleural may be divided into:
- Cervical pleura, apex extending 2.5cm above the clavicle
- Costal pleura
- Mediastinal pleura
- Diaphragmatic pleura, descending below the medial aspect of the 12th rib.

The potential space between the parietal and visceral pleura is called the pleural cavity. The projection of the heart on the left side makes the left pleural cavity smaller than the right one.

Nerve supply

- *Visceral pleura*: autonomic innervation from branches of the vagus nerve.
- *Parietal pleura*: somatic innervation from the intercostal nerves.
- *Diaphragmatic pleura*: phrenic nerve.

Practical hint

- The pleural cavity becomes a real space when the lung collapses. In this case the pleural cavity may contain air (pneumothorax) or blood (haemothorax).
- Central venous catheterisation (internal jugular vein/subclavian vein) or a stab wound above the level of the clavicle may damage the pleura (i.e. pneumothorax).

- The parietal pleural is sensitive to pain. Therefore the intercostal nerves may refer the pain to the abdomen, which explains abdominal pain as a possible symptom of pleuritic and chest wall disease.

The thoracic cage

The thoracic cage is composed of the following structures:
- **Anteriorly:** sternum and costal cartilages
- **Laterally:** 12 pairs of ribs and intercostal spaces
- **Posteriorly:** 12 thoracic vertebrae.

The sternum

This is formed by:
- **Manubrium:** it articulates with the clavicle, 1st cartilage and the upper part of the 2nd cartilage.
- **Body:** its lateral margins articulate with the rest of the 2nd rib and with the 3rd to 7th costal cartilage.
- **Xiphoid process**.

The ribs

The ribs 3 to 10 are 'typical ribs'. They are composed of:
- **Head:** it is wedge-shaped with two articular facets to the corresponding vertebra and the vertebra above.
- **Neck**.
- **Tubercle:** with an articular part (to the transverse process of the corresponding vertebra) and non-articular part.
- **Shaft:** rounded; its anterior part is flattened.
- **Costal groove:** it is located on the lower surface of the shaft. The intercostal artery, vein and nerve are contained in the groove.

The 1st, 2nd, 11th, and 12th ribs are regarded as atypical.
- The 1st rib is the shortest and broadest with a single facet on the head.
- The 2nd rib has an irregular rough tuberosity for the serratus anterior muscle.
- The 11th and 12th ribs are known as 'floating ribs' because their cartilages do not articulate anteriorly.

The ribs articulate as follows:
- **Posteriorly:** each rib articulates with the thoracic spine.
- **Anteriorly:** the superior seven costal cartilages articulate with the sternum; the cartilages from 8th to 10th articulate with cartilage above.

The intercostal space

An intercostal space is composed of three muscles:
- External intercostal
- Internal intercostal
- Innermost intercostals.

A neurovascular bundle contained in the lower surface of the corresponding rib, runs between the internal intercostal and innermost intercostal muscles. It includes from above downwards:
- Vein
- Artery
- Nerve.

Practical hints

Counting ribs may be necessary to identify which rib is injured or if the ribs are used as landmark for procedures such as chest drain insertion. The junction between the manubrium and the body of the sternum is felt like a transverse ridge on palpation. This is known as angle of Louis (sternal angle) and is opposite to the 2nd rib. Ribs are counted from this point.

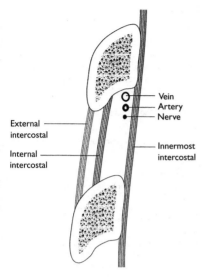

Fig. 3.5 An Intercostal space. A needle passed into the chest immediately above a rib will avoid the neurovascular bundle. From *Applied Basic Science for Basic Surgical Training*, (ed. A. T. Raftery), 2000. Reproduced with permission from Churchill Livingstone

The abdominal wall

The anterior abdominal wall

Fasciae

- *Superficial:* in the lower abdomen this is composed of a superficial fatty layer (Camper's fascia) and a deep fibrous layer (Scarpa's fascia). The latter is attached to the deep fascia of the leg 2.5cm below the inguinal ligament. It also continues into the perineum (Colles' fascia) and extends onto the penis and scrotum.
- *Deep:* a layer of areolar tissue over the muscles.

Muscles

Rectus abdominis and rectus sheath. These run longitudinally on each side of the midline.

Origin: 5th, 6th, 7th costal cartilage.

Insertion: pubic crest. There are also three tendinous insertions which attach the anterior rectus sheath to the xiphisternum, umbilicus, and halfway between.

The *rectus sheath* is mainly composed of the aponeurosis of the lateral abdominal muscles. The composition of the rectus sheath varies at three levels as follow:

1) Above the level of the costal margin, the anterior rectus sheath is composed of the aponeurosis of the external oblique only.
2) From the costal margin to a point half way between the umbilicus, the external oblique aponeurosis and the anterior leaf of the internal oblique aponeurosis form the anterior rectus sheath. The posterior leaf of the internal oblique aponeurosis and the internal oblique aponeurosis composes the posterior rectus sheath.
3) Below a point halfway between the umbilicus and pubic symphysis, all the aponeuroses pass anteriorly forming the anterior rectus sheath. The arcuate line of Douglas marks the inferior border of the posterior rectus sheath. Below this line there is transversalis fascia and peritoneum only.

- **External oblique**

Origin: lower eight ribs.

Insertion: linea alba, which results from the fusion of the rectus sheaths in the midline.

- **Internal oblique**

Origin: lumbar fascia, anterior two thirds of the iliac crest, lateral two thirds of the inguinal ligament.

Insertion: lower six costal cartilages, linea alba, pubic crest.

- **Transversus abdominis**

Origin: lower six costal cartilages, lumbar fascia, anterior two thirds of the iliac crest, lateral third of the inguinal ligament.

Insertion: linea alba and pubic crest.

Abdominal incisions: anatomy

The structures encountered vary depending on the incision used.

- **Midline**

Structures encountered: skin, subcutaneous fat, linea alba, extraperitoneal fat, peritoneum.

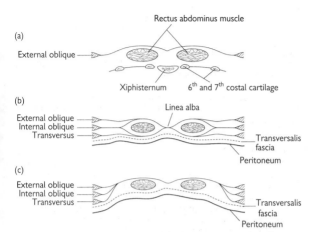

Fig. 3.6 The formation of the rectus sheath. a) above the costal margin; b) above the arcuate line; c) below the arcuate line. From *Applied Basic Science for Basic Surgical Training*, (ed. A. T. Raftery), 2000. Reproduced with permission from Churchill Livingstone

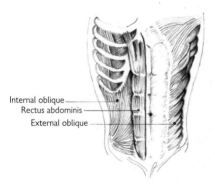

Fig. 3.7 Abdominal wall shows tendindus intersection attachments to anal rectus sheath.

- **Subcostal (Kocher's incision)**
Structures encountered: skin, subcutaneous fat, anterior rectus sheath, rectus muscle, posterior rectus sheath, extraperitoneal fat, and peritoneum.
- **Grid iron**
Structures encountered: skin, subcutaneous fat, Scarpa's fascia external oblique aponeurosis, internal oblique muscle, transversus abdominis muscle, extraperitoneal fat, peritoneum.
- **Paramedian**
Structures encountered: skin, subcutaneous fat, anterior rectus sheath, rectus muscle, posterior rectus sheath. The posterior rectus sheath is a thick structure in its upper part. Below the arcuate line of Douglas it is a thin structure, being composed of the transversalis fascia only.

The inguinal canal

This is a passage about 4cm long in the anterior abdominal wall through which the spermatic cord or round ligament pass. It lies above the medial half of the inguinal ligament and runs downwards, medially and forwards. It is a potential weak spot for the development of inguinal hernia.

It is a series of three openings in the muscles of the anterior abdominal wall which are staggered so that no opening overlies another:
- Deep inguinal ring (the deepest opening): an aperture in the fascia transversalis. Its surface position is about 1.5cm above the mid inguinal point.
- Opening in the combined tendons of transversus and internal oblique muscles (conjoint tendon): the spermatic cord or round ligament traverses this opening.
- Superficial inguinal ring: opening in the external oblique aponeurosis.

Deep inguinal ring

An indirect hernia enters the canal through this ring. It lies lateral to the inferior epigastric vessels. It transmits the round ligament of the uterus, its vessels, and nerve in females. In males the remainder of the processus vaginalis is vestigial superiorly, the cremasteric vessels are medial, and the genital branch of the genitofemoral nerve lies inferiorly. It transmits the spermatic cord and its contents.

Superficial inguinal ring

Is a triangular opening in the external oblique aponeurosis. Its medial and lateral sides are crura, the lateral of which is attached to the pubic tubercle. The medial crus is attached to the pubic symphysis. Therefore when an indirect inguinal hernia emerges from the superficial ring it is above and medial to the pubic tubercle.

Walls of the inguinal canal

- *Anterior*: aponeurosis of external oblique muscle
- *Posterior*: fascia transversalis and conjoint tendon
- *Superior*: lower edge of internal oblique
- *Inferior*: inguinal ligament.

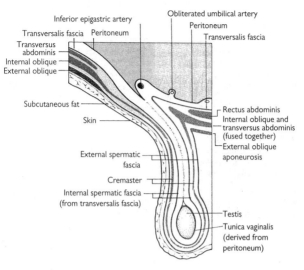

Fig. 3.8 Schematic diagram of the inguinal canal, and the coverings of the testis and spermatic cord. From *Textbook of anatomy*, (ed. A. W. Rogers), 1992. Reproduced with permission from Churchill Livingstone

The femoral canal

A femoral hernia passes through the femoral canal to reach the upper aspect of the thigh below the inguinal ligament.

Features

The femoral artery, vein, and canal are all enclosed in the femoral sheath which is a continuation of the transversalis fascia above the inguinal ligament and that covering iliacus and psoas muscles below. The canal lies on pectineus muscle between the femoral vein and the lacunar ligament. It provides space for the femoral vein to expand when venous return from the leg is increased. It is funnel-shaped, about 2cm long and with an upper opening, the femoral ring, which is 1.5–2cm wide and opens into the abdomen.

The femoral ring

The ring contains:
- Fat—the femoral septum
- A single lymph node (Cloquet's).

Boundaries

- *Anterior:* inguinal ligament
- *Posterior:* pectineal line, pectineus, and its fascia
- *Medial:* lacunar ligament
- *Lateral:* femoral vein

The femoral canal opens below and lateral to the pubic tubercle. The site of appearance of a femoral hernia.

A *femoral hernia* descends through the canal and usually hooks round the anterior margin of the femoral ring to come to lie over the inguinal ligament. Its coverings include fat (the femoral septum), lymph glands, the anterior wall of the femoral canal, cribriform fascia, superficial fascia, subcutaneous fat, and skin.

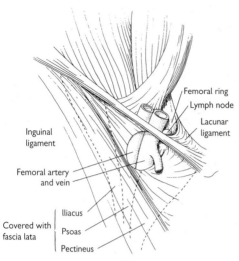

Fig. 3.9 The femoral canal

The digestive system

The oesophagus

The oesophagus is a hollow viscus about 25cm long, which extends from the cricopharyngeal sphincter at the level of the 6th cervical vertebra to the cardia of the stomach. It comprises:

- Cervical oesophagus: extending between the level of the lower border of the cricoid cartilage and the jugular notch.
- Upper oesophagus: extends from the level of the jugular notch to the level of the tracheal bifurcation.
- Middle oesophagus: extends from the carina to the midpoint between the carina and the oesophago-gastric junction.
- Lower oesophagus: this includes the lower thoracic oesophagus and the hiatal segment of the oesophagus (or abdominal oesophagus).

It passes through the lower part of the neck, superior, and posterior mediastinum and pierces the diaphragm at the level of the 10th thoracic vertebra. The lowermost part lies below the level of the diaphragm.

Layers

- Stratified squamous epithelium. A gastric-type mucosa may be present in the lower oesophagus.
- Submucosa.
- Musculature: striated in the upper one third. Smooth muscle in lower two thirds. There is an external longitudinal layer and an internal circular layer.
- There is no serosa.

Relations

In the neck
- Trachea anteriorly, cervical vertebrae posteriorly
- Carotid artery and thyroid on the right and left
- Subclavian artery and thoracic duct on the left at the root of the neck.

In the thorax
- Trachea, left bronchus, left atrium in front
- Right and left pleura and lung
- Aorta mainly behind but on the left at first
- Vagus nerves.

Blood supply

- Arterial: this is through the inferior thyroid artery, the descending thoracic aorta and the left gastric artery.
- Venous drainage: this is through the inferior thyroid veins, the azygos vein and the left gastric vein.

Nerve supply

- Extrinsic and intrinsic nerve plexuses from the vagus nerve (parasympathetic). The vagus nerve is in close relationship with the oesophagus throughout its length.
- Sympathetic supply is from the sympathetic trunks.

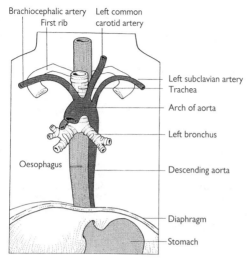

Fig. 3.10 The oesophagus: anterior view. From *Textbook of anatomy*, (ed. A. W. Rogers), 1992. Reproduced with permission from Churchill Livingstone

Sites of anatomical narrowing

There are three sites of constriction. Measuring from the incisor teeth they are at:

- 15cm: cricopharyngeal sphincter
- 25cm: aortic arch and bifurcation of the bronchi
- 40cm: diaphragmatic hiatus.

Foreign bodies may become arrested at these levels. They are also the sites at which strictures (benign or malignant) are most common.

Barrett's oesophagus

Refers to the replacement of the squamous epithelium by a columnar-lined mucosa in the lower oesophagus. This is usually secondary to gastro-oesophageal reflux. Its importance lies in the fact that it is associated with an increased risk of oesophageal adenocarcinoma (up to 30–40 times that of the general population).

The stomach

The stomach extends from the oesophagus to the duodenum. It lies in the upper left quadrant of the abdomen behind the lower ribs and anterior abdominal wall and is separated from the left lung and pleura by the dome of the diaphragm.

It is described as piriform organ which includes:

- An anterior surface.
- A posterior surface.
- A greater curvature, which is convex.
- A lesser curvature, which is concave.

The oesophagus enters the stomach on its right side about 2.5cm below its uppermost part.

The stomach comprises:

- A cardiac orifice at the level of oesophageal opening.
- A fundus proximal to oesophageal orifice.
- A body from fundus to pyloric antrum.
- A pyloric antrum is the dilated part after the incisura angularis.
- A pyloric canal is 2.5cm long. It passes from the antrum to the pyloric sphincter.
- The pylorus, which is continuous with the first part of the duodenum and has thickened muscle—the pyloric sphincter.

Peritoneal folds

The stomach is covered by peritoneum on each surface. These meet at the curvatures to form the lesser omentum above and the greater omentum below. The greater omentum forms three ligaments:

- The gastrophrenic from the fundus to the diaphragm
- The gastrosplenic to the spleen
- The gastrocolic to the transverse colon.

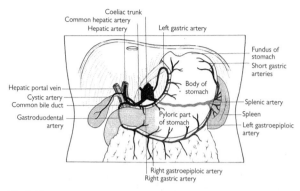

Fig. 3.11. The arterial supply of the stomach: anterior view. From *Textbook of anatomy*, (ed. A. W. Rogers), 1992. Reproduced with permission from Churchill Livingstone

Relations
- Anterior: liver to the right, diaphragm to the left, anterior- abdominal wall.
- Posterior: body of pancreas, part of left kidney, and left suprarenal, splenic artery and spleen. These form the 'bed' of the stomach. The transverse mesocolon passes from the lower border of the pancreas to the transverse colon.

Blood supply
Arterial
- Left gastric from coeliac axis
- Right gastric from hepatic artery
- Gastroduodenal from hepatic artery
- Left gastroepiploic from splenic artery
- Short gastrics (several) from splenic artery
- Right gastroepiploic from the gastroduodenal artery.

Venous drainage
The blood drained from the stomach passes to the portal system.
- Right gastric vein, directly to portal vein
- Left gastric vein, directly to portal vein
- Right gastro-epiploic vein, to portal vein via superior mesenteric vein
- Left gastro-epiploic vein, to portal vein via the splenic vein
- Short gastric veins, to portal vein via the splenic vein.

Nerve supply
The fundus and body of the stomach receive their nerve supply from the proximal vagus. The antrum is innervated by the anterior and posterior nerves of Latarjet also from the vagus.

Lymph drainage
It is to the following lymph node stations:
- Cardiac (right and left)
- Greater and lesser curvature
- Suprapyloric and infrapyloric
- Left gastric artery, common hepatic artery, coeliac artery, splenic artery, middle colic artery
- Hilum of the spleen, posterior of the pancreas, root of the mesentery
- Para-aortic.

The small intestine
This comprises:
- Duodenum
- Jejunum
- Ileum.

The duodenum is retroperitoneal and joins the jejunum at the duodeno-jejunal flexure.

The jejunum and ileum are both suspended from the posterior abdominal wall by a double fold of peritoneum containing the blood supply and venous drainage—the mesentery. Its attachment is about 15cm long and it lies obliquely from the duodenojejunal flexure to the ileocaecal junction. The 20+feet (about 7m) of the small bowel attached to such a small base are therefore convoluted.

As jejunum runs into ileum the features change. Although both have large surface areas internally to aid absorption, the circular folds of mucous membrane decrease in number and size in the ileum and are almost completely absent in the lower ileum so the wall feels thinner. Throughout the small intestine aggregations of lymph follicles are present. These are more marked in the ileum and are called Peyer's patches. They occur on the anti-mesenteric border. Another difference is that mesenteric fat is less abundant near the intestinal wall in the jejunum so that the vessels to the gut can be seen with mesenteric transparent windows between them.

Blood supply

- Arterial: the superior mesenteric artery crosses the third part of the duodenum to enter the root of the mesentery and pass downward towards the right iliac fossa. It gives off several jejunal and ileal arteries, which divide and reunite to supply the small bowel. In doing so, they form a series of arterial arches and arcades. so one or more of the main trunks may be ligated without affecting the blood supply.
- Venous: the veins drain the gut along the arterial pathways and empty into the superior mesenteric vein which joins the portal vein on its way to the liver.

Practical hints

- The duodenojejunal flexure is a site which must always be carefully examined in patients with deceleration injuries because disruption can occur.
- The fact that the blood supply of the small bowel is organised in arches and arcade allows to ligate one of the main trunks without affecting the blood supply. This is done when constructing an ileal pouch for anastomosis to

the rectum in patients with inflammatory bowel disease and familial adenomatous polyposis (see Restorative proctocolectomy).

The large bowel

This is approximately 1.5m long. It comprises of:

- Appendix
- Caecum
- Ascending colon
- Hepatic flexure
- Transverse colon
- Splenic flexure
- Descending colon
- Sigmoid colon
- Rectum
- Anus.

The lumen is wide in the caecum and ascending colon but gradually narrows towards the sigmoid colon.

Structure

It has a peritoneal coat complete over the caecum, appendix, transverse colon and sigmoid colon but incomplete elsewhere. There are small pouches of peritoneum filled with fat over all of the colon—appendices epiploicae.

The outer muscular coat is disposed in three longitudinal bands—the taenia coli. These converge upon the root of the appendix proximally. At the other end they become continuous with the longitudinal layer of the rectum. They are shorter than the colon so its wall becomes puckered into sacculations—colonic haustrations.

Caecum

The ileum terminates in a slit-like opening—the ileocaecal valve. The blind-ending portion below this level is the caecum. It may lie free or be attached to the right iliac fossa by peritoneal folds.

Relations
- Inferior: lateral half of inguinal ligament
- Anterior: greater omentum, coils of ileum, anterior abdominal wall
- Posterior: iliacus and psoas.

Colon

The ascending and descending components are partly retro-peritoneal. The transverse and sigmoid colon are suspended on mesenteries.

Transverse colon

The middle portion lies below the umbilicus. Superiorly lies the greater curvature of the stomach, liver, and gall bladder. Posteriorly from right to left are the second part of the duodenum, the pancreas, loops of small bowel and the spleen. Anteriorly is the greater omentum.

Descending colon

This begins at the splenic flexure and ends at the beginning of the sigmoid colon.

Relations
- Anterior: jejunum, lower part of anterior abdominal wail
- Posterior: left kidney, psoas, quadratus lumborum, iliacus

Sigmoid colon

This begins at the pelvic brim and ends at the level of the 3rd sacral vertebra. It is mobile and variable in length. It is related superiorly to loops of small bowel.

Blood supply

- Caecum and appendix: from the superior mesenteric and ileocolic arteries
- Ascending colon: from ileocolic and right colic arteries
- Transverse colon/flexures: from the right middle and left colic arteries
- Descending colon: left colic artery
- Sigmoid and upper rectum: left colic, superior rectal arteries.

Lymphatic drainage

This is along the arterial supply. Nodes are situated:
- On the bowel surface
- Between the layers of the mesocolon
- Along the branches of the mesenteric arteries
- Along the trunks of the main vessels.

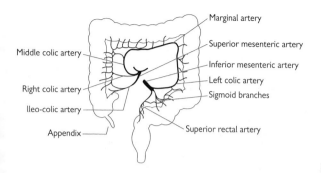

Fig. 3.12 The arterial blood supply of the large intestine. From *Applied Basic Science for Basic Surgical Training*, (ed. A. T. Raftery), 2000. Reproduced with permission from Churchill Livingstone

The appendix

Surface markings

The vermiform (worm-like) appendix is an appendage of the caecum lying in the right iliac fossa. When inflamed, maximum tenderness is classically felt over McBurney's point (one third of the way along a line drawn from the anterior superior iliac spine to the umbilicus).

Features

It is 8–10cm long and 6–8mm in girth. Its base is attached to the caecum at the point of convergence of the three taenia coli on the posteromedial wall (see McBurney's point, above) or responding to McBurney's point on the surface.

It contains numerous aggregations of lymphoid tissue in its wall and has a small lumen. It is covered by peritoneum and has a well-formed mesoappendix derived from the posterior layer of the mesentery of the lower ileum. It is in the mesoappendix that the appendicular vessels lie.

Blood supply

The appendicular artery is a branch of the posterior caecal from the ileocolic artery. It gives off 2–3 branches to the appendix during its course in the free crescentic edge of the mesoappendix.

Variations in position

The appendix may be freely movable. Common variations in order of frequency are:
- Retrocaecal (62%): sometimes extending to the right lobe of the liver, or in the serous coat of the caecum
- Pelvic (34%): rectal examination may produce pain
- Paracaecal (2%)
- Preileal (1%)
- Retroileal (0.5%).

The rectum

The rectum extends from the rectosigmoid junction (at the level of S3) to the proximal part of the anal canal (2.5cm in front of the coccyx). It is 10–15cm long.

Peritoneal covering
- Upper third: the posterior wall is extraperitoneal.
- Middle third: the posterior and lateral walls are extraperitoneal.
- Lower third: is entirely extraperitoneal.

Relations
- Anteriorly:
  Male: rectovescical pouch, bladder, prostate and seminal vescicles. The fascia of Denonvilliers separates these structures from the anterior wall of the rectum.
  Female: recto-uterine pouch of Douglas and the posterior wall of the vagina.
- Posteriorly: sacrum and coccyx.
- Laterally: levator ani and coccygeus.

Blood supply
Arterial
- Superior rectal from the inferior mesenteric artery
- Middle rectal from the anterior division of the internal iliac artery
- Inferior rectal from the internal pudendal artery.

Venous drainage
- Superior rectal vein to the portal vein
- Middle and inferior rectal vein to the internal iliac.

These systems are in communication, forming a potential porto-systemic anastomosis.

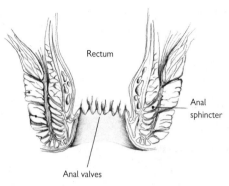

Fig. 3.13 The rectum

The anal canal

The anal canal is the terminal part of the alimentary tract. It is 4cm long.

Embryology
- Upper half: derives from endoderm.
- Lower half: derives from ectoderm.

Epithelial lining
- Upper half: columnar epithelium. Adenocarcinomas usually arise from this area.
- Lower half: squamous epithelium. Squamous carcinomas usually arise from this area.

The line where the lining changes is termed the dentate line.

Blood supply
Arterial
- Upper half: superior rectal artery
- Lower half: inferior rectal artery.

Venous
- Upper half: tributary of the portal system
- Lower half: drains into the systemic venous system.

Lymphatic drainage
- Upper half: to abdominal lymph nodes via the superior rectal vessels
- Lower half: to inguinal lymph nodes.

Nerve supply
- Upper half: autonomic nervous system (insensitive to pinprick sensation)
- Lower half: somatic innervation (sensitive to pinprick sensation).

Anal sphincters
The anal canal is surrounded by:
- Internal sphincter: smooth muscle
- External sphincter: striated muscle.

The external sphincter surrounds the internal sphincter. An intersphincteric groove exists between the two sphincters.

Practical hint
In minor procedures such as injections of haemorrhoids, the needle should be inserted in the upper half of the anal canal that is insensitive to pain.

The liver

This, the largest organ of the body, lies in the right upper quadrant predominantly to the right of the midline and mostly under cover of the ribs. In health it is not normally palpable in the abdomen and extends internally to T8 and the xiphisternum in the midline and almost level with the nipples on each side.

Lobes
- Right
- Caudate
- Quadrate
- Left.

Surfaces
- Anterior
- Posterior
- Superior
- Inferior.

The inferior surface is related to the viscera, the others to the diaphragm.

Ligaments
- Falciform on the anterior and superior surfaces separating the two lobes. It is a fold of peritoneum attached to the peritoneum of the anterior abdominal wall.
- Ligamentum teres (vestigial umbilical cord) runs from the umbilicus in the edge of the falciform ligament, to the inferior surface where it enters a deep cleft—the fissure for the ligamentum teres.
- Ligamentum venosum (vestigial ductus venosus) lies in a fissure on the posterior surface separating the right and left lobes.
- Coronary ligaments are layers of peritoneum reflected on the left side to the diaphragm and enclosing the so-called bare area. Where they join to the right and left bare areas are the right and left triangular ligaments.

Porta hepatis
There is a deep cleft on the inferior surface of the right lobe. The quadrate lobe lies in front, and caudate behind. It transmits the portal vein, the hepatic artery, and the hepatic ducts. The bile ducts lie anterior to the vein and to the right of the artery. Branches of the portal vein, hepatic artery, and bile duct tributaries then run together into the lobes of the liver. These are the portal triad.

Inferior vena cava
- Lies in a deep groove on the posterior surface 2cm to the right of midline. There are three main hepatic veins draining approximately equal proportions of the liver. These drain into the vena cava near the diaphragmatic surface of the liver. Accessory smaller hepatic veins are common.

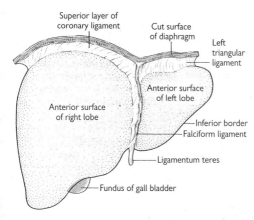

Fig. 3.14 The liver: anterior view. From *Textbook of anatomy*, (ed. A. W. Rogers), 1992. Reproduced with permission from Churchill Livingstone

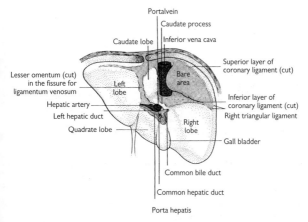

Fig. 3.15 The liver: posterior view. From *Textbook of anatomy*, (ed. A. W. Rogers), 1992. Reproduced with permission from Churchill Livingstone

Segmental anatomy

This is based upon ramifications of the portal triad structures (portal vein, hepatic artery and biliary apparatus). These ramifications accompany each other throughout the liver. The first major divisions of the portal structures divide the liver into a right and left lobe. The division is through a plane that runs from the inferior vena cava to the middle of the gall-bladder fossa. These two lobes are further subdivided in segments:

- Right lobe: anterior and posterior segments (no external features indicate this plane of division)
- Left lobe: medial and lateral segments (plane of division: falciform ligament and fissure of the round ligament)
- Each segment is divided into superior and inferior subsegments.

In total there are eight segments. Their identification permits relatively avascular dissection and minimises the risk of injury of adjacent structures (considerable experience is essential in hepatic resection) during the operations of segmentectomy and lobectomy.

Lesser omentum

The peritoneal coverings converge inferiorly to form a wide fold under the left lobe of the liver. It is attached to the first 2.5cm of the duodenum, the lesser curvature of the stomach, and the diaphragm to the left between the liver and oesophagus. Its right edge is free, being the anterior border of the opening into the lesser sac. The common bile duct, the hepatic artery and portal vein lie in its free edge.

Subphrenic spaces

These are common sites of intra-abdominal abscesses. The right and left subphrenic spaces are between the liver and diaphragm, being separated from each other by the falciform ligament.

- Right subphrenic space (Rutherford Morrison's pouch) is below the liver, anterior to the posterior abdominal wall and related to the gall bladder, duodenum and right kidney
- Left subphrenic space is the lesser omental sac.

Blood vessels

- Hepatic artery and portal vein carry blood to the liver.
- The hepatic veins drain the liver into the inferior vena cava.

Nerves

- Branches of the vagus nerve
- Branches of the coeliac plexus.

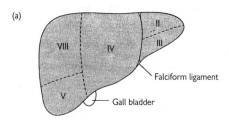

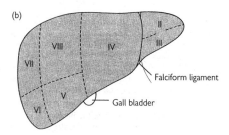

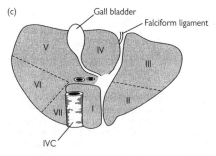

Fig. 3.16 The functional division of the liver into segments. a) anterior view as seen in the patient; b) anterior view with the liver 'flattened' in the ex-vivo position (note that segments VI and VII may now be seen—in vivo they appear more later-ally and posteriorly); c) inferior view. From *Applied Basic Science for Basic Surgical Training*, (ed. A. T. Raftery), 2000. Reproduced with permission from Churchill Livingstone

The gall bladder and bile ducts

The gall bladder

This is a pear-shaped organ attached to the under surface of the right lobe of the liver and projects slightly beyond its free margin. It lies in the right upper quadrant of the abdomen below the upper ends of the linea semilunaris.

It comprises of:
- A fundus
- A body
- A neck.

Features

The gall bladder is about 10cm long and its fundus is completely covered with peritoneum. The body and neck are covered on three sides only, being connected anteriorly to the liver by loose connective tissue from which it is easily separated. The neck has a dilatation called Hartmann's pouch which hangs downwards and may be attached to the duodenum by folds—congenital or inflammatory. The neck becomes the cystic duct which drains into the common hepatic duct to form the common bile duct.

Blood supply

- Arterial: the cystic artery that usually is a branch of the hepatic artery. The cystic artery is contained in a triangular area called Calot's triangle. Its boundaries are: the liver, the cystic duct, and the common hepatic duct.
- Venous: small veins that drain into the liver.

Bile ducts

The right and left hepatic ducts emerge from the liver through the porta hepatis and unite to form the common hepatic duct, which continues as the common bile duct after being joined by the cystic duct.

The common bile duct

This duct, 9cm long, lies in the free edge of the lesser omentum (3cm) then passes behind the first part of the duodenum (3cm) and penetrates its second part obliquely (3cm) behind the head of the pancreas where it lies in a deep groove in front of the right renal vein. Its lower end is dilated to form the ampulla of Vater in common with the main pancreatic duct. It enters the medial wall of the second part of the duodenum.

Relations of the common bile duct

- The hepatic ducts and the supraduodenal part of the common bile duct lie in the free edge of the lesser omentum. The hepatic artery lies on its left side.
- The portal vein lies posteriorly.
- The right hepatic artery passes behind the common bile duct before giving off its cystic branch.
- The lower one third of the common bile duct may actually lie in a tunnel in the pancreas.

Practical hints

- Intermittent compression of the free edge of the lesser omentum can be performed for up to 15 minutes at a time to control hepatic bleeding (Pringle's manoeuvre).
- NB Variations are common. Some are illustrated. Failure to recognise these can spell disaster for the surgeon.

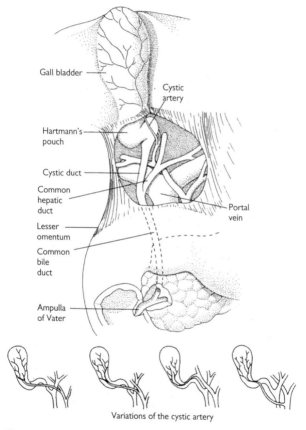

Variations of the cystic artery

Fig. 3.17 The gallbladder and bile ducts

The pancreas

This elongated, lobulated gland lies on the posterior abdominal wall at the level of L1 in the transpyloric plane. It develops from dorsal and ventral buds of endoderm which initially lie diametrically opposite each other. Subsequent duodenal rotation and asymmetric growth lead to fusion of the buds. Their ducts become the accessory and main pancreatic ducts. Abnormal or incomplete rotation produces an annular pancreas, which may cause duodenal obstruction.

Features

It has a *head* in contact with the duodenum on three sides, a *neck* which is indented posteriorly by the portal and superior mesenteric veins, and a *tail* which is contained within the lieno-renal ligament. On cut section the gland is triangular in shape with well-defined superior and inferior borders and a blunt anterior border to which the transverse mesocolon is attached.

Relations

Head
- Posterior: inferior vena cava, right renal vein and artery, terminal portion of common bile duct.
- Anterior: first part of duodenum, transverse colon, gastro duodenal artery.

Body
- Posterior: aorta, branches of coeliac artery on the upper border, superior mesenteric on the lower border, splenic vein, left renal vein and artery, left suprarenal, hilum of left kidney.
- Anterior: transverse mesocolon, stomach, lesser sac.

Pancreatic ducts

The main duct arises in the tail, traverses the body and neck, and then curves downwards to reach the head. It empties into the ampulla of the bile duct on the medial wall of the second part of the duodenum at the greater duodenal papilla. The accessory pancreatic duct opens into the duodenum 2cm above the main duct.

Blood supply

- Arterial: from the coeliac and superior mesenteric arteries. The head and uncinate process are supplied by the superior pancreaticoduodenal artery from the gastroduodenal artery and the inferior pancreaticoduodenal from the superior mesenteric artery. The remainder of the gland is supplied by the splenic artery.
- Venous: drainage is by corresponding veins to the portal vein.

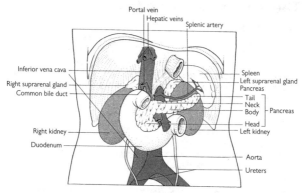

Fig. 3.18 The pancreas: anterior view. From *Textbook of anatomy*, (ed. A. W. Rogers), 1992. Reproduced with permission from Churchill Livingstone

The genitourinary system

The kidneys

The kidneys are retroperitoneal organs. The right kidney is lower than the left one because of the liver, which is above it. Each kidney is surrounded by perirenal fat, which, in turn, is covered by the renal fascia. Especially posteriorly to the kidney, the renal fascia is surrounded by a layer of fat known as perirenal fascia or Gerota's fascia.

Each kidney comprises of:
- A capsule
- Two surfaces: anterior and posterior
- Two borders: medial and lateral
- Two poles: upper and lower
- A hilum where, in antero-posterior direction, the renal vein, artery, and pelvis enter and leave the kidney.

Internal structure
- Medulla: this is composed of 6–10 pyramids. The apex of the pyramids is directed toward the hilum, while the base is facing the outer capsule. The apex opens into a minor calyx. The medulla contains loops of Henle and collecting tubes.
- Cortex: this is situated between adjacent pyramids and separates the base of the pyramids from the renal capsule. It contains glomeruli and convoluted tubes.

Blood supply
The right and left renal arteries are branches from the aorta. Each renal artery divides into segmental arteries. Based on this division the kidney presents five segments:
- Apical
- Anterosuperior
- Anteroinferior
- Inferior
- Posterior.

The right and left renal veins drain straight into the inferior vena cava.

The ureters

The ureters are tubular structures extending from the renal pelvis to the posteroinferior wall of the bladder. Each ureter is 25–30cm long and its diameter varies between 2–8mm. They are retroperitoneal throughout their length.

Relations
- Abdominal part

In the proximity of the pelvis, each ureter crosses anteriorly to the psoas muscle. The upper part of the right ureter is covered anteriorly by the second part of the duodenum. Its inferior part is posterior to the right colic vessels, ileocolic vessels and the root of the mesentery. On the left, the left colic vessels run anteriorly to the upper part of ureter. Inferiorly, the ureter is crossed anteriorly by the sigmoid vessels. In proximity of the pelvis each ureter is crossed anteriorly by the gonadal vessels.

● Pelvic part

Male: each ureter runs medially to the internal iliac artery. At the level of the ischial spine the ureter turns medially, running down with branches of the hypogastric nerves. Just before entering the bladder, the ureter is crossed anteriorly by the vas deferens.

Female: each ureter is lateral to the ovarian vessels. It runs along the lateral wall of the pelvis. It is in close relation with the uterine artery, ovary (the ureter is posterior to it), and broad ligament of the uterus. In proximity of the neck of the uterus, the uterine artery crosses the ureter again, being posterior to it.

Blood supply

● The ureters receive arterial blood supply from the renal artery, branches of the abdominal aorta, gonadal vessels, common iliac arteries, and inferior vesical artery.

● The venous drainage follows the arterial pattern. Veins from the ureter drain into the renal vein and inferior vena cava.

Practical hints

During procedures such as hysterectomy, right and left hemicolectomy, anterior resection, and abdomino-perineal resections the ureters need to be identified to prevent ureteric iatrogenic injuries.

The bladder

This is an extraperitoneal organ, which lies in the pelvis. The empty bladder is below the pubis. When full, it rises in the abdominal cavity.

The bladder comprises of:

● The fundus: postero-superior.

● The apex: antero-superior.

● The body: postero-inferior. Here the two ureteric orifices open.

● The neck: inferior. It contains the internal urethral meatus.

The triangular area described by the two ureteric orifices and the internal urethral meatus is called the trigone.

Relations

● Anteriorly: the space of Retzius separates the bladder from the pubic symphysis.

● Superiorly: peritoneum with coils of small bowel and sigmoid colon. In the female the uterus is in relation with the bladder.

● Posteriorly: in the male, the rectum and the seminal vesicles. In the female, the vagina and the cervix.

● Laterally: the peritoneum covers the bladder down to the level of the umbilical artery. Below this level the bladder is in relation with the lateral walls of the pelvis.

Blood supply

● Superior and inferior vesical arteries, from the anterior branches of the internal iliac artery.

● Short vesical veins. These form a rich venous plexus that is tributary of the internal iliac veins.

Lymphatic drainage

- To the external iliac lymph nodes from the anterior part of the bladder.
- To the hypogastric lymph nodes from the posterior part of the bladder.

Nerve supply

- Extrinsic nerves: from the inferior hypogastric plexuses.
- Intrinsic nerves: from a perivesical plexus which receive both parasympathetic fibres (S2–S4) and sympathetic fibres (T11–L2).

Practical hint

- Because of the relation between sigmoid colon and bladder, diverticulitis may lead to formation of a colo-vesical fistula.
- Since an empty bladder does not rise above the pubis, insertion of a suprapubic catheter must not be attempted unless the bladder is full.

The prostate

Most of the prostate surrounds the posterior and lateral aspects of the prostatic urethra. A minimal amount of prostate lies anterior to the urethra.

The prostate comprises of:

- Lateral lobes: they are continuous anteriorly, but separated posteriorly by a midline sulcus)
- Median lobe: it lies posteriorly between ejaculatory ducts and the urethra
- Posterior lobe: atrophic
- Isthmus: anterior to urethra.

It is composed of two main components:

- Glandular component
- Smooth muscle component.

Relations

- Superiorly: neck of the bladder and seminal vesicles.
- Inferiorly: urogenital diaphragm.
- Anteriorly: lower part of the pubic symphysis.
- Posteriorly: rectum (separated by the fascia of Denonvilliers).
- Laterally: levator ani.

Blood supply

- The inferior vesical artery (branch of the internal iliac artery) is the main source of blood supply.
- Venous blood is drained through the prostatic venous plexus into the vesical and hypogastric veins.

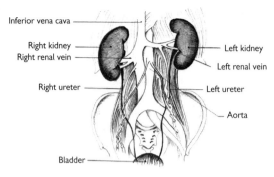

Fig. 3.19 The kidneys and ureters

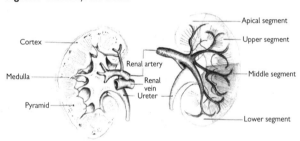

Fig. 3.20 The segments and blood supply of the kidneys

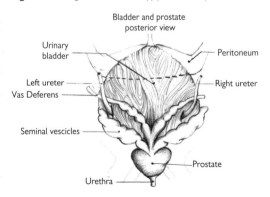

Fig. 3.21 The bladder and prostate: posterior view

Surgical instruments, materials, and the acquisition of surgical skills

G. O'Dair, G. R. McLatchie, and
David J. Leaper

Introduction

There is considerable variation in the types of instruments used in different hospitals and the manufacturing companies who produce them. Instruments carry both generic and eponymous names which can lead to confusion. It is important for the surgeon and theatre staff to have a mutual understanding of the names of surgical instruments.

The basic surgical trainee, in order to assist and perform surgical operations, needs to be familiar with several basic types of general surgical instruments. These fall under the following categories:

- Scalpel handles
- Needle holders
- Scissors—suture and dissecting
- Tissue dissecting forceps
- Tissue holding forceps
- Artery forceps
- Hand-held retractors
- Self-retaining retractors
- Bowel clamps
- Vascular instruments
- Suckers
- Endoscopic equipment
- Laparoscopic equipment.

Scalpel handles

Scalpel holders are numbered and accommodate a variety of sizes of scalpel blades. Care should be taken to mount and remove scalpel blades using an artery clip (Fig. 4.1).

Needle holders

Most needle holders are ratcheted and have a specially designed surface between the jaws to allow a firm grasp of the needle and prevent it twisting. They should be placed halfway along the needle to avoid damage to the needle point and the swage (which would cause detachment from the suture). (Fig. 4.2)

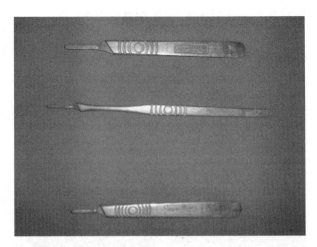

Fig. 4.1 Scalpel holders no. 3, 4, and 5

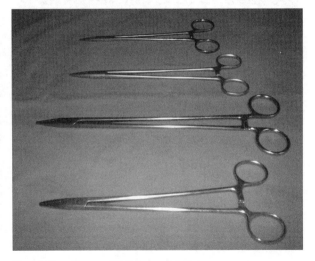

Fig. 4.2 Mayo, Masson, and DeBlakey needle holders

Scissors—suture and dissecting

Scissors are either straight or curved and used to cut sutures or for dissection. Longer curved scissors are useful for dissection deep within body cavities. (Figs. 4.3–4.5)

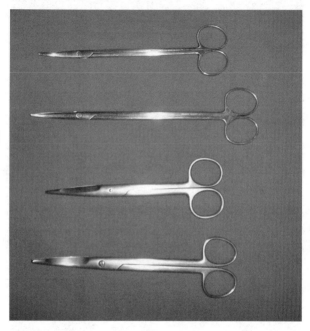

Fig. 4.3 Short and long McKindoe scissors

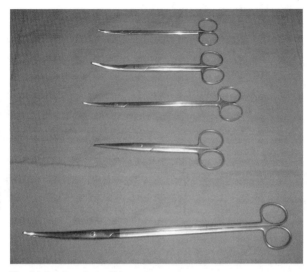

Fig. 4.4 Straight and curved Mayo scissors

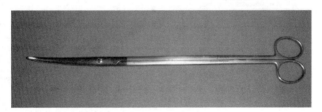

Fig. 4.5 30cm Metzenbaum/Nelson scissors

Tissue dissecting forceps

Dissecting forceps aid surgical dissection. Delicate structures such as bowel, arteries and veins etc. are handled with non-toothed forceps, while more robust structures can be handled with toothed forceps, for example the skin or abdominal wall. The teeth can be used as a hook with avoidance of tissue damage. (Fig. 4.6)

Tissue holding forceps

Atraumatic tissue holding forceps, such as Duval and Babcock, can be used to manipulated bowel and visceral structures. Lane and Allis forceps cannot be used this way as they are relatively traumatic and hence used to hold the skin and abdominal wall. Rampley sponge holders can also be used as tissue forceps such as retracting on the gallbladder fundus during open cholecystectomy. (Fig. 4.7)

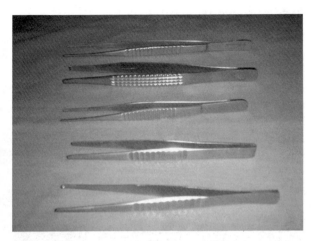

Fig. 4.6 Tissue dissecting forceps

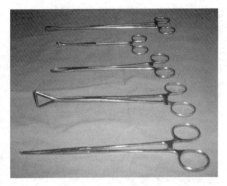

Fig. 4.7 From top: Rampley, Babcock, Littlewood, Duval, and Allis tissue holding forceps

Artery forceps

Artery forceps vary in size and are either straight or curved. They are used to clamp vascular structures prior to division and ligation. (Fig. 4.8)

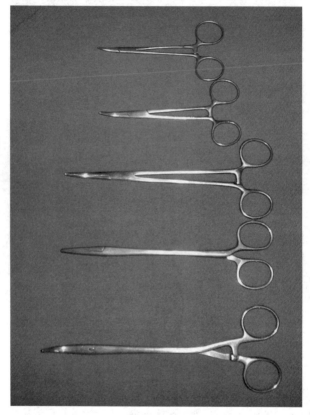

Fig. 4.8 From top: Mosquito, Criles, 7 inch Spencer Wells, Rochester-Penn, and Moynihan artery forceps

Hand-held retractors

Hand-held retractors are used by assistants during operative procedures in order to provide the surgeon with a clear field of vision of the operative field. (Figs. 4.9–4.11)

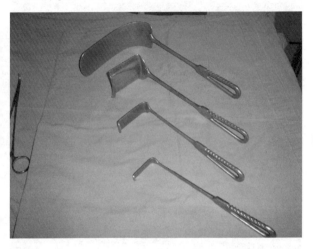

Fig. 4.9

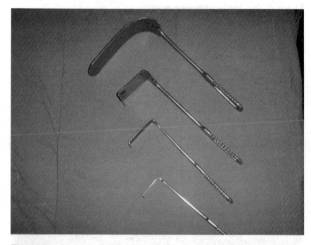

Fig. 4.10

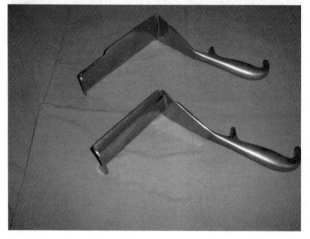

Fig. 4.11

Self-retaining retractors

These allow assisting surgeons to be used for other tasks by retracting open the surgical wound. (Figs. 4.12–4.17)

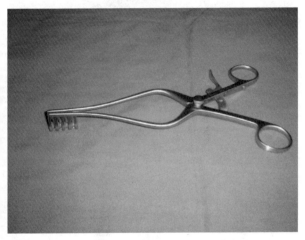

Fig. 4.12 Travers self-retaining retractors

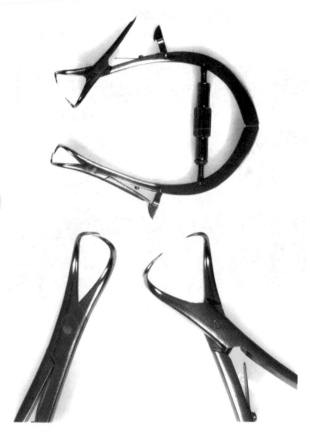

Fig. 4.13 Jolles retractor (thyroid surgery)

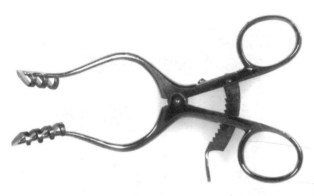

Fig. 4.14 West retractor

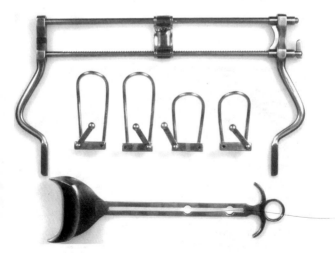

Fig. 4.15 Balfour set

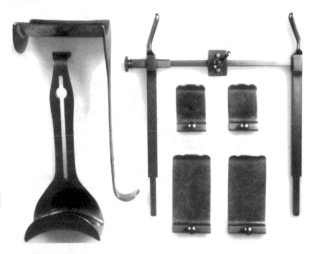

Fig. 4.16 Goligher set

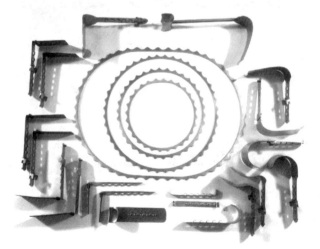

Fig. 4.17 Turner Warwick set

Bowel clamps

Crushing bowel clamps are either curved or straight. Traumatic clamps occlude bowel that will be removed with the resection specimen. Non-crushing bowel clamps atraumatically occlude bowel that is not resected to prevent spillage of bowel content prior to anastomosis or stomal formation. (Figs. 4.18–4.21)

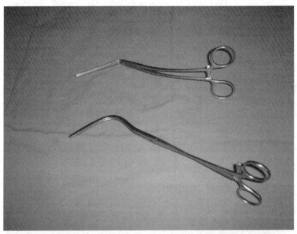

Fig. 4.18 Hayes (top) Zachary-Cope (bottom) (closed)

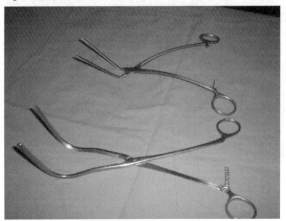

Fig. 4.19 Hayes (top) Zachary-Cope (bottom) (open)

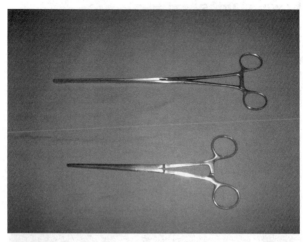

Fig. 4.20 Doyen bowel clamps (closed)

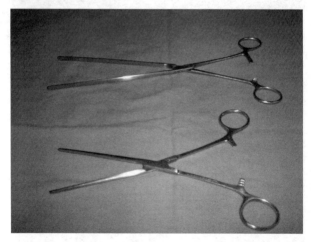

Fig. 4.21 Doyen bowel clamps (open)

Vascular instruments

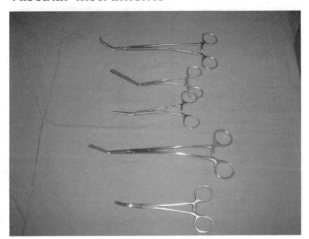

Fig. 4.22 Satinsky (top)

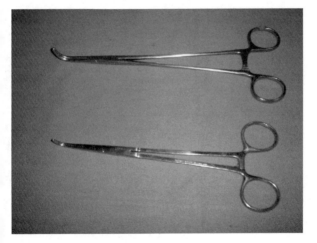

Fig. 4.23 O'Shaughnessy (top) Lancy (bottom)

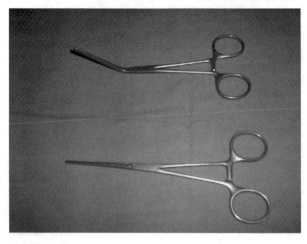

Fig. 4.24 Ringed Bulldog (top) Debakey (bottom)

Suckers

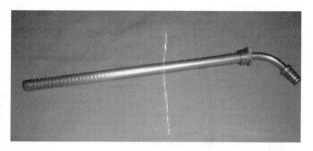

Fig. 4.25 Poole Sucker. Low pressure, internal/external sheath.

Endoscopic equipment

Gastroscopy set
Components
Light source
Water bottle (air feed system)
Mouth guard
Biopsy forceps
Gastroscope—lens
tip control
air/suction buttons
biopsy channel
suction/air feed connectors.

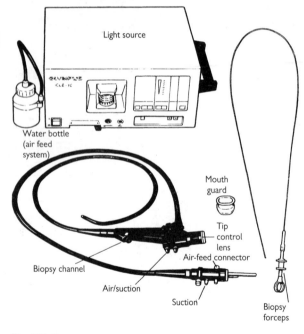

Fig. 4.26 Gastroscopy set

Proctoscopy/sigmoidoscopy set

Components
Light source
Light lead
Bellows and eyepiece
Biopsy forceps
Light attachment
Proctoscopes (adult and paediatric)
Sigmoidoscopes (rigid).

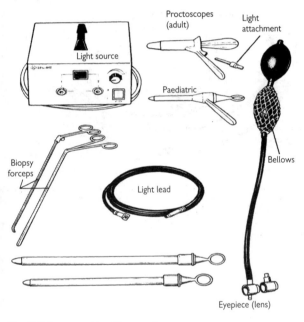

Fig. 4.27 Proctoscopy/sigmoidoscopy set

Flexible sigmoidoscopes

Components
Light source
Light connection
Suction valve
Biopsy forceps
Flexible sigmoidoscope—tip control
air/suction buttons
biopsy channel.

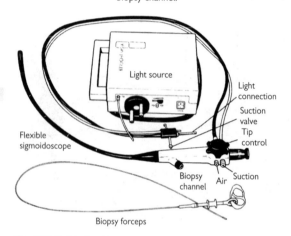

Fig. 4.28 Flexible sigmoidoscope

Colonoscope

Components
Light source
Light connection
Colonoscope—tip controls
water/wash pipe
suction valve
light connection.

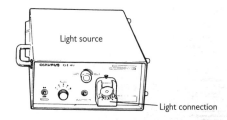

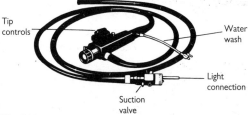

Fig. 4.29 Colonoscope

Laparoscopic equipment

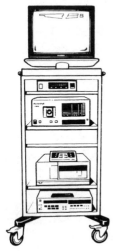

Fig. 4.30 Laparoscope. Monitor (*top*), light source, Mavigraph (video printer), and VCR

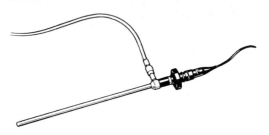

Fig. 4.31 Laparoscope. Light cable and camera

Fig. 4.32 Camera

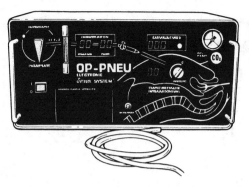

Fig. 4.33 Insulator

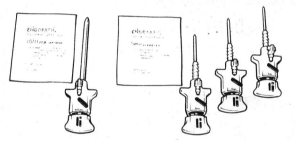

Fig. 4.34 Endopath. Disposable surgical trochars

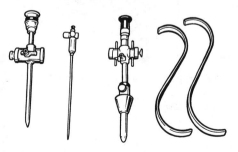

Fig. 4.35 10mm trochar, Veress needle, Hasson trochar, and 'S' refractors

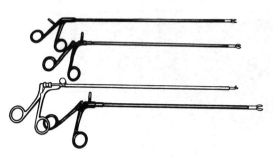

Fig. 4.36 5mm instruments

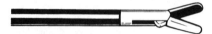

Fig. 4.37 5mm grasper

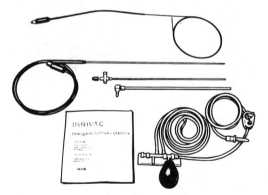

Fig. 4.38 Laser fibre (*top*), laser scalpel, irrigator aspirator and Irrivac®

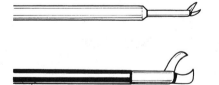

Fig. 4.39 Laparoscopic scissors. Designed as either curved, hooked, or straight, there is a variety available

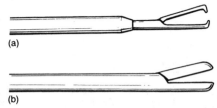

Fig. 4.40 (a) 10mm claw grasper; (b) 10mm spoon forcep

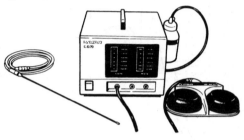

Fig. 4.41 Heater probe

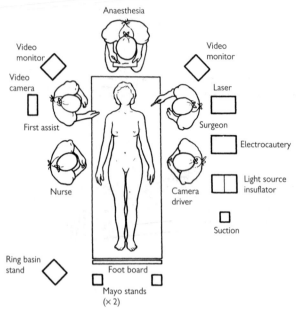

Fig. 4.42 Room set-up (appendicectomy)

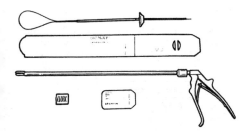

Fig. 4.43 ENDOLOOP ligature with reducer (*top*), LIGACLIP endoscopic clip applier and clips

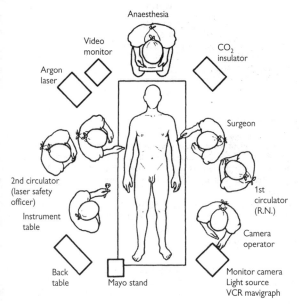

Fig. 4.44 Room set-up (cholecystectomy)

Suture materials

Suture materials in surgery can be categorised as absorbable and non-absorbable and are composed of either natural or synthetic materials. The gauge or calibre are usually expressed using the US Pharmacopoeia sizes (USP).

USP	Diameter (mm)
8/0	0.05–0.069
7/0	0.07–0.099
6/0	0.10–0.14
5/0	0.15–0.19
4/0	0.20–0.24
3/0	0.25–0.29
2/0	0.3–0.39
0	0.4–0.49
1	0.5–0.59
2	0.6–0.69
3	0.70–0.79

Absorbable sutures

Natural

Traditionally, catgut was popular—derived from sheep or cow intestine. Its use has largely been abandoned given the theoretical risk of transmission of infections such as new variant Creutzfeld-Jacob disease (CJD) and its unpredictability has virtually excluded its current use.

Synthetic

Polyglactin (Vicryl), polydioxanone (PDS) and polyglycolic acid (Dexon) are all absorbable suture materials, Vicryl and Dexon are braided. They handle, tie and are stronger than catgut.

Non-absorbable sutures

Natural (silk, cotton)

These braided sutures tie and handle well but perpetuate infection by the capillary action caused by the braiding. Only silk remains in popular use as synthetic sutures are superior but they do contribute to infection and are best avoided.

Synthetic

These may be monofilament or braided. Examples include polyproylene (Prolene), polyamide (Nylon), polytetrafluoroethylene (PTFE) and polyester (Dacron). They cause little tissue reaction but are a little more difficult to handle than silk. Their use is common for abdominal wall closure, hernia repair and skin closure. As they are not absorbed they retain their tensile strength. *Suture sinus formation*, such as at the site of the knot in abdominal wall closure, are recognised complications of non-absorbable sutures.

Stainless steel wire

This suture may be mono- or multi-filament, and may be used in cardiothoracic surgery for the closure of median sternotomy wounds. It is very strong but difficult to handle and rarely leads to sinus formation.

Needle types

Needles are either straight or curved. Half-circle needles are most commonly used. Deeper tissues require a larger circle arc.

- **Straight or linear needles** are for suturing easily accessible tissues such as skin.
- **Cutting needles** are triangular in cross section with the apex of the triangle in the concavity of the needle. Reverse cutting needles have the apex on the convexity and are less traumatic. They are used for skin, tendons and scarred tissue.
- **Round bodied needles** (taper point) are oval or round in cross section. They are used for intestinal and vascular anastomosis and suturing muscle and peritoneum.
- **Round bodied** J-shaped needles are useful for closing defects in the abdominal wall such as those created during laparoscopic procedures or inserting synthetic mesh for incisional hernias. The 'heel' of the needle pushes deeper structures, such as bowel, away to allow safer suturing of the abdomen.
- **Blunt needles** are popular as they decrease the risk of needle-stick injuries. They are commonly used for mass closure of the abdomen. They are, however, more difficult to used than sharp needles.

Knot tying

Safe knot tying is fundamental to good surgical practice and one of the first challenges faced by the basic surgical trainee. There are a number of ways in which the surgical trainee can acquire competence. Exposure to surgical procedures allows the observation of knot tying and initial practice. Local anaesthetic minor operation lists are often an excellent place to develop basic skills. All of the Royal Colleges of Surgery offer widely available Basic Surgical Skills courses. They are a recognised mandatory part of basic surgical training and should be attended as soon as possible during the training programme.

Principles of knot tying

- Tie knot firmly so it does not slip.
- Carry the knot down to the tissues with the tip of the index fingers and make sure that the strands of the ligature are flat by drawing then in opposite directions. This prevents twisting and the knot slipping.
- Do not use undue force otherwise the knot will cut through the tissue or fracture.
- Tie knots in anticipation of postoperative tissue swelling to prevent necrosis.
- Do not clamp the knot to complete your tie. This will weaken the suture, particularly monofilament sutures.
- Avoid friction or sawing between strands when tying as the suture may weaken.
- The knot should be as small as possible to exclude foreign material.
- Do not add extra knots 'to make sure'.

Basic knotting techniques

Basic surgical trainees should be familiar with the following knots:
- The one-handed reef knot
- Instrument tying
- The surgeon's knot
- The slip or granny knot
- The Aberdeen knot.

Guidelines for obtaining a fine scar

Try to place the incision in Langer's contour lines. Use atraumatic techniques and avoid tension. Non-absorbable sutures may be removed as follows:
- Face and neck: 2–4 days
- Scalp: 5–7 days
- Abdomen and chest: 7–14 days
- Limbs: 5–10 days
- Feet: 10–14 days.

Sutures can be removed earlier than these times for cosmetic reasons. If removed early additional support to the wound can be facilitated with Steri-strip adhesive skin strips. These may also be used as an alternative to skin sutures, particularly in children. Skin clips are an alternative to skin sutures. They have low infection rates and similar cosmetic results. However they are more expensive.

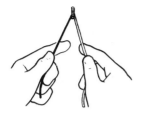

Fig. 4.45(a) With the palms up and the strands running over the index fingers, hold the strands against your palms with the fourth and fifth fingers. Perform all manipulations with the thumb, index and third fingers

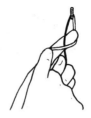

Fig. 4.45(b) Bring the right-hand strand over to make a *loop* around the left index finger

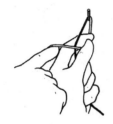

Fig. 4.45(c) Form a *pinch* with the left thumb and index finger

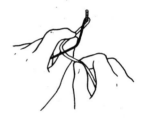

Fig. 4.45(d) Push the left-hand pinch through the loop with the thumb

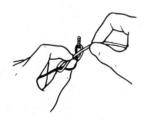

Fig. 4.45(e) Bring the right-hand strand over and grasp it with the pinch

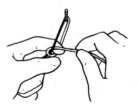

Fig. 4.45(f) Push your pinch with the strand through the loop with index finger and grasp the strand on your side with the right thumb and index fingers

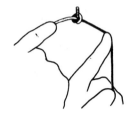

Fig. 4.45(g) Draw the strands in opposite directions with right hand, crossing over the left side

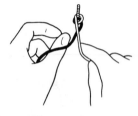

Fig. 4.46(a) Hook left thumb pushing the left strand up over the thumb

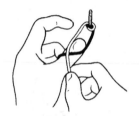

Fig. 4.46(b) Form a loop around the left thumb by bringing the right-hand strand from left side to the right, over the left thumb and left-hand strand

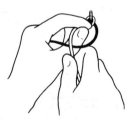

Fig. 4.46(c) Form a pinch with the left thumb and index finger

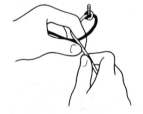

Fig. 4.46(d) Push the pinch through the loop with the index finger and grasp the right-hand strand with the pinch

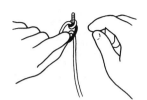

Fig. 4.46(e) This time, push the pinch with strand through the loop with the left thumb

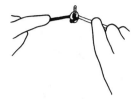

Fig. 4.46(f) Again grasp the strand with the right thumb and third finger and carry the knot down with the index fingers to complete the square knot

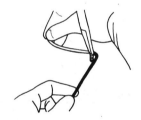

Fig 4.47(a) Swing the right-hand strand behind and around the clamp

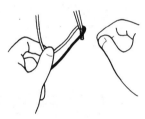

Fig 4.47(b) Grasp the right-hand strand with the left thumb and index finger

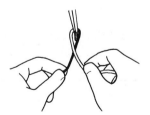

Fig. 4.47(c) Catch the right-hand strand (black) again with right hand. Now the right-hand strand is crossing over the left-hand strand

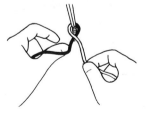

Fig. 4.47(d) Push the left-hand strand with the left thumb, the tip riding over the left-hand strand

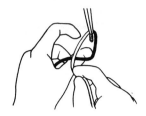

Fig. 4.47(e) Make a loop by bringing the right-hand strand over the thumb, crossing over the left-hand strand

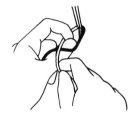

Fig. 4.47(f) Make a pinch with the left index finger and the thumb

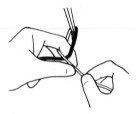

Fig.4.47(g) Push the pinch through the loop with the index finger and then grasp the right-hand strand with the pinch

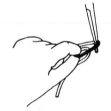

Fig. 4.47(h) Push the pinch and the strands through the loop with the thumb

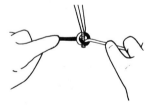

Fig. 4.47(i) Regrasp the right-hand strand with the right hand and carry down the knot with the index fingers

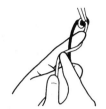

Fig. 4.48(a) Make a loop around the left index finger

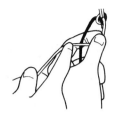

Fig. 4.48(b) Make a pinch with thumb and index finger

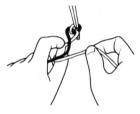

Fig. 4.48(c) Push the pinch through the loop with the thumb

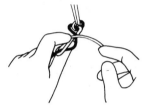

Fig. 4.48(d) Grasp the right-hand strand by the pinch

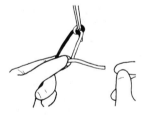

Fig. 4.48(e) Push the pinch with the strand through the loop

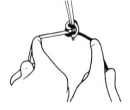

Fig. 4.48(f) Regrasp the right-hand strand and carry the knot down, with the right hand crossing over the left hand

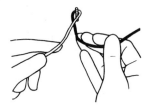

Fig. 4.49(a) With the right-hand strand *crossing under* the left, hold the strands with the thumb and index finger. Tie around clamps, with the right-hand strand grasped from under the left

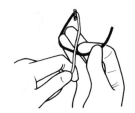

Fig. 4.49(b) Place the right third and fourth fingers over the right-hand strand and loop the left-hand strand around them. After mastering this, you need use only the third finger

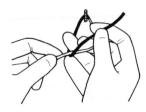

Fig. 4.49(c) Flex the distal phalanx of the right third finger over the black left strand of the loop

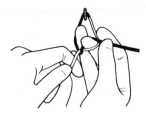

Fig. 4.49(d) Swing the white right strand through the loop with the back of the third finger

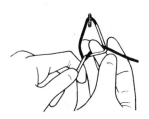

Fig. 4.49(e) Pull the white strand through the loop with the right third and fourth fingers

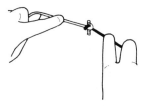

Fig. 4.49(f) Carry the knot down with the index fingers and lay the knot flat

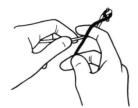

Fig. 4.50(a) Push the right-hand strand up and over the right index finger and bring it over to form a *loop* over the left-hand strand

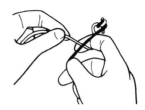

Fig. 4.50(b) Flex the right index finger around the left black strand of the loop

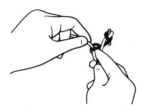

Fig. 4.50(c) Swing the right-hand strand with the back of the right index finger and pull it through the loop with the help of the third finger

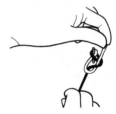

Fig. 4.50(d) Cross the left-hand strand up and over to the right while right hand pulls towards the left

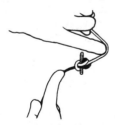

Fig. 4.50(e) Carry the knot down with the index fingers and lay it flat

Surgeon's or friction knot

This knot is used as a tension tie, usually in repairing tendons or approximating the fascial planes. It can also be used when closing skin incisions. The steps are described in the illustrations.

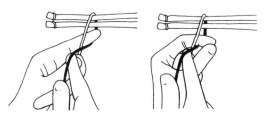

Fig. 4.51(a) A loop is formed around the left index-thumb pinch

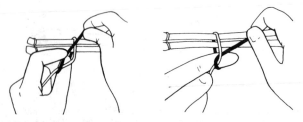

Fig. 4.51(b) The pinch is put through the loop and the right-hand strand is grasped by the pinch and pushed through with the left index finger

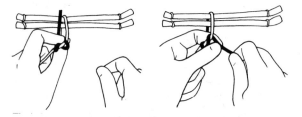

Fig. 4.51(c) The index-thumb pinch is once again put through the loop and the right-hand strand is again grasped by the pinch and pushed through the loop with the index finger for the second time

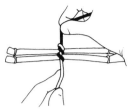

Fig. 4.51(d) The knot is carried down by the index fingers and kept flat. The knot can be completed with the second half of the two-hand tie

The instrument tie

This is frequently used when closing skin incisions and also during GI or vascular anastomosis.

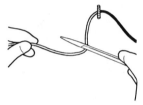

Fig. 4.52(a) With the needleholder in the right hand, hold one end of the string with the left hand

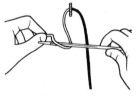

Fig. 4.52(b) Form the first loop around the needleholder by passing it over and then under the left strand

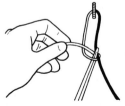

Fig. 4.52(c) Pick up the free end with the needleholder and pull it throuth the loop

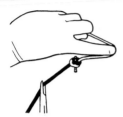

Fig. 4.52(d) Lay the knot flat by crossing the left hand over the right

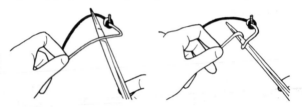

Fig. 4.52(e) Make a loop around the needleholder, this time, by pushing it under and then over the left-hand strand

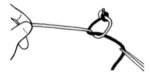

Fig. 4.52(f) Pick up the free end with the needleholder and pull it through the loop. Lay the knot flat by pulling on the strands in opposite directions

Surgical drains

The use of surgical drains has always been controversial and opinions vary considerably. Postoperative drainage may be indicated to aid evacuation of pus, blood, bile, or fluid and help abolish dead space or remove anticipated collections. Most drains consist of latex based material or polyvinylchloride (PVC), silastic and polyurethane polymers.

Types

Active drains employ suction devices

Closed systems These comprise either reusable or disposable systems. The reusable systems provides high pressure suction with a reservoir capacity but are less commonly use than disposable drains. Disposable drains provide low pressure suction (100mmHg) by way of a compressible bottle. The system can be charged and recharged by emptying the bottle, compressing, and reconnecting the drainage tube. Non-return valves should be used to prevent reflux and inward migration of bacteria. Colonisation of the reservoir contents can occur.

Open systems Sump drains contain an air inlet lumen which prevents blockage by soft tissue. Although more efficient than closed suction systems, they have the disadvantage of requiring a non-portable suction system and may permit the entry of bacteria although this can be reduced by filters.

Passive drains work by siphonage or gravity. These may also be open or closed. Closed systems drain into a bag by low pressure suction working on the siphon principle. Open systems drain by capillary action or gravity into dressing or stoma bags. Therefore their efficiency depends on the position of the patient and the volume and site of the collection.

If a fistulous track is necessary to provide a long period of drainage, such as bilary drainage after exploration of the common bile duct latex drains are preferable as fibrosis is stimulated.

Complications

- Secondary infection (more common with open drains)—this can be reduced by the presence of non-return valves.
- Primary haemorrhage at the site of insertion of the drain and secondary haemorrhage if internal vascular structures are damaged via suction or on removal.
- Pressure or suction necrosis of bowel leading to injury, anastomotic dehiscence, and intra-abdominal sepsis.
- Migration within or without the body cavity.
- Blockage is common and can distract from covert haemorrhage or body space fluid collection.

The timing of drain removal is not readily definable. In principle they should be removed when their purpose is fulfilled.

- Low daily output—when draining for bile and serous collections.
- Draining for blood should depreciate, as good operative technique will minimise postoperative haemorrhage. However in situations when a drain is placed after bleeding, the change from a bloody fluid to haemoserous with cardiovascular stability should encourage removal.

- The toleration of oral intake, absence of distension, return of bowel sounds, passage of flatus, and bowel motion are indications for removal of drains placed adjacent to an intestinal anastomosis.
- Thoracostomy tubes can be removed from the chest when daily output is low, when there is no further air leak on coughing and a non-swinging fluid level in the closed underwater drainage system when treating a pneumothorax, haemothorax or pleural effusion.

Preparations for surgery

Scrub-up technique

The aim of preoperative scrub up is to remove surface organisms from the hands and the forearms. The technique does not remove deeper organisms from the hair follicles or sweat glands, and recolonisation usually occurs within 20–30min. However modern washing agents such as povidone iodine (Betadine) and chlorhexidine (Hibiscrub) will kill organisms for up to 2 hours after scrubbing. There is no advantage to excessive or lengthy scrubbing, and only nails need scrubbing. Hand and wrist jewellery should be removed. Three minutes is adequate for the first scrub of the day. Between cases hands can be washed with a spirit solution or rewashed for 1–2min. Staff with an infective lesion of the skin should not be in theatre until recovery is complete.

- Adjust the temperature of the water until acceptable. Lightly wash the hands and forearms. Take a sterile brush, apply washing agent and clean fingernails.
- Wash hands and forearms for about 2min allowing water to run downward towards the elbows.
- Dry each hand and forearm separately with disposable towels provided, dry from wrist to forearm.
- Put on your gown first and then glove your non-dominant hand followed by dominant. This can be achieved by picking up the inner sleeve of the glove with the fingers of the opposite hand, directly or through the sleeve of the gown, ensuring that the outer (patient side) of the glove is not touched.

Punctured gloves

Gloves are punctured regularly during surgical procedures, this should be borne in mind particularly for prolonged and contaminated cases and replaced when recognised. Soiled gowns should likewise be replaced.

Shaving

Shaving should only occur directly before surgery, ideally on the operating table by an appropriate person. Shaving before this time can cause damage to the epidermis and folliculitis increasing the risk of infection.

Skin preparation

Prepare the skin with either Betadine or Chlorhexidine in alcohol. Two applications are usually made. Operating on mucous membranes should involve removal or debris first then cleaning with normal saline. The eyes should be closed with adhesive tapes for head and neck surgery.

Drapes

The operative field is draped with disposable or non-disposable drapes prior to commencement of surgery. Disposable drapes are preferable as they are waterproof and avoid the use of towel clips; however they are expensive.

Abdominal incisions

Abdominal incisions should be large enough to permit the intended procedure to be performed safely and efficiently.

Vertical incisions

Upper midline This permits access to the stomach, duodenum, gallbladder, liver, spleen and transverse colon. The incision may extend from the xiphisternum to the umbilicus and can be extended distally if necessary. It is continued through the skin, subcutaneous tissue and linea alba to the peritoneum. This is held between artery forceps away from the abdominal contents and then incised with a scalpel. Two fingers are then inserted to allow safe division of the peritoneum and abdominal wall upwards and downwards with scalpel, point diathermy or dissecting scissors.

Lower midline The incision extends from the umbilicus to the symphysis pubis. This permits access to the infra-colic compartment and pelvis. The bladder should be catheterised prior to incision to avoid injury when full given its close relationship to the anterior abdominal wall.

Full length midline This incision extends from the xiphisternum to the symphysis pubis and is useful for aortic and complex colorectal procedures.

Mass closure

This is the technique of choice for closing midline wounds. All layers of the abdominal wall are taken except skin and subcutaneous fat. One or more single or loop sutures are used with an over and over technique taking at least 1cm bites of abdominal wall 1cm apart, with a ratio of suture to incision length of 1:4 or more. This allows tension free closure and accommodates postoperative tissue oedema. Absorbable sutures such as PDS or non-absorbable such as Prolene or Nylon can be used with blunt needles to avoid needle-stick injury. The subcutaneous tissue may or may not be closed and skin closed with absorbable or non-absorbable suture or skin clips as for any other abdominal incision.

Paramedian incision

This incision is in the upper or lower abdomen parallel to and 2cm from the midline. It permits access to the organs of each quadrant of the abdomen according to its site but tends to have been replaced by the fast open-close midline. The anterior rectus sheath is divided and the muscle dissected laterally to expose the posterior sheath. This is divided vertically, together with the transversalis fascia and peritoneum. The peritoneum and posterior rectus sheath are closed together in one layer of non-absorbable sutures followed by the anterior sheath and skin. There is a lower risk of wound dehiscence or incisional hernia if the lateral paramedian approach is used because of the overlying rectus muscle when the wound is closed.

Oblique incisions

Kocher's (subcostal) incision This allows access to the contents of the right and left upper quadrants and is particularly indicated for operations on the gall bladder and spleen in patients with a wide costal angle. The incision may extend from the midline to the lateral edge of the rectus into the oblique muscles. It lies parallel to and about 2–2.5cm below the costal margin. All tissues are divided in the line of the incision. Closure is by the mass technique or in layers in the following order: peritoneum and posterior sheath together and then anterior sheath (with non-absorbable or delayed absorption sutures, e.g. Prolene, Nylon, or PDS) and skin closure.

Rooftop incision This exposure allows access to the upper abdomen incorporating bilateral subcostal incisions continuous below the xiphisternum to permit access to the stomach, pancreas, spleen and adrenal glands. Either masse closure or closure in layers of the anterior and posterior rectus sheath with Prolene, PDS, or Nylon is acceptable. The wound is associated with a sound scar and less postoperative pain.

Thoracoabdominal incision A left thoracoabdominal incision involves the patient positioned on their right side and the use of a double-lumened endotracheal tube. An oblique abdominal incision is extended alone the line of the 8th or 9th rib dividing the intercostals muscles and pleura. This is used for access to the distal oesophagus, cardia of the stomach and diaphragm. Closure of the abdomen is as for other oblique incisions. The chest is closed by approximating the ribs with strong interrupted Prolene sutures over a chest drain.

Rutherford-Morrison incision This allows access to the lower ureter, the colon and the iliac arteries. The approach can be trans- or extraperitoneal. The incision extends laterally from just above the anterior superior iliac spine to a point about 2.5cm above the pubic tubercle medially. All tissues are divided in the same line and the inferior epigastric vessels are ligated. The peritoneum can then be reflected anteriorly to access retroperitoneal structures such as the ureter, inferior vena cava, iliac vessels or lumbar sympathetic chain.

Gridiron incision This is the traditional appendicectomy incision extending obliquely from a point two-thirds of the way along the imaginary line drawn from the anterior superior iliac spine to the umbilicus. The incision is made at right angles to this line. Skin, subcutaneous fat, and fascia are divided in the same line, the external oblique, internal oblique, and transverses abdominis are either split in the line of their fibres or cut to expose the peritoneum, which is then opened between artery forceps. Closure is in layers, with Vicryl to peritoneum and muscular layers.

Any doubt over diagnosis is an indication for diagnostic laparoscopy, however, occasionally the preoperative diagnosis of appendicitis is wrong. In this situation the incision can be extended medially and laterally if disease of the terminal ileum or right colon requires resection. Alternatively or for pathologies of the left or upper abdomen the incision should be closed and midline incision performed.

Transverse incisions

Transverse skin crease incisions can be made in Langer's lines in the upper or lower abdomen. They can be used to approach the gall bladder, stomach, duodenum, aorta, kidneys, right colon, or for defunctioning loop stomas etc. Exposure and drainage are better. Chest complications (particularly in patients with pre-existing respiratory disease) and postoperative pain are less common and incisional hernias unusual.

Lanz incision

This is a right lower-quadrant transverse skin crease incision which gives better cosmetic results. It is similar to the gridiron.

Pfannenstiel incision

This suprapubic transverse incision allows access to the pelvic cavity predominantly for gynaecological purposes. The incision is 8–12cm long superior to the pubis. It divides skin, fat, external oblique, internal oblique, and transversalis fascia from one inferior epigastric artery to the other. The rectus abdominis muscles are split vertically in the midline for several centimetres to expose the peritoneum, which is then opened between artery forceps. If greater access is required, the rectus may also be divided transversely and retracted cranially.

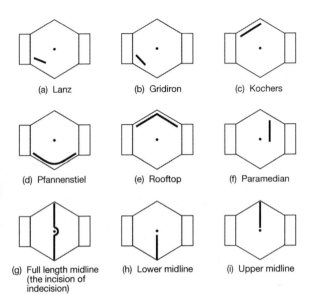

(a) Lanz

(b) Gridiron

(c) Kochers

(d) Pfannenstiel

(e) Rooftop

(f) Paramedian

(g) Full length midline
    (the incision of
    indecision)

(h) Lower midline

(i) Upper midline

Fig. 4.53 Abdominal incisions

Upper gastrointestinal endoscopy

Check list

1 Ensure that the patient is fully prepared, has received an adequate explanation, and has given consent.
2 Ensure that the endoscope is working properly.
3 Ensure that the endoscope has been cleaned.

Insertion technique

Wear gloves during the procedure. Insert a butterfly needle or small venflon into a vein on the dorsum of the hand. Spray the fauces with anaesthetic. Ask the patient to lie in the *left lateral* position. Insert a mouth guard and administer oxygen with pulse oximetry with nursing supervision. If requested give the patient sedation with reversal agents readily available. This varies according to preference but midazolam in 1–2mg increments usually up to 5–10mg is appropriate. Hold the instrument controls in the left hand. Insert the tip of the endoscope with the right hand into the mouth. Gently advance the endoscope passing it over the tongue with the tip flexed. When the laryngx and vocal cords are visualised anteriorly the endoscope is directed posteriorly, and ask the patient to swallow. *Do not force the instrument.*

Inspection of upper GI tract

Oesophagus Look for webs or carcinoma in the upper third. Gently inflate after clearing mucus by suction. The gullet usually distends so that a clear view can be obtained. Look for landmarks like the cardiac impulse. In the lower oesophagus check the mucosal folds for inflammation due to oesophagitis and note the distance from the incisor teeth. Check also for hiatus hernia. Deep inspiration by the patient is helps to identify the position of the diaphragm. If there is an obvious lesion pass the biopsy forceps down the biopsy channel and take a specimen for histology (preferably brushings for cytology, which is safer).

Stomach Follow the lumen at all times. Inflate as required. On entry note obvious abnormalities like abnormal folds, tumours, blood, bile, retained fluids or foods. Aspirate excessive fluid to prevent inhalation. Now inspect the whole lumen, the greater and lesser curves, the incisura and roof of the pyloric antrum. The fundus can be visualised at this point by flexing the tip of the instrument by 180° (J manoeuvre). Alternatively this can be done after examination of the duodenum if access was convenient earlier. Carry out biopsy or CLO test if indicated. Now advance the endoscope to inspect the pylorus. Note its mobility and the presence of deformity or inflammation.

Duodenum Enter the duodenum by keeping the pylorus in the centre of your view. The 'up-and-down' control with the left hand assists advancement. Once inside the duodenal cap carry out a full inspection, withdrawing the tip and depressing it to achieve this. To examine the remainder of the duodenum the endoscope usually has to be rotated 90° to the right using the up-and-down control to see the lumen.

Withdrawal Re-inspect the lumina of the duodenum, stomach and oe-sophagus on withdrawal by rotating the tip. Aspirate excessive air from each area once you are satisfied with the examination. Ensure the patient has appropriate instructions and prescriptions after the procedure.

Examination of the anus and rectum

Tell the patient what you intend to do. Ask them to lie on their left side with their knees drawn up towards their abdomen and their buttocks at the edge of the bed. Stand with your left side next to the patient's back.

Action

Separate the buttocks and inspect the anus. Note whether there are changes of excoriation, erythema, moistness, or soiling of the perianal skin and underwear. Identify anal tags, prolapsed haemorrhoids or peri-anal warts.

Digital examination

Wear rubber gloves and apply lubricating jelly to the tip of the right index finger. Place the pad of your index finger on the anal orifice posteriorly and apply enough pressure to permit entry. At this stage the patient may complain of pain and discomfort and you may note spasm of the sphincter. This suggests an anal fissure. Do not persist with the digital rectal examination. Note if there is a sentinel at the lower end of the fissure, usually situated posteriorly. Lubrication of the finger with ligno-caine gel may permit digital examination. However if there is spasm and pain it is better to examine the patient under anaesthetic.

Once the finger is in the anus, change its direction so that the tip 'points' into the rectum. With the pad of the finger feel the posterior and lateral walls. Are there any abnormalities—mass, ulcer, polyp?

Now bend your knees and rotate the finger so that you can feel the anterior rectal wall. Is there a mucosal abnormality? Can you feel the prostate anteriorly in a male patient? Note its consistency. In female patients you can feel the cervix through the anterior wall as a knob-like projection. Note whether movement of the cervix leads to pain or discomfort.

Proctoscopy

The proctoscope is a short instrument consisting of an obturator enclosed in a viewing barrel with a handle and a light source.

Action

Apply lubricating jelly to the tip of the obturator and press it on to the anal orifice until it has penetrated. Once the instrument has been completely inserted, remove the obturator, attach the light source and gently but slowly withdraw the instrument. Note the state of the rectal mucosa. Is it pink (normal)? Does it bleed easily? Does it completely fill the barrel (prolapse)? As you withdraw the instrument note whether there are haemorrhoids. They can appear as purple projections at the 3, 7, and 11 positions or circumferentially. Band or inject them if indicated. Note also whether there are polyps or an anal fissure anteriorly or posteriorly (proctoscopy is usually painful in the presence of a fissure but it may be made possible by applying lubricating jelly containing a local anaesthetic.)

Sigmoidoscopy

The sigmoidoscope is a rigid steel or plastic hollow tube about 25–30cm in length and up to 2cm in diameter. It comprises an outer hollow tube, an obturator, which is withdrawn after the instrument has been inserted, and a light source, which is fibre-optic in modern instruments. There is an attachment on the lens piece for the insufflation of air to open up the lumen ahead of the instrument.

Preparation of patient

The patient should have the procedure explained fully and give consent. Preparation of the bowel is often unnecessary. A disposable enema may help in cases of difficulty, but sometimes may have the reverse effect.

Position

The patient lies in the left lateral position with the hips flexed and the buttocks raised.

Procedure

- Carry out a digital examination of the rectum. If it is loaded, defer sigmoidoscopy until the bowel has been prepared with a disposable enema.
- Lubricate the sigmoidoscope. Disposable plastic sigmoidoscopes are lubricated under running warm tap water. With the obturator in place, introduce the sigmoidoscope gently through the sphincter to about 5cm by pointing it towards the umbilicus.
- Remove the obturator and advance under direct vision after attaching the eyepiece, insufflator and light source. Keep the lumen in view at all times as you pass the instrument upwards to its full length. Negotiation of the rectosigmoid junction requires considerable experience and skill. If the patient suffers discomfort, do not persist.
- Note the appearance of the mucosa and the presence of contact bleeding, ulceration or neoplasm. Take biopsies of suspected abnormalities for histological examination using the specialised biopsy forceps provided. Polyps can be removed by snaring and diathermy. It requires considerable experience to interpret what you see.

NB If a biopsy has been taken the patient should not have any type of enema for at least a week because of the risk of perforation of the bowel or air embolus. Carry out proctoscopy last; this is best for banding and injection procedures.

Flexible sigmoidoscopy

This fibre-optic instrument is now in routine use. It is longer than the rigid sigmoidoscope allowing views as far as the proximal descending colon. Bowel preparation is required. As with OGD, considerable training is required to become skilful.

Colonoscopy

The colonoscope is longer than the flexible sigmoidoscope. The entire colon to the caecum and terminal ileum can be inspected. It has diagnostic and therapeutic uses.

Indications
- Assessment of the colon in patients with suspected malignant disease (can be passed to the caecum).
- Follow-up assessment of patients with resected malignancy.
- Assessment and biopsy of inflammatory bowel disease.
- Screening of patients with adenomas (and their removal).
- Assessment and biopsy of diverticular disease (which may mimic carcinoma on occasions).
- Removal of polyps.
- Decompression of sigmoid volvulus.
- Investigation and decompression of pseudo-obstruction.

Breast and endocrine surgery

T. Lennard and S. Aspinall

Fine needle aspiration cytology

FNAC is a quick, atraumatic and inexpensive diagnostic test for the investigation of symptomatic or screen-detected breast lesions. Interpretation requires an experienced cytopathologist and aspirates can be reported at a one-stop clinic, which allows inadequate aspirates to be repeated.

Fine needle aspirates are graded as follows:
- AC1 inadequate
- AC2 benign
- AC3 indeterminate
- AC4 suspicious of malignancy
- AC5 malignant.

There is a false negative rate of approximately 5%. Failure to confirm the diagnosis by FNAC in breast lesions with clinical or radiological signs of malignancy requires further investigation. Fine needle aspiration cytology of impalpable lesions may be performed under image guidance—ultrasound or mammography (stereotactic).

Indications
- Triple assessment of breast lumps
- Screen-detected breast abnormalities
- Assessment of suspected recurrence or lymphadenopathy.

Consent

Verbal consent only is required. Warn the patient that bruising might follow the procedure. Pneumothorax is a complication.

Technique

Use a 21–23G needle, 20ml syringe, syringe holder, glass slides and slide holder. Local anaesthetic is generally not required.
- Fix the breast lump between the thumb and index finger and clean the skin over the lump with an alcohol swab.
- Insert the needle into the centre of the lump, apply suction with the syringe with a freehand or with a syringe holder, pass through the lesion 4–5 times. It is not necessary to continue until aspirate appears in the hub of the needle.
- Release the suction with the tip of the needle in the lesion and withdraw the needle. Expel the contents of the needle onto a slide. Disconnect the syringe from the needle. Fill the syringe with air. Re-connecting the needle expel the contents onto a second slide (repeat).
- Spread the aspirate evenly over the slide with a clean slide held perpendicular. Dry the slides, label them, and place them in the slide holder.
- Ask the patient to apply pressure to the aspiration site to prevent haematoma formation.

Complications
- 7Haematoma—may make interpretation of the mammogram difficult.
- Pneumothorax—rare, may be avoided by inserting the needle parallel to the chest wall.

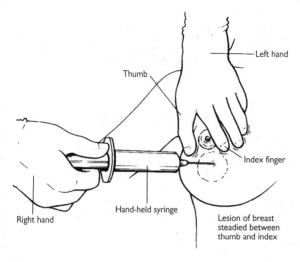

Fig. 5.1 Fine-needle aspiration of the breast. As an alternative to the hand-held syringe a Cameco gun can be used

Core biopsy

Core biopsy removes a core of breast tissue for histopathological examination. Confirmation of malignancy on core biopsy before definitive treatment avoids the need for excision biopsy of suspicious lesions. Core biopsy can be performed freehand for palpable lesions or under image-guidance—mammographic (stereotactic) or ultrasound—for impalpable lesions.

Indications

- Suspicious breast lesions (palpable or impalpable).
- Lesions indeterminate or suspicious of malignancy on fine needle aspiration cytology.
- Alternative to fine needle aspiration cytology, especially if cytopathological expertise is not available.
- Tumours being considered for neo-adjuvant or primary endocrine therapy.

Position

Supine with the head of the examination couch raised for freehand biopsy of palpable lesions.

Consent

Only verbal consent is required. Explain the risks of haematoma and infection.

Technique

- Clean the skin with an alcohol swab. Raise a wheal under the skin with 2ml of 1% lignocaine and infiltrate in the subcutaneous tissue.
- Incise the skin sufficiently to introduce the tip of the biopsy needle. Core biopsy gun, such as the Bard Magnum™, is a spring-loaded two-step firing device, which uses a large-bore (14 gauge needle).
- Advance the tip of the needle to the edge of the lesion, keeping it parallel to the chest wall. Firing the gun advances a notched needle through the lesion followed by a cutting cannula. The specimen is collected in a notch on the side of the needle.
- Withdraw the needle, inspect the adequacy of the core and place it in formalin fixative (an adequate core often sinks).
- Repeat this procedure to obtain 4–5 cores of tissue.
- Apply pressure to the biopsy site. A small dressing only is required.

The vacuum-assisted biopsy device (Mammotome™)

A vacuum-assisted biopsy system such as the Mammotome™ can be used as an alternative to the core biopsy gun. This device differs from the core biopsy gun in that it is inserted into the breast only once. Multiple tissue samples are then obtained by means of a vacuum, which draws tissue into the sample notch. The indications for Mammotome™ may extend to excising small breast lesions.

Breast conservation surgery—wide local excision

The aim is to excise a breast tumour with a margin of normal tissue. Breast conservation surgery for invasive breast cancer is usually performed with an axillary procedure. Radiotherapy is given to the remaining breast tissue following surgery. Overall survival following treatment for breast cancer is not affected by the choice between breast conservation and mastectomy, however, the incidence of local recurrence may be greater following breast conservation.

Indications
- Breast cancer <4cm (pre-invasive or invasive).

Contraindications
- Centrally placed tumours
- Breast cancer >4cm
- Multi-focal tumours.

Consent
Present information to the patient so that a fully informed decision between breast conservation plus radiotherapy and mastectomy can be made. Warn the patient that further surgery may be required if excision margins are not clear.

Preoperative preparation
- Mark the site of any palpable breast lumps preoperatively with the patient supine.
- There is no need to screen detected or impalpable lesions preoperatively. This is performed on the morning of the operation. A hood guidewire and sheath are inserted under image guidance into the breast lesion. Cranio-caudal and lateral mammograms are taken to accompany the patient to theatre.

Position
Supine with arm abducted on an arm board. Prepare and drape the breast and arm as for a mastectomy.

Procedure
Palpable breast lesions
- Incise over the breast lesion, bearing in mind the direction of Langer's lines in the breast. Unless the tumour is superficial, do not excise the skin over the tumour.
- Raise skin flaps on either side of the lesion. Use the index finger of the non-dominant hand on the lesion and excise the tumour with a margin of normal breast tissue down to pectoralis fascia.
- Continue dissection posteriorly in the plane between the breast and pectoral fascia and excise a cylindrical specimen containing the breast tumour with a margin of normal breast tissue.

- Then orientate the specimen by placing a stitch marked with ligaclips in the anterior, inferior and medial surfaces of the specimen, using the **AIM** technique (1 = **a**nterior, 2 = **i**nferior, 3 = **m**edial). Take tumour bed biopsies from the walls of the cavity.

Impalpable breast lesions

The patient comes to theatre with the guidewire in situ protected by a dressing.

- Review the mammograms, palpate of the end of the guidewire sheath and make an incision over it. Proceed as outlined above, being careful not to dislodge the guidewire.
- Placing a Babcock over the breast tissue containing the guidewire and carry out local excision of the lesion. Orientate the specimen and take a radiograph of it with the wire still in situ, to confirm adequate excision of the target lesion. Tumour bed biopsies are performed as above.

Closure

- Ensure haemostasis. Insert a Redivac drain in the cavity. Close the subcutaneous tissue with 2/0 Vicryl and skin with 3/0 Monocryl.

Complications

- Haematoma
- Infection
- Further surgery.

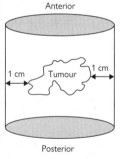

Anterior

1 cm   Tumour   1 cm

Posterior

Fig. 5.2 Specimen excised at breast conservation surgery

Mastectomy

Several types of mastectomy have been described for breast cancer. Halsted described wide excision of the breast tumour with, in addition, the pectoralis minor and major. Patey modified the radical mastectomy excising the pectoralis minor only, to facilitate axillary lymph node clearance. A simple mastectomy, usually combined with axillary lymph node clearance for invasive breast cancer is described. More recently skin-sparing and subcutaneous mastectomies, which preserve the skin envelope and inframammary fold have been developed to facilitate breast reconstruction.

Indications

- Breast cancer >4cm
- Patient preference for breast cancer <4cm
- Centrally placed tumours
- Multi-focal disease.

Preoperative preparation

Mark the side of the mastectomy preoperatively.

Position

Supine with the arm abducted on an arm board. Prepare the skin from the sternal notch to costal margin and from sternum to mid-humerus.

Incision

- Mark an ellipse of skin orientated horizontally (or obliquely) to include the nipple areolar complex and skin over the tumour (if superficial).
- Hold the breast tissue to be excised and confirm that the skin flaps can be approximated at the end of the procedure.
- Incise skin and subcutaneous tissue along the marked ellipse.

Procedure

- Use dissecting scissors or pencil diathermy, develop the plane between breast tissue and superficial fascia. Place Allis or Littlewood's forceps on the subcutaneous tissue of the skin flaps and ask your assistant to hold the skin flap vertically. Countertraction on the breast may help identify the correct tissue plane.
- Continue the dissection down to the pectoralis fascia, taking care not to buttonhole the skin. In this manner the superior skin flap is elevated to the level of the second intercostals space and the inferior flap to the inframammary fold.
- Lift the breast laterally to develop the plane between the posterior surface of the breast and pectoralis fascia from the medial edge. Use a combination of blunt and sharp dissection, diathermising any internal mammary artery perforating branches, crossing this tissue plane. Continue the dissection lateral to the free border of pectoralis major to include the axillary tail of the breast.
- Perform an axillary procedure with the mastectomy for invasive breast cancer (see Axillary surgery).

Closure
- Place a Redivac suction drain under the skin flaps.
- Close subcutaneous tissue with 2/0 Vicryl and skin with 3/0 Monocryl.

Postoperative care
Drains are left in situ until drainage is minimal.

Complications
- Seroma
- Haematoma
- Infection
- (see also Complications of Axillary surgery)

Skin sparing mastectomy
This operative is performed in conjunction to an immediate reconstructive procedure for early stage breast cancer. The breast tissue, nipple areolar complex and skin overlying superficial tumours are excised.
- Make an incision through skin and subcutaneous tissue around the areolar. Extend this laterally to improve the access for the mastectomy.
- Make a separate incision in the axilla if an axillary procedure is to be performed (see Axillary surgery).
- Excise the breast as described for simple mastectomy proceeding in a centripetal direction to improve exposure.
- Remove the breast through the axillary incision enabling the specimen and axillary contents to be removed en bloc, once axillary node dissection has been completed. The complications are similar to simple mastectomy and axillary surgery. Skin flap necrosis is a complication particular to skin sparing mastectomy.

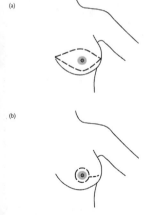

(a)

(b)

Fig. 5.3 Incisions for simple and skin sparing mastectomy (a) Simple mastectomy (b) Skin sparing mastectomy

Axillary surgery

Removal of axillary lymph nodes in invasive breast cancer has two roles:
1. Determination of the axillary lymph node status provides important prognostic information upon which decisions about adjuvant therapy are based.
2. Removal of metastatic lymph nodes treats axillary disease.

Sentinel lymph node biopsy

This is a minimally invasive technique to predict the nodal status of the axilla base on the histological examination of the first node to receive lymph from the breast cancer (sentinel node). An unnecessary axillary lymph node clearance can be avoided in patients with a node negative axilla.

Procedure

- Inject blue dye and radio-labelled colloid into the breast parenchyma surrounding the tumour or under the skin overlying the tumour.
- Use preoperative lymphoscintigraphy, intra-operative gamma detection probing or dissection along blue dye stained lymphatics to identify the sentinel node. Often a combination of these procedures is performed.
- Make a 2–3cm incision over the sentinel node, excise it and send it for histological examination.
- If metastasis is in the sentinel node this is an indication for axillary lymph node clearance. The absence of metastases in the sentinel lymph node indications a node negative axilla. Current problems with this technique are a false-negative rate of 5% and uncertainty of the significance of micrometastases.

Axillary node clearance

The extent of axillary node clearance performed in invasive breast cancer is dependent on the likelihood of finding involved lymph nodes. Three levels of axillary node clearance are described:
- Level I—up to lateral border of pectoralis minor
- Level II—up to medial border of pectoralis minor
- Level III—up to apex of the axilla.

Level III axillary clearances is usually reserved for instances where there is a high probability of extensive axillary node involvement or there are palpable lymph nodes in the axilla.

Indications

- Invasive breast cancer
- Positive sentinel lymph node biopsy.

Consent

Warn the patient of the risk of frozen shoulder, lymphoedema, numbness of the skin under the arm and seroma.

Position

Supine with the arm abducted on an arm board. Prepare and drape the breast for mastectomy or breast conserving surgery, including the axilla and arm down to the mid humerus.

Incision

If axillary surgery is performed with mastectomy or breast conserving surgery for a tumour in the upper outer quadrant of the breast, a separate incision for the axilla may not be necessary. Otherwise, make a transverse incision from the lateral border of pectoralis major anteriorly to latissimus dorsi posteriorly.

Procedure

- Identify the lateral border of pectoralis major. Continue up the lateral border identifying pectoralis minor beneath until the axillary vein is reached. This is the superior limit of the dissection.
- Retract pectoralis minor and major upwards and medially. Alternatively, for a level III clearance, detach the pectoralis minor from its attachments to the ribs and coracoid process, then clean the anterior aspect of the axillary vein sweeping the contents of the axilla downwards from the inferior surface of the axillary vein with a pledget or dissecting scissors held open.
- Identify the thoraco-dorsal trunk laterally and the long thoracic nerve of Bell medially and preserve them. Identify the intercostobrachial nerve, which passes across the axilla from medial to lateral, it may be sacrificed.
- Place ligaclips on other small vessels and divide them. Then remove the axillary contents en bloc with the mastectomy specimen.

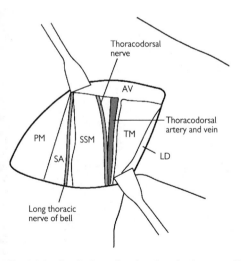

Fig. 5.4 Landmarks for axillary lymph node clearance. AV: axillary vein; LD: latissimus dorsi; PM: pectoralis major; SA: serratus anterior

Closure
- Leave a Redivac drain in left axilla.
- Close the subcutaneous tissue with 2/0 Vicryl and skin with 3/0 Monocryl.

Postoperative care
- Teach the patient to practise shoulder movements to prevent frozen shoulder.
- Leave the axillary drain in place until there is minimal drainage over 24 hours.

Complications
- Frozen shoulder
- Nerve damage:
  - Intercostobrachial—numbness and paraesthesia of the skin under the axilla
  - Long thoracic nerve of Bell—winging of the scapula
  - Thoracodorsal nerve—weakness of shoulder extension/adduction.
- Lymphoedema
- Seroma.

Breast reconstruction

Tissue expansion and insertion of an implant

The principle of this form of breast reconstruction is expansion of the soft tissues of the chest wall to a larger than desirable size by a temporary tissue expander, which is later replaced by a permanent implant. This is the simplest form of breast reconstruction. Minimal extra scarring is incurred. However, the cosmetic results may not be as natural as an autologous tissue breast reconstruction and revisional surgery is frequently required.

Indications
• Immediate or delayed breast reconstruction.

Contraindications
• Radiotherapy to chest wall
• Concurrent infection.

Consent
Discuss the advantages and limitations of each method of breast reconstruction with the patient, so that she can make an informed decision. Warn the patient of the short and long term complications of breast implants, i.e. infection, skin flap necrosis, extrusion and deflation of the implant and capsular contraction.

Preoperative preparation
• Determine the type, shape and dimensions for the implant
• Mark the position of the submuscular pocket for the temporary tissue expander on the chest wall preoperatively
• Give prophylactic antibiotics at the start of the procedure.

Procedure
• Make an incision through the previous mastectomy scar, continuing dissection to expose the underlying pectoralis major. Create access to the submuscular pocket by splitting pectoralis muscle along the line of fibres or by dissecting between pectoralis major and serratus anterior. Fill-up the submuscular pocket by blunt dissection. This should extend from the clavicle to the rectus sheath medially to the sternal attachment of the pectoralis major.
• Aspirate air from the tissue expander. Place it in the submuscular pocket and fill it with the largest possible volume of normal saline.
• Place the lower border of the expander 2–3cm below the level of the contralateral inframammary fold. Site the reservoir valve subcutaneous in a lateral or inferior pocket.
• Close the incision in layers (subcutaneous tissue and skin).

Normal saline is then injected at the out-patient department into the reservoir until the temporary expander is 150–250ml larger than the size of the permanent implant. This can be facilitated by measuring the volume of the specimen at mastectomy. Over-expansion is maintained for about three months. The expander is then deflated to the desired volume.

At a second procedure the temporary expander and reservoir are exchanged for the implant, which consists of an outer textured silicone envelope containing either saline or gel. It is placed in the submuscular

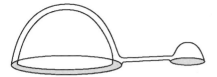

Fig. 5.5 Temporary tissue expander, connecting tube and reservoir dome

pocket and the incision is closed in layers. A Becker implant acts as both a tissue expander and permanent implant. The reservoir port only needs to be removed with this implant.

Complications
- Early—haematoma, infection, skin necrosis
- Late—pain, extrusion and deflation of the implant, capsular contraction (especially after radiotherapy).

Latissimus dorsi flap

Indications
- Immediate or delayed breast reconstruction—may be autologous or accompanied by a tissue expander/implant.
- Salvage procedures such as failed TRAM flap, locoregional recurrence and radionecrosis of the chest wall.

Contraindications
- Smoking, obesity and diabetes mellitus (relative)
- Thoracotomy
- Transection of thoracodorsal pedicle.

Consent
Inform the patient of possible partial or complete flap loss. Explain any complications specifically related to an implant.

Preoperative preparation
- Determine the size of the skin and tissue components of the flap preoperatively
- Mark the skin ellipse and borders of latissimus dorsi on the patient's back. The skin ellipse is usually placed under the brassiere strap as orientation to fill the mastectomy defect after rotation of the flap.

Position
Supine with the arm abducted for the mastectomy/excision of mastectomy scar and axillary surgery. Then place the patient in the lateral position to harvest the latissimus dorsi, and finally reposition the patient supine to reconstruct the breast.

Procedure
- Excise the mastectomy scar, raise skin flaps superiorly to the second intercostals space and inferiorly to the inframammary fold.

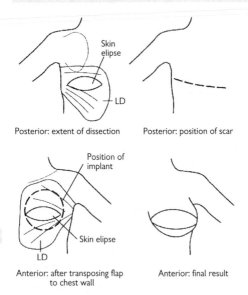

Posterior: extent of dissection

Posterior: position of scar

Position of implant

Skin elipse

LD

Anterior: after transposing flap to chest wall

Anterior: final result

Fig. 5.6 Latissimus dorsi flap

- Dissect in the axilla to identify the thoracodorsal pedicle. Divide the branches of the thoracodorsal trunk to serratus anterior.
- Identify the anterior border of latissimus dorsi. Cover the mastectomy defect with a dressing.

Turn the patient to the lateral position and incise the skin ellipse. Develop the plane below Scarpa's fascia and identity the borders of latissimus dorsi. Divide the attachments of latissimus dorsi to the thoracolumbar fascia and iliac crest and elevate the musculocutaneous flap. Tunnel the flap through the axilla to the mastectomy defect. Divide the latissimus dorsi tendon and the thoracodorsal nerve if required.

- Close the donor site over suction drains.

Reconstruct the breast after returning the patient to the supine position. Attach the latissimus dorsi to pectoralis major superiorly and insert the expander/implant into the submuscular pocket. Then complete the inset of the flap.

Closure
Close both wounds in layers over suction drains.

Complications
- Functional impairment at the extremes of shoulder extension

Partial or total flap loss, infection and haematoma.

Transverse rectus abdominis myocutaneous (TRAM) flap

The transverse rectus abdominis myocutaneous (TRAM) flap uses tissue from the lower abdominal wall, which is supplied by perforators from the superior and deep inferior epigastric vessels, to reconstruct the breast. The pedicled TRAM flap uses the rectus muscle isolated on its superior epigastric vascular pedicle, which is rotated up to fill the mastectomy defect. The free TRAM flap uses rectus muscle and sheath, harvested with the deep inferior epigastric vessels, which are detached from their origin and anastomosed to vessels in the axilla or the internal mammary artery.

Indications

Immediate or delayed breast reconstruction.

Contraindications

- Previous surgical division of the inferior epigastric vascular pedicle
- Obesity, diabetes mellitus, smoking (relative).

Consent

The patient should be aware of the specific complications of partial or complete flap loss and incisional hernia at the donor site. Though an excellent cosmetic result can be achieved with a TRAM flap, the procedure is lengthy, incurring additional scarring and a longer convalescence.

Preoperative preparation

- Examine the abdomen for the presence of hernias, divarication of the recti, abdominal incisions, and weakness of the anterior abdominal wall.
- Mark the inframammary fold and upper margin of excision of the mastectomy scar.
- Mark the TRAM flap on the lower abdomen. This is an ellipse extending from the anterior superior iliac spines to the umbilicus superiorly and the suprapubic region inferiorly.

Position

Supine on the operating table with both arms abducted. Place a sandbag under the scapular region on the mastectomy side to facilitate exposure of the axillary vessels. Insert a urethral catheter and place an intermittent venous compression device on the legs.

Operative technique

- Excision of mastectomy scar
  - Mark the inframammary fold and the upper margin of the mastectomy scar preoperatively.
  - Excise the mastectomy scar. Elevate the upper skin flap extending the incision laterally to allow exposure of the axillary vessels.
- Raising the TRAM flap
  - Excise skin and subcutaneous tissue down to fascia along the lines marked preoperatively.
  - A lateral and medial row of myocutaneous perforators emerges through the rectus sheath. Raise the flap from lateral to medial in the plane above the deep fascia. Preserve the medial row of perforators on the pedicled side to supply the subcutaneous tissue and skin of the flap.

- Harvest the medial portion of rectus sheath and muscle below these perforators and extend this from the umbilicus to the arcuate line. Continue the rectus sheath incision inferiorly and laterally towards the origin of the deep inferior epigastric vessels. Identify the deep inferior epigastric vascular pedicle, divided flush at its origin from the external iliac vessels to raise the flap.
- Closure of donor site
  - Advance the free lateral edge of the rectus sheath to the midline and suture it to the linea alba with continuous non-absorbable sutures, reinforce the repair by double-breasting the lower medial sheath to its lateral counterpart.
- Flap inset and creation of breast mound

The most commonly used recipient vessels are the thoracodorsal or circumflex scapular vessels.

  - Secure the flap to the chest wall with temporary sutures while a microvascular anastomosis is performed. The creation of a breast mound involves replacement of the breast volume, shape, skin deficit and re-establishment of the inframammary fold.
  - Attach the flap to the chest wall under the upper skin flap.
  - Inset the skin ellipse and suture it to the mastectomy defect.
  - Leave drains in the inframammary fold and axilla, but avoid suction in the region of the microvascular anastomosis.

Postoperative care

Nurse the patient in a warm room with analgesics and keep her well-hydrated. Any compromise of flap perfusion may necessitate urgent surgical exploration.
- Remove the drains when drainage is minimal
- Remove the urethral catheter once the patient is ambulatory.

Complications

- Seroma
- Partial and total flap loss
- Fat necrosis (which may mimic recurrence of breast cancer)
- Incisional hernia at the donor site.

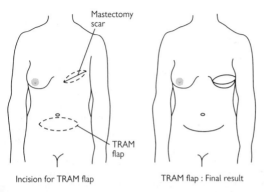

Incision for TRAM flap

TRAM flap : Final result

Fig. 5.7 TRAM flap

Incision and drainage of breast abscess (intermediate)

Breast abscesses are most likely to occur during pregnancy, the early post-natal period, or during lactation, although they can also occur at anytime. When not occurring in the context of lactation or pregnancy, the infection is usually sited in the main part of the breast and is usually related to mammary duct ectasia when close to the nipple areolar complex or, occasionally, an infected tubercle of Montgomery. The latter is not a true breast abscess but rather an infection in one of the large modified sweat glands around the areolar, and should be treated as any skin abscess or infected epidermoid cyst.

In mammary duct ectasia simple incision and drainage of the abscess may result in mammillary fistula and a more formal excision of the duct system may be required to treat the underlying problem. Aspiration of the abscess may also be possible and causes the risk of fistula.

Incision

Place this over the fluctuant abscess, circumferential to the nipple areolar complex.

Procedure

• Incise the abscess. Take a swab of the pus for culture and sensitivity.
• Breakdown any loculi with your finger and send part of the cyst wall to histology, as occasionally inflammatory breast carcinoma can mimic an abscess. Curette or lavage the cavity to remove adherent debris.
• Pack the cavity. Occasionally a tube drain will be required in large abscesses that are not in the dependant part of the breast.
• Use wide bore needle aspiration, either freehand or under ultrasound guidance in small abscesses.
• Antibiotic cover and repeat aspiration has been shown to be successful. This avoids anaesthesia and in-patient say, which is particularly important for the breast-feeding mother.

Closure

• Leave the wound open with a small pack in situ. This is particularly important if there is surrounding cellulitis or skin damage. Remove the antiseptic-soaked packs under general anaesthetic (if required) 24–48 hours later. Once the infective process is controlled, closure is rapid and may not need further packing.
• Consider delayed primary closure.

Excision biopsy of breast lump (intermediate)

Indications
- When fine needle aspiration or Trucut biopsy has failed to exclude malignancy.
- When the patient elects to have the lesion removed for symptomatic reasons.

Preoperative preparations
- Confirm the side and the site of the breast lump and ask the patient to indicate it to you.
- Mark the lump and the forearm on the affected side with an indelible marker.
- Ensure the patient is lying in the position she will be on the operating table when the marking is made.

Position of patient
Supine with the arm abducted on a side board.

Incision
Use Langer's lines and make the incision, circumferential to the areola if possible.

Procedure
- Incise the skin and fat underlying it, deepen the incision down to the breast tissue. Use diathermy for haemostasis as the operation progresses. With circumscribed benign lesions stay close to the lesion itself, avoiding unnecessary excision of otherwise healthy breast tissue. In more diffuse areas when a diagnostic biopsy is being performed, aim to reduce less than 20g tissue to optimise cosmetic outcome.
- Do not remove skin or lymph nodes at the time of a diagnostic excision—this is only appropriate during a therapeutic operation.
- If there is a significant risk of malignancy, place the incision in such a position that any subsequent surgery can be carried easily to include the first scar. Some breast lumps are very mobile and it may be necessary to hold and stabilise them with Allis forceps during dissection.
- Dissect the breast tissue using the scalpel, scissors or diathermy, depending on preference.

Closure
- Aim for complete haemostasis with diathermy by inspecting all quadrants of the biopsy before closure begins. If there is a large cavity or dead space or if there is oozing from the cavity, then bring out a small suction drain through a separate stab wound.
- Close the breast tissue and subcutaneous tissues with Vicryl on a cutting needle and use subcuticular Monocryl or Prolene for the skin.
- Infiltrate the wounds with local anaesthetic at the end of the closure and dress them with an adhesive waterproof dressing, so that the patient can bathe in the early postoperative period.

Microdochectomy (intermediate)

Indications
Discharge from a single duct in the nipple. Spontaneous discharge which has repeatedly stained clothing should be treated in this way.

Preoperative care
Under anaesthesia and before making the incision, press the breast in a radial fashion around the nipple areolar complex to try and palpate the thickened duct beneath it or induce the discharge. The anticipated site of the abnormal duct dictates the line of the incision.

Consent
Warn the patient that any operation on the duct system may make subsequent breast feeding difficult or impossible. Occasionally there may be reduced nipple sensation after surgery.

Position of the patient
Supine with the arm abducted.

Incision
Radial in the line of the suspected abnormal duct, just lateral to the edge of the pigmented skin of the areola.

Procedure
- Identify the duct on the nipple using a fine lachrymal probe. Using a size 15 blade, cut down from the nipple along the line of the probe to the edge of the areola. Dissect the duct with a small margin of breast tissue around it.
- Using fine forceps and iris scissors, remove the probe with the operative specimen.

Closure
Secure haemostasis. Close the incision with a subcuticular 3/0 absorbable suture such as Vicryl, leaving the nipple slightly open distally allows drainage of any further blood or serum without the need for a formal drain.

Hadfield–Adair operation (intermediate)

Indications
- Complicated mammary duct ectasia (particularly when there has been a mammillary fistula).
- Subareolar biopsy of a breast lump.
- Nipple inversion relating to duct ectasia or previous surgery.

Consent
Patients should be warned that breast feeding will not be possible after this operation and that there may be reduced sensation in the nipple. Very rarely nipple necrosis occurs.

Position of patient
Supine with the arm by the patient's side or an arm rest.

Incision
- Make a circumferential incision around the inferior half of the areola.
- Take care to prevent undercutting of the skin and avoid going more than halfway around the circumference to minimise the risk of nipple necrosis. The edge of the areola can be lifted up with skin hooks.

Procedure
- Continue the dissection from the back of the areola to the under surface of the nipple, disconnecting the nipple from the underlying terminal ducts and breast tissue.
- Be careful not to buttonhole the skin or the nipple in doing this.
  In duct ectasia, large ducts may be seen and these will exude secretions. If there is concern that the material secreted is infected, send a swab for microbiology analysis.
- Once the ducts have been disconnected from the nipple, excise a pyramid of tissue from underneath the nipple reaching back into the breast tissue, the base of which will be 3–4cm.
- Send the excised tissue for histology.
- If the nipple was inverted now evert and maintain it in position by using a fine Vicryl purse-string suture.

Closure
- Ensure meticulous haemostasis.
- Use a 3/0 Vicryl suture to close the breast tissue or subcutaneous fat in the defect left by the excision. Close the skin with a subcuticular absorbable or non-absorbable suture and place a waterproof dressing over the whole nipple areolar complex.
- Infiltrate the skin with local anaesthetic at the end of the procedure.

Complications
- Persistent infection. Rarely, if persistent infection and discharge is a problem, it may be necessary to excise the nipple areolar complex.
- Fistula formation.
- Recurrent inversion of the nipple.

Fine needle aspiration cytology of the thyroid gland

Indications

- Cytology diagnosis of a thyroid swelling
- Drainage of a thyroid cyst.

Preoperative preparation

- Explain to the patient what you are going to do.
- Inform the patient that bleeding occasionally occurs but that this very rarely leads to further complications and consent is not required.
- There is no known risk of disseminating malignancy by fine needle aspiration biopsy.

Procedure

- Use a sterile, disposable 20ml syringe with a 17 gauge (blue) venupuncture needle, holding the syringe in a syringe holder, which gives better manoeuvrability of the biopsy apparatus.
- Local anaesthetic is not required. Clean the skin and arrange biopsy glass slides adjacent to the patient. Pierce the skin and the thyroid swelling with the needle and aspirate. Make two or three passes through the thyroid in the direction of the biopsy. Multiple passes made at different angles through the gland tends to increase the risk of haemorrhage and a 'bloody' tap.
- Release suction on the needle once the sampling is completed but before the needle is removed from the biopsy target. Ask an assistant to press on the skin with a cotton wool swab while the slide is prepared.
- Detach the needle containing the aspirated material from the syringe, suck air into the syringe and then blow the contents of the needle on to the previously prepared slides. These slides should be air-dried and then sent to the Cytology Department for analysis.
- Place a small adhesive dressing on the site of puncture in the neck. In multiple nodules or difficult cases, ultrasound-guided biopsy may be preferable.

Thyroid lobectomy (major)

(see Chapter 3—Anatomy for surgeons)

Indications

- To remove a proven thyroid malignancy, usually as part of a total thyroidectomy.
- To remove a suspicious thyroid swelling to confirm a diagnosis for malignancy.
- To remove a large benign goitre, causing compressive or cosmetic symptoms as part of a unilateral or total thyroidectomy.
- To treat thyrotoxicosis, either as a unilateral lobectomy for a single toxic nodule or as a bilateral procedure for Grave's disease.

Preoperative preparation

- Avoid nodulectomy or partial lobectomy as a diagnostic procedure. Avoid operating on any nodule without a preoperative needle aspiration diagnosis.
- Biopsy the thyroid nodule before removal (see Fine needle aspiration cytology of the thyroid). Check the patient's thyroid function tests, thyroid antibodies and serum calcium before admission. Patients with thyrotoxicosis need preoperative blockage and replacement therapy (typically Carbimazole and Lugol's iodine to reduce vascularity). In thyroid malignancy or bilateral benign disease, total thyroidectomy will be the appropriate operation but for all other procedures, thyroid lobectomy should be carried out.
- Estimate any retrosternal extension preoperatively with X-rays of the thoracic inlet, CT, or MRI scanning.

Consent

- Inform the patient that there will be a scar and a small risk of permanent voice change, and difficulty in swallowing if damage to the recurrent laryngeal nerve occurs (around 1%). Use indirect laryngoscopy to record preoperative cord function.
- Inform the patient of the risk (15–20%) of temporary hypocalcaemia (haemorrhage rare) postoperatively.
- Inform patients undergoing diagnostic lobectomy of the possible need for a second operation to remove the contra-lateral lobe.
- Inform patients undergoing less than total thyroidectomy for thyrotoxicosis of the risk of recurrent hyperthyroidism and lateral chance of hypothyroidism, and the need for thyroid replacement therapy and/or calcium supplements together with the need for occasional drainage (around 10% of patients).

Position of the patient

- Supine with the neck extended at 20–25% and the table foot down to empty the neck veins. Place the head in a padded ring with a pillow or pad beneath the shoulders.
- Seal the drapes around the neck with a plastic adhesive sheet, such as Opsite. This prevents blood trickling down the neck and into the hair.
- Use general anaesthetic with a secure cuffed endotracheal tube.

Incision

- Mark the incision beforehand with a marking pen or suture garrotte midway between the sternal notch and thyroid cartilage.
- Make sure the incision does not extend beyond the medial border of the sternomastoid on each side. Infiltrate the neck with local anaesthetic containing adrenaline, which reduces skin bleeding.

Procedure

- Deepen the incision through the skin into the fat and the platysma muscle. Raise superior and inferior flaps in the subplatysmal plain, using either the diathermy or scalpel.
- Use Joll's retractor to hold the skin flaps apart, exposing the strap muscles. These should be divided in the midline and retracted laterally. In large goitres, divide the strap muscles transversely at the latter end to avoid branches from the ansahypolossi rather than retracting them.
- Palpate both lobes to ensure the 'normal' contra-lateral lobe is free of disease.
- Sweep away the structures to the lateral aspect of the thyroid lobe (the common carotid artery and the internal jugular vein) allowing the hilum of the gland to be seen. This is easier once the middle thyroid vein is identified, divided and ligated. Now the superior and inferior parathyroids can usually be seen. Keep the operative field as dry as possible to minimise blood staining, which makes identification of the parathyroids and the recurrent laryngeal nerve difficult. The parathyroids are normally located within a 1cm radius of the inferior thyroid artery.

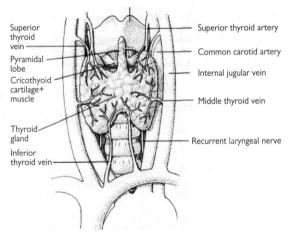

Superior thyroid vein
Pyramidal lobe
Cricothyoid cartilage+ muscle
Thyroid gland
Inferior thyroid vein

Superior thyroid artery
Common carotid artery
Internal jugular vein
Middle thyroid vein
Recurrent laryngeal nerve

Fig. 5.8

- An assistant should apply counter traction, which is essential for identifying the tissue planes. Use pledgelet dissection to mobilise the lobe.
- Take inferior thyroid artery branches close to the capsule with small clips and draw down the superior pedicles, ligate them in continuity or secure between clips and tie them doubly. Secure the inferior thyroid veins between ties or ligaclips, allowing the lobe to be reflected off the trachea.
- Identify the superior laryngeal nerve external branch when mobilising the upper pole and securing the superior thyroid artery.
- Now remove the lobe by dividing the isthmus and oversewing this with Vicryl.
- Carry out total thyroidectomy by performing the same procedure on the contra-lateral side.

Closure

- Use a suction drain if there is a large dead space or oozing.
- Reapproximate the strap muscles with 3/0 Vicryl (continuous). Close the skin with 4/0 subcuticular Monocryl. Skin clips can also be used but they can prove difficult to remove in an emergency unless they are Michel type with a specific removal device.

Postoperative care

- Ask the anaesthetist to identify the cords postoperatively, although their appearance may be misleading.
- Return the patient to the recovery area without a dressing on the wound so that any neck swelling can be rapidly identified and the patient returned to theatre for the evacuation of the haematoma.
- Remove suction drains after 24–48 hours.
- Check serum calcium daily and commence thyroid replacement therapy immediately. Patients can usually be discharged within 48 hours, for total thyroidectomy at 72 hours.

Complications

- Thyrotoxic storm—uncommon if the patient has been satisfactorily blocked prior to surgery.
- Haemorrhage—(rare) take the patient back to theatre if there is any difficulty in breathing or swelling in the early postoperative period and evacuate the haematoma.
- Unilateral recurrent laryngeal nerve palsy presents as a voice change postoperatively. If bilateral, presents as a compromised airway, which may need to be treated by tracheostomy urgently.
- External laryngeal nerve damage presents as a change in the timbre of the voice.
- Wound infection.
- Hypocalcaemia (carry out calcium check). Administer calcium supplements, either oral or intravenous, with or without vitamin D medication if indicated.

Late complications

- Recurrent thyrotoxicosis
- Tracheal malacia.

Sub-total thyroidectomy

Most surgeons now perform a total lobectomy or total thyroidectomy for virtually all thyroid disease. It is desirable to leave a small remnant of thyroid tissue and this can be achieved by placing a ring of haemostats around the edge of the thyroid and incising into it with a scalpel to remove the desired volume of tissue. Then leaving approximately one eighth of the lobe on each side, the remnant can then be oversewn with continuous 3/0 Vicryl.

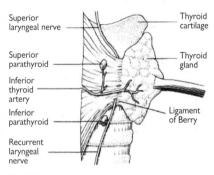

Superior laryngeal nerve

Superior parathyroid

Inferior thyroid artery

Inferior parathyroid

Recurrent laryngeal nerve

Thyroid cartilage

Thyroid gland

Ligament of Berry

Fig. 5.9 Anterior dislocation of the right thyroid lobe to show recurrent laryngeal nerve and parathyroids

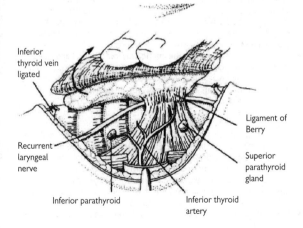

Inferior thyroid vein ligated

Recurrent laryngeal nerve

Inferior parathyroid

Ligament of Berry

Superior parathyroid gland

Inferior thyroid artery

Fig. 5.10 Anterior dislocation of the left thyroid lobe to show recurrent laryngeal nerve and parathyroids

Parathyroidectomy (major)

Indications
- Hyperparathyroidism
- Parathyroid carcinoma
- Secondary hyperparathyroidism
- As part of multiple endocrine neoplasia syndromes.

Preoperative preparation and consent
- Inform the patient that in primary hyperparathyroidism the usual pathology is that one gland is overactive. Use localisation scans (ultrasound and MIBI) to localise the parathyroid if carrying out a focused approach or laparoscopic approach.
- In gland exploration, local studies are not necessary.
- Have frozen section facilities available to confirm the presence of parathyroid tissue in the resected samples.

Position of the patient
Supine with the head in a neck ring, the neck extended and a 20–25° upward tilt.

Incision and access
As for thyroidectomy.

Procedure for open operation
- Divide the middle thyroid vein and mobilize the gland by lifting it forwards into the wound. Using a pledgelet, push away the loose areolar tissue to the lateral aspect of the thyroid, including the common carotid artery and the internal jugular vein. The parthyroids lying close to the inferior thyroid artery will expand into any dead space when they are enlarged.
- Start to look for them near the inferior thyroid artery. Each gland is a yellowish-brown colour, will have a definitive vascular pedicle, in most instances it will be easy to see. In a focused approach or laparoscopic approach, remove only the previously identified gland.
- Use PTH measurements perioperatively to assist in confirming that the target has been successfully identified. Expect a 50% fall in PTH level within 10 minutes if the offending adenoma has been removed.
  If more than one gland is diseased, carry out careful search in all the conventional sites on both sides. If the gland is not in the normal position inspect the thyrothymic ligament, the upper thymus, the carotid sheath, behind the upper pole of the thyroid and palpate the thyroid lobe itself carefully in case the adenoma is intrathyroidal. It is more common to fail to find an adenoma in the conventional position than to have an ectopic gland and an anatomical variant of the norm.
- If in doubt about the nature of the tissues removed, send biopsies for frozen section.

- Once identified, the adenoma is removed by securing its vascular pedicle with diathermy or clips, taking care not to breach the capsule—damage to which can cause spillage of contents producing multiple seedlings of parathyroid tissue throughout the neck (parathormatosis).
- Use laparoscopic approach or a focused scan in preoperatively localised adenomas. Target the dissection over the site of the adenoma and proceed directly to it. Laparoscopic or minimally invasive removal or parathyroid tissue is gaining position in the armamentarium of parathyroidectomy, but it is essential to have two concordant localisation studies to direct the surgeon to the appropriate site.

Closure

- Drainage is seldom required.
- Following an open operation, close the strap muscles and platysma with 3/0 Vicryl and the sin with 4/0 Monocryl.
- In focused approach, only the skin need be closed.

Postoperative care

- In the recovery room, leave the wound undressed to permit checking for any swelling and bleeding.
- Carry out calcium checks.
- Swallowing difficulties or hoarseness may indicate evidence of unilateral recurrent laryngeal nerve injury.
- Stridor usually indicates bilateral nerve injury and Horner's syndrome, damage to the cervical sympathetic chain.

Adrenalectomy (major)

Indications
- Functioning adrenal tumour, Cushing's syndrome, Conn's syndrome or phaeochromacytoma
- Incidentaloma over 3.5cm in size
- Suspected adrenal carcinoma.

Preoperative care
- Carry out intensive work-up to exclude or confirm the presence of a functioning adrenal tumour. In Cushing's syndrome this will require estimation of cortisol in the plasma and urine and ACTH levels. In Conn's syndrome, measurements of aldosterone, renin, and potassium. In phaeochormocytoma, this will require estimations of urinary catecholamines and plasma catecholamine levels.
- Imaging the adrenal glands using CT scan, MRI, or MIBG (meta iodo benzyl guanidine). Additionally, octreotide scanning may be helpful.
- In functioning tumours, the principle of block and when required, replacement therapy. The active hormone should be blocked pharmacologically, e.g. phaeochromacytoma block with alpha blockade, hyper-aldosteronism blocked with spironolactone.

Consent
- Obtain consent for a laparoscopic or open procedure.
- Inform the patient of the possible need for postoperative steroid replacement therapy.

Position of patient
- Anterior, patient supine, foot down 30°, lateral tilt.
- Lateral, patient in full lateral position, table broken to 30° over ribs 10 and 11 (also used for laparoscopic approach). Strap the patient to the table for both approaches.

Incision
- Anterior, long midline incision, extend it laterally through trans-pyloric plane if access difficult.
- Laparoscopic (open approach) over rib 11 from the lateral border of sacro-spinalis to abdominal wall.

Procedure
- Anterior approach.
  Left adrenal: pack the small intestine downwards, retract the costal margin upwards, place the left hand over the spleen and divide the posterior parietal peritoneum from the splenic flexure to the oesophageal hiatus. Apply several pairs of forceps to retract the peritoneum downwards. Identify the kidney with the adrenal gland above it. Identify and divide between ligatures the adrenal vein, which drains into the left renal vein, mobilize and remove the gland by blunt dissection, cauterise bleeding vessels.

Right adrenal: retract the liver upwards and the hepatic flexure downwards. Note the vena cava and kidney. Divide the posterior parietal peritoneum along the upper pole of the kidney to the vena cava. Identify the gland, divide the two or three adrenal veins, which drain into the vena cava between ligatures, remove the gland by blunt dissection. Secure haemostasis.

- Laparoscopic approach.

Divide the lieno renal ligament on the *left side* allowing the spleen to be mobilised medially. The adrenal gland will be seen lying close to the lower pole of the spleen between it and the kidney. Mobilise the gland using an ultracision harmonic scalpel and secure the adrenal vein with ligaclips.

Right side: Mobilise the right lobe of the liver and retract it in a headwards direction. The adrenal gland lies just lateral to the inferior vena cava above the right kidney. Identify the adrenal vein early and ligate it with ligaclips to mobilise the gland. Place the gland in a retrieval system and remove it through one of the port sites.

Postoperative care

- Blood pressure and blood sugar in patients with phaeochromacytoma in high dependency or intensive care unit. Monitoring of fluid requirements as there may be further vasodilation once the phaeochromocytoma is removed.
- Use steroid replacement therapy in Cushing's syndrome as the contralateral gland is usually suppressed. Patients with Cushing's syndrome usually have associated myopathy and obesity which make postoperative recovery slow.
- Suspected adrenal carcinomas, remove a pad of fat around the adrenal gland to ensure adequate tumour clearance.

Complications

- Hypotension due to volume disturbance
- Acute Addison's disease
- Wound infection
- Haemorrhage
- Chest infection as a result of subphrenic operation.

Pancreas (complex major)

(Refer to Hepatobiliary Surgery)

Pancreatic endocrine tumours may be solitary or part of a multiple neoplasia syndrome (MEN1).

Indications

- Removal of functioning endocrine tumours (e.g. insulinoma, glucagonoma, somatostatinoma, gastrinoma and tumours which are secreting pancreatic polypeptide).
- Non-functioning pancreatic tumours which may or may not be malignant.

Upper gastrointestinal surgery

Y. K. S. Viswanath and S. Dresner

Bleeding peptic ulcer disease

Patients with major upper gastrointestinal haemorrhage require urgent resuscitation and careful monitoring followed by early endoscopic assessment. This is essential to identify the site and cause of bleeding and to initiate appropriate endoscopic therapy. IV omeprazole 80mg bolus followed by 8mg/hour infusion for 72 hours is beneficial but does not stop active bleeding.

Indication

Failure of endoscopic control (including significant re-bleeding after initial successful endoscopic therapy).

Incision

Upper midline.

Position of patient

Supine.

Bleeding duodenal ulcer

- Kocherise the duodenum. Apply 2/0 Vicryl stay sutures and perform a longitudinal duodenotomy with diathermy. With the advent of PPI medication, definitive ulcer surgery (such as vagotomy) is not indicated and therefore the pyloric ring is preserved.
- Clear the stomach and duodenum of clotted blood with suction. Achieve bleeding point haemostasis with digital pressure.
- Secure any bleeding or exposed vessel (either a branch or the main trunk of the gastroduodenal artery) by under-running with interrupted 2/0 Vicryl /2/0 PDS or 2/0 Prolene on a small needle avoiding underlying structures such as the common bile duct. Irrespective of the material employed, sutures inevitably slough off as the ulcer heals, long after the vessel has thrombosed. If the ulcer cavity has a tough fibrous base it may be feasible to exclude it from the lumen using interrupted 2/0 Vicryl or PDS.
- Close the duodenotomy transversely with interrupted 2/0 Vicryl or PDS, as longitudinal closure may cause stenosis. If transverse closure is not possible due to a long duodenotomy, carry out longitudinal closure with Roux-en-Y gastroenterostomy (see Radical surgery for gastric caner, this chapter). An alternative is a Finney pyloroplasty (side-to-side gastroduodenostomy in two layers with interrupted 2/0 Vicryl or PDS. Use this approach also if the pyloric ring has been transgressed although it is more common to close such a gastroduodenotomy transversely with interrupted 2/0 Vicryl or PDS as a Heineke–Mickulicz pyloroplasty.

With giant ulcers the first part of the duodenum may completely disintegrate and once opened prove difficult to close. Retrieve this situation with an antrectomy with Roux-en-Y reconstruction (see Radical surgery for gastric cancer, this chapter). Close the duodenal stump primarily with a linear stapler or interrupted 2/0 Vicryl or PDS. Alternatively, suture the margins to the fibrous ulcer cavity overlying the pancreas (Nissen technique). To prevent duodenal stump leak, drain the duodenum with a Foley catheter inserted through the closure line or, preferably, by a T-tube in the healthy lateral wall of the second part of the duodenum.

Perforated peptic ulcer disease

Although the incidence of peptic ulcer disease has declined dramatically, perforation continues to affect significant numbers of elderly and medically unfit patients. Delay in diagnosis beyond 24 hours is associated with a 7-fold increase in mortality, 3-fold risk of morbidity and double the hospital stay.

Indication

- Clinical diagnosis of a perforated viscus with diffuse peritonitis, varying degrees of shock and (usually) free sub-diaphragmatic gas on erect CXR.
- Deterioration in the condition of patients with localised signs initially selected for conservative management.

Preoperative preparation

- Naso-gastric decompression decreases further spillage of gastroduo-denal contents and peritoneal contamination.
- Careful fluid resuscitation with placement of urinary catheter ± central venous access.
- Broad spectrum IV antibiotics and IV anti-secretory medication.

Position of patient

Supine.

Incision

Upper midline.

Procedure

On opening the peritoneal cavity a variable quantity of gas and bile-stained fluid will be encountered, confirming the diagnosis. Foul smelling faeculent fluid and gas indicate a colonic perforation. Depending on the duration of the peptic perforation there may be extensive fibrinous exudate and omental adhesions in the sub-hepatic space overlying the duodenum. The commonest site of perforation is the anterior wall of the first part of the duodenum. If this is clear then the anterior and posterior aspects of the stomach should be inspected and if no perforation is found the remainder of the GI tract must be thoroughly assessed.

- Close small perforations by oversewing interrupted full thickness 2/0 Vicryl sutures along the margins of the ulcer, leaving the ends long, so that a well vascularised omental patch can be lightly oversewn onto the primary repair.
- Often the ulceration is chronic and the defect large with a friable margin. Attempts at primary closure may cause sutures to cut out or result in duodenal stenosis. In this situation place interrupted 2/0 Vicryl sutures away from the ulcer margins and simply use them to secure the omental patch directly onto the perforation.

- Repair gastric perforation in a similar fashion. Biopsy the ulcer to exclude malignancy (approximately 6% of cases). With the advent of powerful antisecretory medication, definitive ulcer surgery (such as a vagotomy) is now no longer indicated.
- Thoroughly wash the peritoneal cavity with 3 litres of warm saline. Drainage is unnecessary and may increase morbidity.

Closure
Mass closure with 1 PDS and clips to skin.

Complications
- 10% mortality
- Multi-organ dysfunction syndrome
- Pelvic/sub-phrenic abscess formation
- Wound infection
- On-going leak and duodenal fistula formation.

Discharge
- 7–10 days if uncomplicated recovery.
- >90% have *Helicobacter pylori* infection. Discharge with eradication therapy and an 8 week course of proton pump inhibitor to prevent ulcer recurrence.
- Follow-up endoscopy to check healing/biopsy gastric ulcers.

Laparoscopic surgery
Laparoscopic omental patching has now widely been reported with comparable results to open surgery with the apparent established advantages of decreased pain, wound infection, incisional herniation and hospital stay. However, the procedure is technically demanding and time-consuming and at present should be confined to enthusiasts within the context of a clinical trial.

Oesophageal rupture and perforation

Indications
- Boerhaave's syndrome (post-vomiting/barogenic spontaneous rupture)
- Iatrogenic perforation (endoscopic or operative)
- Traumatic injury (penetrating gun/stab wounds or blunt compression injury)
- Ingestion of corrosive agent or foreign body.

Preoperative evaluation
- CXR (surgical emphysema/pneumo-mediastinum/hydro-pneumothorax)
- Video endoscopy to assess site/size of injury and associated pathology
- Contrast radiography to assess extent of any leak
- CT.

General considerations
- Contained or small perforations with minimal contamination can usually be treated conservatively as long as there is no distal obstruction. These usually occur after instrumental perforation in a starved patient. Insert an NG tube endoscopically if recognised early.
- Treat malignant perforation in the presence of advanced disease with a covered endo-prosthesis.
- Carry out surgery on injuries with heavy contamination, free uncontained leakage or distal luminal obstruction.

T-tube drainage
This is the standard approach to those perforations or ruptures that are associated with heavy contamination, tissue necrosis and local sepsis.
- After initial debridement, wash-and myotomy, insert a large bore T-tube into the oesophageal defect and secure in place by longitudinal closure with interrupted 2/0 Vicryl. This creates a controlled oesophago-cutaneous fistula. Remove the T-tube after 3–4 weeks.
- Insert large bore intercostal drains and close the chest.
- Insert a feeding jejunostomy via a mini laparotomy for prolonged enteral nutrition.

Primary repair
This is suitable only for injuries recognised early prior to infection and necrosis of local tissues.
- Boerhaave's syndrome usually affects the lower left oesophagus. Explore chest via a left low (8th or 9th interspace) postero-lateral thoracotomy. Extensive lavage of food material and debridement of devitalised tissue is required. Open the mediastinal pleura widely, perform a long myotomy to expose the whole length of the mucosal tear which is longer than the muscular breach.
- Carry out repair in two layers with interrupted 3/0 PDS. Use an intercostal flap for further reinforcement to prevent on-going leakage.
- Insert large bore intercostal drains and close the chest.
- Insert a feeding jejunostomy for prolonged enteral nutrition via a mini laparotomy.

Gastro-oesophageal reflux disease

The principle of surgery is to construct and/or accentuate the barrier function between the oesophagus and stomach to prevent gastro-oesophageal reflux.

Indications for anti-reflux surgery
- Failed medical therapy
- Recurrent stricture formation whilst medical therapy
- Patient (who is fit) preference for surgery over long term medical therapy
- Reflux induced malnutrition in children/mentally handicap
- In association with Heller's myotomy for achalasia cardia
- Reflux induced episodic aspiration with risk of pulmonary fibrosis.

Position of patient
Supine.

Surgical approaches
- Transthoracic
- Transabdominal
- Open method
- Laparoscopic method.

Types of surgery
Complete fundoplication with formation of 360° wrap is the most popular and is known by the name Nissen fundoplication. Various modifications have been made to the original surgery described by Nissen in order to reduce postoperative side effects such as gasbloat syndrome, dysphagia etc. Short and floppy wrap is one such modification that is performed commonly with division of short gastric vessels. In Nissen–Rossetti fundoplication the short gastric vessels are not divided and the wrap is fashioned using anterior fundus.

Surgical outcome
The anti-reflux surgery is successful in 85–90% of patients. The overall postoperative mortality is <1 in 1000 (0.1%). Perioperative complications comprise pneumothorax, splenectomy in <1% and oesophageal perforation. Late complications can occur in 10–15%, including gasbloat, temporary dysphagia and increased flatulence.

Para-oesophageal hiatus hernia repair

Indication
Acute presentations
- Oesophageal or gastric obstruction
- Upper GI bleeding
- Acute organo-axial or mesentero-axial gastric volvulus
- Gastric strangulation or perforation.

Chronic symptoms
- Post-prandial pain (70%)
- Nausea and vomiting (40%)
- Dysphagia (40%)
- Gastro-oesophageal reflux (mixed sliding/rolling hernia) 30%.

Preoperative preparation
- CXR and contrast radiography
- Attempted NG decompression
- Upper GI endoscopy.

Position of patient
Supine.

Open technique
Upper midline with self-retaining and sternal elevating retractors.

Procedure
The para-oesophageal defect contains most of the herniated viscus (usually stomach).
- Reduce the stomach and other herniated organs such as omentum, spleen or colon with gentle downward traction and by tilting the table head-up.
- Dissect the peritoneal hernia sac free from its mediastinal attachments and excise it.
- Ligate the posterior aspect of the sac.
- In the acute situation, carefully assess organ damage and carry out resection if necessary.
- In the presence of an associated sliding hiatus hernia, mobilize the oesophagus into the abdomen and carry out a posterior crural repair with non-absorbable sutures as for a standard fundoplication.
  Then close the hernial defect with interrupted 1 Nylon or Prolene, buttressing the sutures with PTFE patches so that they do not cut out of the diaphragm.
- If the defect is large a tension free suture repair my not be possible. In this situation, suture a PTFE or polypropylene mesh or special pre-shaped hiatus hernia mesh (Fig. 6.1) is sutured to the margins of the defect using interrupted 2/0 Prolene and then covered with omentum to prevent inflammatory damage or migration into adjacent organs. At the end of the repair the hiatus should allow the passage of an index finger adjacent to the oesophagus.

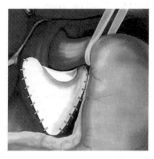

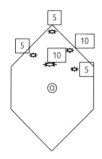

Fig. 6.1 Mesh repair of hiatus hernia

Fig. 6.2 Port sites for laparoscopic repair (5 = 5mm, 10 = 10mm) (courtesy CR Bard, Inc.)

Even in the absence of any sliding component or history of reflux symptoms, many surgeons perform a fundoplication to further fix the stomach within the abdomen. This is usually a full 360° posterior wrap (see section on anti-reflux surgery). An alternative approach, particularly in elderly frail patients, is to perform a gastropexy or percutaneous gastrotomy. A gastropexy is carried out by suturing the gastric fundus to the diaphragm and the greater curve to the left side of the anterior abdominal wall using a series of interrupted non-absorbable sutures. A gastrotomy is fashioned around a Conflo™ PEG tube and sutured to the anterior abdominal wall using 2/0 Vicryl, with subsequent removal 6–8 weeks later.

Closure
Mass closure with 1 PDS and clips to skin.

Laparoscopic repair
The main principles of the operation are as that of the open procedure. The procedure is carried out with the patient in modified lithotomy and anti-Trendelenberg position with operating surgeon standing between the legs. The port sites are shown in Fig. 6.2.

Open (Heller's) cardiomyotomy for achalasia

Indication

Achalasia is characterised by a hypertensive non-relaxing lower oeso-phageal sphincter (LOS) associated with non-coordinated spastic oeso-phageal peristalsis. Pneumatic balloon dilatation of the LOS and myotomy have similar results, although concomitant fundoplication at the time of surgery can prevent gastro-oesophageal reflux.

Transabdominal cardiomyotomy

Incision

Upper midline.

Procedure

- Carry out a preoperative endoscopy which will allow clearance of any retained debris in the oesophagus and deflation of the stomach. If an anti-reflux procedure is planned, leave the endoscope in situ or replaced with a bougie passed over a guide-wire. Self-retaining and sternal elevating retractors provide good access to the hiatus.
- Retract the left lobe of the liver after division of the triangular ligament. Divide the phreno-oesophageal ligament and develop the peri-oesophageal plane up into the posterior mediastinum preserving the vagi. Insert 2/0 Vicryl muscular retraction stay sutures to facilitate an antero-lateral oesophageal myotomy >8cm using McIndoe scissor dissection through the circular and longitudinal muscle fibres.
- Spread the muscle fibres widely apart using tissue forceps to prevent reconstitution, causing the mucosa and submucosa to bulge outwards. Continue the myotomy 1–2cm across onto the stomach with the scalpel to ensure complete LOS division.

Controversy exists whether all patients require anti-reflux surgery, al-though it is common to perform a partial anterior fundoplication over the abdominal area of the myotomy. The antero-lateral aspect of the fundus is sutured in 3 longitudinal rows to each muscular edge of the myotomised segment and then to the right crus (Dor procedure) using interrupted absorbable sutures.

Closure

Mass closure with 1 PDS and clips to skin.

Transthoracic cardiomyotomy

Thoracic surgeons favour a postero-lateral 6th interspace thoracotomy. This approach provides superior exposure of the oesophagus allowing a longer myotomy up to the level of the aortic arch. Recent innovations include minimally invasive thoracoscopic myotomy although long-term results are not yet available.

Complications

- Perforation
- Recurrent dysphagia due to inadequate myotomy or an over-tight fundoplication
- Gastro-oesophageal reflux
- Diverticulum formation
- Malignant change (surveillance endoscopy may be indicated).

Laparoscopic cardiomyotomy

Position and preoperative preparation

- Patients are placed in lithotomy position with the operator between the legs.
- Apply intermittent pneumatic compression stockings to minimise DVT risk.
- Undertake preoperative endoscopy as for open cardiomyotomy.

Procedure

- Insert a 10mm midline port 5–10cm above the umbilicus using the open technique and create 12–14mmHg capno-pertioneum.
- Use the 30° laparoscope. Insert a Nathanson retractor 5mm port site just below the xiphisternum to elevate the left lobe of the liver.
- Insert two further 5–10mm left and right subcostal ports for the hiatal dissection and subsequent suturing together with an additional 10mm left upper quadrant port for gastric retraction using an atraumatic Babcock.
- Divide the proximal gastro-hepatic ligament using the harmonic scalpel, preserving the hepatic branch of the vagus and exposing the right crus.
- Divide the phreno-oesophageal ligament around its antero-lateral aspect. Mobilise the dilated oesophagus by blunt mediastinal dissection preserving the vagi. Then free the oesophagus from the left crus and retract at least 5–6cm into the abdomen. If an anterior fundoplication is planned then a large retro-oesophageal window in front of the crura is not required. A crural repair is not carried out unless the hiatus is widened.
- Create a 6cm myotomy over the right antero-lateral aspect of the oesophagus using bipolar scissors or the harmonic scalpel, preserving the anterior vagus. Continue the myotomy over the 2cm of the cardia and suture a Dor partial anterior fundoplication intra-corporeally as described in the open repair. It is not usual to divide the short gastric vessels to allow an adequate mobilization of the fundus. Check for haemostasis and perforation. Drains are not usually required.

Closure

- 1 PDS on J-shaped needle to rectus sheath.
- Subcutaneous 3/0 Monocryl to skin.

Complications

As for open cardiomyotomy.

Open splenectomy

Indications
- Trauma
- Haematological conditions.

Position of patient
Supine.

Incision
- Long midline for trauma
- Extended left subcostal for elective procedures.

Procedure
- Draw the splenic flexure of the colon and any associated omental attachments inferiorly and separate from the spleen.
- Open the lesser sac and divide the gastro-splenic ligament with ligation of the short gastric vessels along the greater curve and fundus of the stomach with 2/0 Vicryl.
- Identify the splenic artery along the superior border of the pancreas and control distally with a vascular sling.
- Gently retract the spleen medially and divide the posterior peritoneal attachments of the phrenico-splenic and lieno-renal ligaments. Separate the tail of the pancreas from the spleen and doubly ligate the splenic vein and artery separately in continuity with a non-absorbable 2/0 suture. Then remove the spleen.

Emergency situation
- Mobilise the spleen forward by dividing the posterior peritoneal attachments and clamping the pedicle early to prevent further blood loss. Then continue the procedure as above.
- Preservation of the spleen is desirable. Repair small tears or achieve haemostasis with selective ligation of the splenic vessels at the hilum. Control splenic capsular tears by diathermy or application of collagen impregnated packs. If splenectomy is performed some surgeons may re-implant splenic tissue into the omentum, particularly if there are no splenuculi. A large bore drain is left in the splenic bed.

Closure
In two layers with 1 PDS. Clips to skin.

Complications
- Haemorrhage
- Subphrenic haematoma/abscess
- Pancreatitis/pancreatic leak from ischaemia or trauma
- Overwhelming post-splenectomy infection
- A-V fistula formation between splenic vein/artery if ligated together.

Prophylaxis
- Pneumoccal/Hib/mennigococcal vaccines
- Life-long penicillin.

Laparoscopic splenectomy

With the advent of harmonic scalpel and ligasure, small to large spleens can be removed through the laparoscopic method. Some surgeons employ hand assisted techniques using a pneumosleeve to preserve the pneumoperitoneum. Usually at least four ports are necessary and the procedure can be carried out in right lateral/supine or modified lithotomy position depending on the surgeons preference.

Weight reduction surgery for morbid obesity

People with a Body Mass Index (BMI) equal to or exceeding 40kg/m², or between 35kg/m² and 40kg/m² with significant comorbid conditions satisfy the criteria as having morbid obesity. In England and Wales it was estimated in 1998 that 0.6% of men and 1.9% women were morbidly obese amounting to 2500 people/200,000 population.

Surgery is recommended as a management alternative for morbidly obese people providing the following criteria are accomplished:

• They should have been receiving multidisciplinary intensive management in a specialised weight management clinic.
• There should be no specific clinical or psychological contraindications.
• They should be aged 18 years or over.
• They should demonstrate all appropriate non-surgical measures have been sufficiently tried and failed.
• They should be fit for anaesthesia and surgery.
• They should be self-motivated and understand the need for long term follow-up.
• Secondary causes such as hypothyroidism, Cushing's syndrome etc. should be identified and treated by a specialist endocrinologist.

Preoperative preparation

Comprehensive, multidisciplinary assessment involving various professionals such as an endocrinologist, dietician, physiotherapist, upper GI surgeon, psychologist, and anaesthetist is necessary. All patients need sleep capnography to exclude apnoea, as they require post surgery intensive therapy unit (ITU) and/or or high dependency unit (HDU) management.

Position of patient

Supine.

Surgical principles

The principal aim of surgery is to improve the quality of life through significant reduction of weight and maintaining that weight loss on a longer term. Broadly, surgical interventional procedures are classified into two categories; restrictive and malabsorptive. In the former the size of the stomach is restricted so the patient feels full with less food and in the later segments of GI tract are bypassed so as to limit the absorption of food.

Vertical gastroplasty (restrictive procedure)

This involves creation of a long narrow gastric tube along the lesser curve of the stomach. A stapling device is used to carry out the vertical partition.

Horizontal gastroplasty (restrictive procedure)

This entails creation of a small proximal gastric reservoir and establishes continuity through a small anterior gastro-gastrostomy. The horizontal partition is usually achieved through four rows of staples across the stomach.

Gastric bypass (restrictive and malabsorptive procedure)

Following creation of a small gastric reservoir, a good length (usually 100cm) of the proximal small intestine is bypassed. This is achieved by Roux-en-y anastomoses. The bypass induces a state of malabsorption and aid further weight loss.

Gastric banding (restrictive procedure)

A purpose made prosthesis such as the Swedish adjustable gastric band (SAGB) is inserted around the proximal stomach just below the cardia. The prosthesis is connected through the tubing to a reservoir that is deposited in subcutaneous tissue. The balloon on the inner aspect of the prosthesis can be inflated or deflated so as to affect the gastric reservoir outlet size.

Radical surgery for gastric cancer

Preparation for gastric surgery

All patients require thorough fitness assessment and exclusion of distant/unresectable disease using CT, endoscopic ultrasound and staging laparoscopy. In general palliative resection or bypass is not indicated unless there is obstruction or significant bleeding.

Position of patient

Supine.

Extent of gastric resection

The stomach can be divided into thirds (lower—L, middle—M, upper—U). Distal third (L) tumours require subtotal gastrectomy (approximately 80% of the stomach) with preservation of the fundus and short gastric arterial supply. Middle third (M), proximal third (U) and whole stomach tumours (LMU) require total gastrectomy. Tumour at the cardia requires total gastrectomy with excision of 5cm of distal oesophagus. The GI continuity is established through Roux-en-Y anastomosis. Early tumours of the proximal stomach may be treated by proximal subtotal gastrectomy and jejunal interposition. T4 disease into pancreas, spleen, colon or liver may require additional organ resection in young fit patients without distant disease.

Lymphadenectomy

Radical excision of the stomach and associated lymph nodes is widely practiced in Japan and specialist Western Centres. Gastric cancer with lymph node metastases may remain a loco-regional disease and radical excision with lymphadenectomy can be justified on the following grounds:

- Optimal pathological disease staging and estimate of prognosis
- Improved loco-regional control
- Prolonged survival and possible cure.

The pattern of lymphatic spread has been carefully documented in relation to the primary tumour and divided into three tiers based on the relative incidence of nodal disease.

- N1 (perigastric tier)
- N2 (nodes along main arterial supply to the stomach)
- N3 (distant nodal stations away from the stomach).

The amount of nodal dissection performed is represented as D1, D2 or D3 depending on how many tiers are removed. There is strong supporting evidence that a D2 gastrectomy should be the standard surgical procedure for gastric cancer, although the case for this approach remains unproven in randomised trials. The morbidity of more extensive D3 resections, particularly if the distal pancreas or spleen needs to be resected, appears to outweigh the potential benefits. The N1, N2, N3 and metastatic (M) nodes for gastric cancer subsites are shown in Table 6.1.

Table 6.1 Nodes for gastric cancer subsites

No.	Location	LMU/MUL MLU/UMU	LD/L	LM/M/ML	MU/UM	U
1	Right paracardial	1	2	1	1	1
2	Left paracardial	1	M	3	1	1
3	Lesser curve	1	1	1	1	1
4sa	Short gastric	1	M	3	1	1
4sb	Left gastroepiploic	1	3	1	1	1
4d	Right gastroepiploic	1	1	1	2	2
5	Suprapyloric	1	1	1	3	3
6	Infrapyloric	1	1	1	3	3
7	Left gastric artery	2	2	2	2	2
8a	Anterior common hepatic artery	2	2	2	2	2
8b	Posterior common hepatic artery	3	3	3	3	3
9	Coeliac artery	2	2	2	2	2
10	Splenic hilum	2	M	3	2	2
11p	Proximal splenic artery	2	2	2	2	2
11d	Distal splenic artery	2	M	3	2	2
12a	Left hepatoduodenal ligament	2	2	2	3	3
12b,p	Posterior hepatoduo- denal lligament	3	3	3	3	3
13	Retropancreatic	3	3	3	M	M
14v	Superior mesenteric vein	2	2	3	M	M
14a	Superior mesenteric artery	M	M	M	M	M

L, lower; M, middle; U, upper; D, distal.

Gastroenterostomy

A Roux-en-Y gastro-enterostomy is almost always employed, as it is associated with lowest degree of bile reflux. Bilroth 1 reconstruction after subtotal gastrectomy produces maximal bile reflux into the gastric remnant. Bilroth II and Polya (retro-colic loop gastro-jejunostomy) re-constructions were frequently carried out for benign peptic ulcer surgery but also produce bile reflux and in symptomatic patients require revision to a Roux-en-Y configuration. Loop gastro-jejunostomy continues to be employed for palliative bypasses, as there is only one anastomosis. It may be combined with a division of the stomach above the site of the malignant obstruction to prevent future in-growth into the anastomosis as a 'Divine exclusion'.

Indications
- Reconstruction after gastric resection
- Drainage procedure after peptic ulcer surgery
- Obstructing/inoperable gastric/duodenal/pancreatic malignancy
- Revision of previous peptic ulcer surgery
- By-pass surgery for morbid obesity.

Roux-en-Y reconstruction

- Divide the proximal jejunum just beyond the DJ flexure. Divide the mesenteric vessels to provide a mobile well-vascularised distal segment. Create a retro-colic window in an avascular part of the transverse mesocolon.
- Perform a stapled oesophago-gastrostomy if reconstruction is carried out after total gastrectomy. Place a 2/0 Prolene purse string in the oesophagus either by hand application between stay sutures or by using a purse string instrument. Secure an appropriate size circular gun head (usually 28mm diameter) in place. Insert the gun into the open end of the Roux loop from the left hand side of the patient and create an end-side anastomosis taking care not to twist the mesentery or catch additional tissue in the anastomosis.
- Keep the blind end of the jejunum as short as possible and closed with a linear stapler. Oversewn with 2/0 Vicryl. Occasionally, the blind end is deliberately kept long so as to create a side-to-side pouch reconstruction.
- Employ a hand sewn continuous two-layer anastomosis after subtotal gastrectomy between the lowest part of the gastric remnant and the Roux loop using 2/0 PDS or Vicryl. An end-side anastomosis is usually too narrow and a side-side anastomosis is preferred.
- Close the blind end of the Roux loop with a linear stapler and oversew it. In constructing the anastomosis this blind end is positioned on the patient's right hand side (in contrast to total gastrectomy) so that there is dependent drainage from the stomach.
- After completing the gastro-jejunostomy, secure it beneath the colon and incorporate closure of the window in the transverse mesocolon.
- Perform the distal Roux anastomosis 40–50cm distally as a side-to-end jejuno-jejunostomy using one or two layers of 2/0 PDS or Vicryl.

Loop gastro-jejunostomy

- Identify a mobile proximal jejunal segment. The retrocolic route is the shortest and associated with the best position for drainage.
- Perform the anastomosis along the lower greater curve in two layers with 2/0 Vicryl or PDS with 5–10cm of iso-peristaltic jejunum. Then secure the gastro-jejunostomy below the transverse mesocolon.

Preoperative preparation for oesophagectomy

Indications
- Malignancy
- End-stage benign disease
- Occasionally emergency resection required for corrosive injury/perforation or spontaneous rupture.

Staging malignant disease
Endoscopy
- Site/size of tumour
- Dilatation for improved nutrition
- Insertion of feeding naso-gastric tube
- Histological diagnosis
- Suitability of oesophageal replacement (stomach/colon).

Exclude distant/unresectable disease
- CT thorax/abdomen
- Endoscopic ultrasound
- PET scanning
- Bone scintigraphy
- Laparoscopy
- Bronchoscopy.

Re-stage after neo-adjuvant treatment
- Assess fitness for surgery
- Full blood count/electrolytes/liver function tests
- Pulmonary function tests
- Arterial blood gases
- Exercise test
- ECG
- Cardiological/respiratory consultation
- Nutritional assessment and hyperalimentation
- Anaesthetic assessment—single lung anaesthesia/thoracic epidural.

Preparation for surgery
- Stop smoking
- Control of dental caries
- Thrombo-embolic prophylaxis
- Intravenous broad-spectrum antibiotic cover
- Cross match four units of blood
- Intensive care/high dependency bed availability
- Colon preparation if required for a conduit
- Psychological preparation and counselling.

Rationale for radical surgery and lymphadenectomy
- Optimal staging
- Improved loco-regional control
- Improved cure rate.

Left thoracic subtotal oesophagectomy

Some thoracic surgeons favour this approach for lower and middle third oesophageal tumours. It is contraindicated for malignancy above the aortic arch for which a right-sided three-phase approach is required. The theoretical advantage is that tumour operability is assessed as the initial part of the procedure, although with modern imaging inoperability in the chest is rare. Disadvantages include poor access to the abdomen and insufficient mediastinal access to nodal tissue and the thoracic duct.

Left thoraco-laparotomy

Position of patient
Right lateral position.

Procedure
Make an oblique incision from the left hypochondrium over the costal margin along the 7th rib to its posterior angle. Divide the thoracic wall muscles with diathermy and open the pleural space at the upper border of the 7th rib.

- Collapse the lung.
- Divide the costal margin and detach the diaphragm from the ribs peripherally, avoiding phrenic nerve damage.
- Open the peritoneum along the main incision from rectus sheath to costal margin and exclude distant/unresectable disease (Fig.6.3).
- Mobilise the oesophagus and adjacent tissue from the hiatus upwards.
- Preserve the left recurrent laryngeal nerve as the oesophagus is freed by blunt dissection around the aortic arch.
- Pass a tape around the oesophagus at this point to aid retraction and dissect into root of the neck, identified by the 1st rib.
- Mobilise the stomach in a similar fashion to that described for the abdominal Lewis-Tanner approach (see following section).
- Divide the gastro-splenic, gastro-colic and gastro-hepatic ligaments with preservation of the right gastric and gastro-epiploic vessels.
- Ligate the left gastric vessels and divide separately and carry out a pyloroplasty.
- Kocherise the duodenum to gain length.
- Divide the upper oesophagus above the aortic arch after stay sutures have been applied.
- Divide the proximal stomach with a linear stapler across the lesser curve towards the fundus to create a gastric tube and deliver the specimen.
- Oversew the gastrotomy line with 2/0 PDS.
- Pass the high point of the fundus up to the apex of the thorax and suture it to the oesophageal stump.
- Repair the diaphragm and costal margin with continuous 1 Nylon.
- Insert apical and basal underwater seal chest drains and re-expand the lung.
- Approximate the ribs with interrupted 0 Vicryl and close the muscle in layers with 1 PDS and clips to skin.

Left cervical incision

Mobilise the oesophagus as previously described and fashion an end-to-side oesophago-gastric anastomosis with interrupted 2/0 PDS. Insert a 24Fr Wallace–Robinson drain adjacent to the anastomosis. Close the wound in layers with 2/0 Vicryl and subcutaneous 3/0 Monocryl to skin.

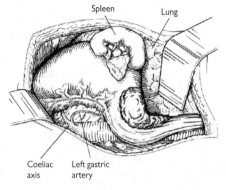

Fig. 6.3 Thoraco-abdominal approach for lower-third oesophageal carcinoma

Transhiatal oesophagectomy

Rationale

Transhiatal oesophagectomy has fewer pulmonary complications when compared to the transthoracic approach, although with no significant reduction in mortality. The oesophagus is resected by blunt dissection with anastomosis of the conduit through a neck incision. Major blood loss can occur and there is sub-optimal lymphadenectomy producing a higher local recurrence rate. Modern retractors facilitate more dissection under direct vision and many thoracic surgeons favour this approach, particularly for benign disease.

Abdominal phase

Exclude distant or unresectable disease through a midline incision. Carry out routine gastric or colonic mobilisation as previously described to allow tension free passage up to the neck. Divide the phreno-oesophageal ligament. Mobilise the lower 5–10cm of oesophagus and tumour checking that there is no fixation to the aorta or tracheo-bronchial tree. Stop the mediastinal dissection and perform a pyloroplasty.

Cervical phase

- Make a 5cm oblique left cervical incision parallel to the sterno-cleidomastoid centred at the level of the cricoid cartilage.
- Divide the platysma and omohyoid and ligate the inferior thyroid artery and divide it.
- Retract the carotid sheath laterally and the larynx and trachea medially avoiding damage to the recurrent laryngeal nerve in the tracheo-oesophageal groove.
- Mobilise the oesophagus posteriorly by blunt dissection from the pre-vertebral fascia into the superior mediastinum. Dissect the oesophagus free by sharp dissection from the trachea avoiding damage to the posterior membranous aspect. Once encircled with a sling, the cervical and upper thoracic oesophagus can be mobilised to the level of the carina by further blunt dissection.

Mediastinal phase (Fig. 6.4)

- Now pass a hand through the hiatus and free the oesophagus by blunt finger dissection. Carry out sequential division of the posterior attachment to the aorta and the anterior connection to the tracheo-bronchial tree. Finally, mobilise the oesophagus from its lateral pleural adhesions. Much of this can be achieved under direct vision with adequate retraction and synchronous dissection from the neck.
- If there is uncontrollable blood loss pack the area and convert to an open thoracotomy.
- Penetration of either pleural space necessitates tube thoracotomy.
- Divide the proximal oesophagus in the neck and suture a drain to the distal cut end and bring this out in the abdomen. Then excise the specimen and prepare the colonic or gastric conduit, suturing it to the drain and passing it up into the neck. Anchor the conduit to the pre-vertebral fascia in the neck.
- Insert a feeding jejunostomy and close the abdomen with 1 PDS and clips to skin.

Anastomosis (Fig. 6.4)

- Fashion an end-to-end oesophago-gastric or oesophago-colic anastomosis with interrupted 2/0 PDS as previously described.
- Insert a 24Fr Wallace–Robinson drain adjacent to the anastomosis and close the wound in layers with 2/0 Vicryl and subcutaneous 3/0 Monocryl to skin.

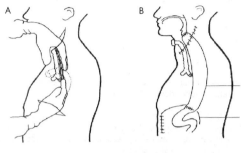

Fig. 6.4 Transhiatal mobilisation of oesophagus

Abdominal and right thoracic subtotal oesophagectomy

This is the Ivor Lewis or Lewis–Tanner procedure, commonly used for middle and lower third of the oesophageal tumours. Reconstruction is usually carried out with a gastric pull-up anastomosed at the apex of the thorax.

Abdominal phase

Position of patient

Supine.

Procedure

- Exclude distant and unresectable disease via an upper midline incision. Use modern fixed retracting devices to enhance gastric and hiatal exposure.
- Mobilize the stomach as previously described with preservation of the right gastric and gastro-epiploic vessels. Carry out a varying degree of lymphadenectomy. No drains are usually required. Close the abdomen with mass closure with 1 PDS and clips to skin.

Thoracic phase

Position of patient

Left lateral position.

Procedure

- Perform a postero-lateral thoracotomy with diathermy. Retract the inferior aspect of the scapula upwards and enter the thorax through the 5th or 6th intercostal spaces (the 2nd rib is at the apex of the sub-scapula space). Divide the intercostal muscles above the rib and collapse the lung. Excise the neck of the lower rib to allow a controlled fracture and better exposure. Ligate the intercostal vessels and destroy the nerve to decrease postoperative pain.
- Exclude distant or unresectable disease. Divide the right pulmonary ligament up to the inferior pulmonary vein. Ligate the arch of the azygous vein and divide it in continuity with 2/0 Vicryl. Develop the plane between the azygos vein and the aorta with en bloc excision of the thoracic duct and para-aortic nodes. Ligate oesophageal aortic branches with 3/0 Vicryl and skeletonise the antero-lateral descending thoracic aorta. Dissect the oesophagus medially from the lung hilum and pericardium taking all nodes en bloc. Pass a tape around the oesophagus to aid retraction. Expose proximally the right and left main bronchi with en bloc excision of carinal, bronchial, and para-tracheal nodes, avoiding damage to the posterior membranous aspect of the tracheo-bronchial tree.
- Ligate the thoracic duct just above the diaphragm to prevent chylothorax. Excise para-oesophageal tissue en bloc with mediastinal pleura posteriorly and inferiorly, exposing the left lung. Continue oesophageal mobilisation to meet the trans-abdominal dissection (Fig. 6.5A, B). Divide the final pleural attachments to allow entry of the stomach into the thorax.

- Withdraw the NG tube. Apply oesophageal stay 2/0 Vicryl sutures and transect the oesophagus at the apex of the thorax. Divide the proximal stomach along the lesser curve with associated abdominal nodes and fashion a gastric tube. Carry out a gastro-oesophageal anastomosis as previously described (Fig. 6.5C).
- Insert apical, basal and left pleural (sometimes) underwater seal drains. Approximate the ribs and close the wound with interrupted 0 Vicryl. Close the muscle in two layers with 1 PDS and apply clips to skin.

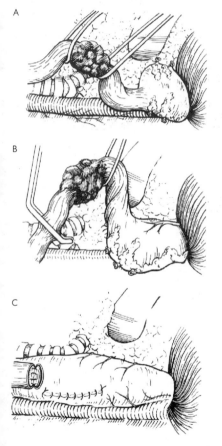

Fig. 6.5 Right thoracic resection of the oesophagus with gastric interposition

Three stage oesophagectomy

Some surgeons prefer to expose/divide and anastomose the oesophagus in the neck. The additional resection of the oesophagus is not much more than that achieved by the Ivor Lewis technique although this technique is required for proximal tumours so that an adequate proximal resection margin can be achieved. The procedure is commonly referred to as a 'McKeown' oesophagectomy. It involves the same initial approach as an Ivor Lewis oesophagectomy but with complete dissection of the thoracic oesophagus up to the thoracic inlet. The additional of a left or right neck approach is then carried out for the additional resection.

In Japan a bilateral cervical approach is employed for middle third and upper third squamous cell carcinomas in order to perform radical cervical lymphadenectomy. This latter approach is seldom used in the West based upon the lower incidence of cervical nodal disease for lower third adenocarcinomas and the associated additional morbidity mainly from recurrent laryngeal nerve injury.

Carcinoma of the hypopharynx and upper cervical oesophagus are usually dealt with by head and neck surgeons employing a pharyngo-laryngo-oesophagectomy with free jejunal graft interposition.

Gastric interposition as an oesophageal substitute

Indication

The stomach is usually the first choice as an oesophageal substitute. It is well vascularised, simple to mobilise into the thorax or neck with good functional results. Additionally, only one anastomosis is required. It is common to use the posterior mediastinal route through the oesophageal bed. Retro-sternal (anterior mediastinal) or pre-sternal (subcutaneous) routes are longer, non-anatomical and seldom employed.

Incision

Upper midline.

Procedure

- Exclude distant or unresectable disease.
- Retract the greater omentum/transverse colon from the stomach and divide the gastro-colic omentum below the right gastro-epiploic arcade centrally, entering the lesser sac. Continue dissection towards the fundus and left gastro-epiploic pedicle and then inferiorly to expose the origin of the right gastro-epiploic vein after division of the crossover vessel to the middle colic vein. Separate the hepatic flexure from the duodenum and Kocherise it to the midline exposing the IVC and aorta. This allows the pylorus to swing up to the hiatus providing maximum gastric length.
- Divide the lesser omentum close to the liver and preserve the right gastric artery inferiorly as it emerges from the common hepatic artery. Ligate the hepatic branch of the vagus as there may be a significant associated vessel. Preserve any large aberrant hepatic artery. Now divide the gastro-splenic ligament, ligate the short gastric vessels away from the fundus with 3/0 Vicryl. Elevate the stomach and divide the lesser sac adhesions over the pancreas. Ligate the left gastric vein in continuity with 3/0 Vicryl and divide it. Divide the origin of the left gastric artery and transfix it with 3/0 Vicryl. Carry out an en bloc partial D2 nodal clearance of the left gastric, common hepatic and splenic arteries. Resect the coeliac nodes with skeletonisation of the abdominal aorta up to the hiatus. Take the crura and cuff of diaphragm en bloc with the oesophagus. Carry out further transhiatal dissection into each pleural space to allow the correct planes for thoracic en bloc excision of the mediastinal pleura.
- The stomach should now be completely mobile. Carry out a Heineke–Mikulicz pyloroplasty with interrupted Gambee 2/0 Vicryl sutures. Skeletonise the lesser curve in the abdomen by dividing the lesser omentum and left gastric tissue above the right gastric pedicle. It is common practice to fashion a feeding jejunostomy. Close the abdomen with monolayer PDS.

- Once resection of the oesophagus is complete, pull the stomach through to the apex of the thorax or neck for anastomosis. Depending on the extent of gastric involvement, excise a varying degree of the lesser curve and proximal stomach to create a gastric tube. Perform the anastomosis in the posterior fundus at the high point of the stomach, well away from the resection line to ensure no compromise of blood supply as previously described.

Colonic interposition for oesophageal replacement

Indications

- When the stomach is absent, rendered ischaemic, or damaged by caustic injury
- Where tumour extent requires resection of whole stomach
- For extra-anatomical bypass (sub-sternal or subcutaneous routes)
- Surgical preference (particularly vagal preserving procedures).

Preoperative preparation

- Colonoscopy to exclude inflammatory bowel disease/severe diverticulosis/malignancy or multiple polyp formation
- Mesenteric angiography to assess adequacy/pattern of colonic blood supply and identify which section of colon to use (usually an iso-peristaltic left colonic segment based upon the left colic pedicle)
- Colonic preparation with Picolax/Kleenprep.

Position of patient

Supine.

Incision

Long midline.

Procedure

- Exclude distant or unresectable disease and detach the omentum from the transverse colon. Mobilize the splenic and hepatic flexures and the ascending and descending colon to the midline so that the whole colon is free on its mesentery. Bring the apex of the left colonic loop based upon the ascending branch of the left colic artery to the xiphisternum and marked it with a 2/0 Vicryl stitch. Measure the distance from the xiphisternum to the mandible and mark this length proximal to the first stitch. Ligate the marginal vessels and divide them at this point. Divide the transverse mesocolon by ligating the middle colic pedicle below its bifurcation to preserve any arcade.
- Prepare the site of the proximal oesophageal anastomosis (usually in the left neck) and divide the right colon with a linear stapler. Tie the resection line to a long drain and insert the colon into a bowel bag for atraumatic traction up into the neck. Perform the proximal anastomosis with interrupted 2/0 Vicryl full-thickness sutures. Straighten the colon without mesenteric twisting and secure it inferiorly to the diaphragm.

- Now divide the distal colon 10cm below the diaphragm. If the vagi are divided and the stomach denervated then a better functional outcome is gained by an additional proximal two thirds gastrectomy and end-to-end colo-gastric anastomosis to the antrum in two layers with 2/0 PDS (Fig. 6.6). Carry out a Heineke–Mikulicz pyloroplasty. If a vagal preserving procedure has been performed then the stomach is retained with a posterior end-to-side colo-gastric anastomosis using a circular stapling device through a small anterior gastrotomy. Insert an NG tube in either event. Restore colonic continuity with an end-to-end colo-colic anastomosis in two layers with 2/0 PDS. Insert a feeding jejunostomy for nutritional support.

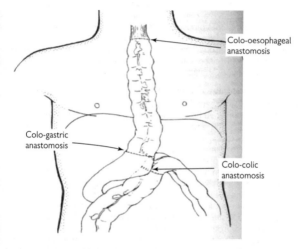

Fig. 6.6 Right colonic interposition from cervical oesophagus to antrum with colo-colic anastomosis

Oesophageal anastomosis after subtotal oesophagectomy

The oesophageal remnant is anastomosed to the conduit used for reconstruction, usually stomach or occasionally colon. Jejunum is rarely used for replacement except as free graft after pharyngo-laryngo-oesophagectomy for hypo-pharyngeal and proximal cervical tumours.

Oesophago-gastric or oesophago-colic anastomoses are hand sewn or stapled in the neck or upper thorax. The outcome is similar and surgical preference/approach dictates the selection of anastomotic technique. Cervical anastomoses have a higher leak rate, although a neck leak may not produce as severe clinical consequences as an intra-thoracic leak. Circular stapled anastomoses produce a higher stricture rate than sutured anastomoses, particularly if guns smaller than 25mm are used. Irrespective of technique, anastomoses should be tension-free, have good blood supply with close application of epithelial margins. Trauma from non-crushing clamps should be avoided.

Stapled oesophageal anastomosis

- Prepare the oesophageal remnant by NG tube withdrawal, aspiration, and insertion of a 2/0 Prolene purse string. Pass a double-ended straight needle suture through a purse string clamp (Fig. 6.7) applied across the oesophagus before transection. Divide the oesophagus close to the margin of the clamp. Alternatively, use a small round-bodied needle to place the Prolene purse string by hand at 5–7mm intervals with 5mm bites circumferentially, the oesophagus being held open by multiple full thickness 2/0 Vicryl stay sutures. Insert the head of the gun and the purse string secured around its neck (Fig. 6.8).
- If a gastric tube is used, insert the staple gun through the proximal resection margin and site the anastomosis posteriorly at the high point of the stomach, away from the gastrotomy line so as not to compromise the blood supply. Pass the spike through and secure the gastric wall with a 2/0 Vicryl purse string suture around the neck of the gun. After firing the gun inspect the completeness of the donuts (Fig. 6.9). Advance the NG tube and close the gastrotomy line with a linear stapler and oversew with 2/0 PDS. Variations of this approach can be used to produce end-to-end or end-to-side oesophago-colic anastomoses in the thorax or neck.

Sutured oesophageal anastomosis (Fig. 6.10)

- The simplest approach is a single layer of interrupted full-thickness 2/0 Vicryl or PDS sutures.
- First form the gastric tube completely and make a 2cm incision at the site where a stapled anastomosis would be fashioned. Place lateral stay sutures and suture the posterior wall initially with the knots internally. In the thorax the whole row is placed first and then the oesophagus parachuted down with sequential ligation of the sutures. Then complete the anterior row with knots externally and avoid redundant tissue from size discrepancy. A similar technique can be used to fashion end-to-end oesophago-colic anastomoses.

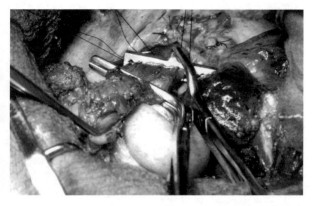

Fig. 6.7 Purse string clamp across the oesophagus 5–6cm proximal to the tumour

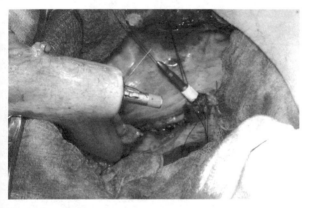

Fig. 6.8 Staple gun in the gastric conduit with the staple head in the proximal cut end of the oesophagus

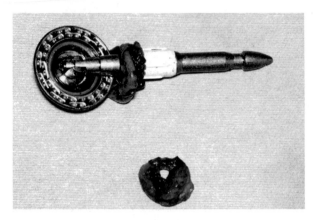

Fig. 6.9 Gastric and oesophageal donuts with the staple head

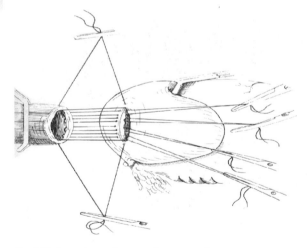

Fig. 6.10 Sutured oesophago-gastric anastomosis

Complications following oesophagectomy

Early complications
- Haemorrhage
- Pneumonia/acute respiratory distress syndrome (ARDS)
- Pneumothorax/pleural effusion
- Thrombo-embolic complications
- Anastomotic leak
- Chylothorax
- Recurrent laryngeal nerve palsy
- Gastric outlet obstruction (if no pyloroplasty performed)
- Mortality (5–10%).

Late complications
- Anastomotic stricture (particularly for stapled anastomoses)
- Post-thoracotomy pain
- Dumping
- Post-vagotomy diarrhoea
- Reflux
- Cancer recurrence (loco-regional and/or metastatic).

Colorectal surgery, appendix, and small bowel

A. K. Agarwal, J. Shenfine,
H. El-Khalifa, and David J. Leaper

Fissure-in-ano

A linear ulcer occurring below the dentate line. May be due to increase in anal resting pressure from overactivity of the internal anal sphincter causing hypoperfusion and fissuring at sites of 'watershed' vascular supply. They occur in the anterior and posterior midline and are more common in the posterior midline. Consider possible underlying pathology such as Crohn's disease, infection, trauma, or malignancy.

Use of bulk laxatives, stool softeners, and topical application of local anaesthetic assist in the spontaneous healing of most acute fissures. Topical glyceryl trinitrate 0.2% or Diltiazem 2% applied locally, reduce anal pressure and achieve healing in 50–70% of all fissures.

Lateral internal sphincterotomy

Indication

Surgery is indicated when medical therapy fails. Anal dilatation has been abandoned in favour of lateral internal sphincterotomy because the latter process is more controlled and incontinence is less common.

Position of patient

Lithotomy.

Procedure

This is done as a day procedure under general anaesthesia.

- Perform a digital rectal examination and sigmoidoscopy.
- Introduce a bivalve anal speculum. Open it gradually to put the fibres of the internal sphincter on the stretch.
- Ask the assistant to apply traction to perianal skin.
- Palpate the intersphincteric groove in the 3 o'clock position.
- Infiltrate local anaesthetic with 1:200 000 adrenaline in the groove and make a 1cm incision along the groove.
- The lower border of the internal sphincter is identified as a white band. Using blunt ended scissors develop the intersphincteric and submucosal planes. Divide the internal sphincter to the level of the dentate line.
- Excise any skin tag or hypertrophied internal papilla.
- Apply pressure to achieve haemostasis. Leave the wound open.

Flap repairs may be used for recurrent fissure after sphincterotomy and where risk to continence is high.

Postoperative complications

- Incontinence
- Recurrence/persistence
- Bleeding/haematoma.

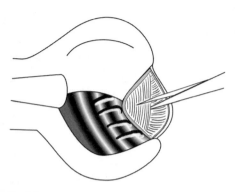

Fig. 7.1 Lateral internal sphincterotomy

Divided internal sphincter

Posterior fissure

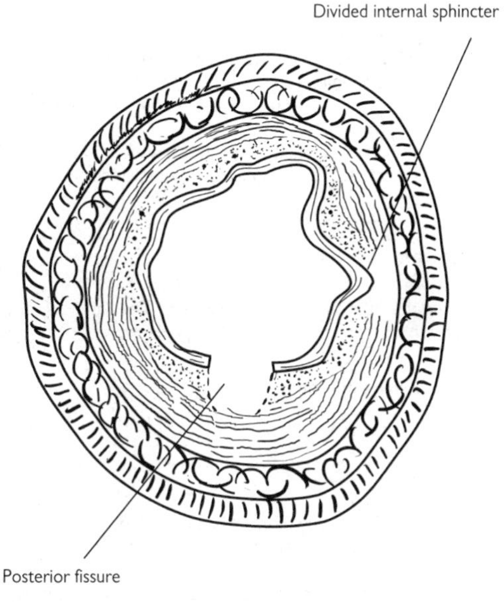

Fig. 7.2 Lateral internal sphincterotomy: technique and result

Haemorrhoids

Degeneration of the supporting structures of the three anal cushions causes them to prolapse leading to development of haemorrhoids. The majority of patients present with intermittent, small rectal bleeds and require no treatment other than reassurance and dietary advice but thorough evaluation is necessary to exclude other pathologies such as inflammatory bowel disease and malignancies. Examination should include inspection of the perineum, digital rectal examination, proctoscopy and sigmoidoscopy, and full colonic examination may be required by colonoscopy or barium enema.

Injection sclerotherapy

Indication

Persistent haemorrhoidal bleeding or small anterior mucosal prolapses. The aim of the procedure is to cause submucosal fibrosis.

Position

Left lateral.

Procedure

Done as an outpatient procedure.

- Draw up 10–15ml of 5% phenol in almond oil into a Luer lock syringe with a shouldered Gabriel needle.
- Pass a proctoscope and identify the left lateral, right anterior, and right posterior internal haemorrhoids.
- Inject 3–5ml of the solution under vision into the submucosa above each haemorrhoid. The correct plane of injection is indicated by elevation of the mucosa.

Review the patient at six weeks and repeat the procedure if necessary.

Rubber band ligation

Indication

Persistent haemorrhoidal bleeding and prolapsing. The aim of the procedure is to fix the mucosa thereby preventing prolapse.

Contraindication

Anticoagulation and immunocompromise.

Position

Left lateral.

Procedure

Done as an outpatient procedure.

- Pass a proctoscope and identify the internal haemorrhoids. Non-suction banders require an assistant to keep the proctoscope in position.
- Grasp the mucosa above the haemorrhoid and draw it into the barrel of the loaded ligator. Suction banding frees the surgeon's left hand to hold the proctoscope in position whilst applying suction to draw the mucosa into the bander. It is important to make sure before releasing the band that the grasping or suction on the mucosa does not cause pain. If it does, apply the banding to a more proximal position above the anorectal ring.

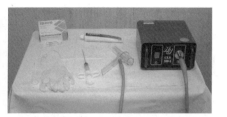

Fig. 7.3 Equipment for injection sclerotherapy

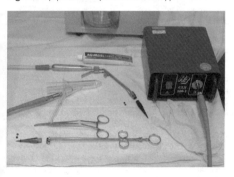

Fig. 7.4 Equipment for rubber band ligation

Site for injection/rubber band ligation

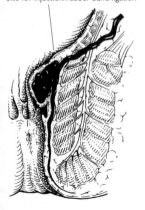

Fig. 7.5 Site for injection/rubber band ligation

Warn the patient that it is usual to feel some rectal discomfort and a desire to defaecate for the next 2–3 days and that a small amount of bleeding or the passage of a 'blackberry-like' thrombosed pile is common between 4–10 days. Review the patient at six weeks and repeat the procedure if necessary.

Haemorrhoidectomy

Indication
- Prolapsing haemorrhoids with symptomatic external haemorrhoids (pain, swelling).
- Second degree haemorrhoids (reduce spontaneously) and third degree haemorrhoids (needing to be reduced manually) that do not respond to out-patient procedures.
- Fourth degree haemorrhoids (which remain prolapsed permanently).

Position
Lithotomy or prone jack-knife with general anaesthetic.

Procedure
Usually done as an inpatient.
- Prepare the skin, towel up and shave the perineum. Insert a bivalve anal speculum and assess the position and size of the haemorrhoids. Start with the most posterior lying haemorrhoid so that blood does not obscure vision.
- Apply artery forceps to the skin at the edge of the external haemorrhoid and incise the skin with cutting diathermy.
- Continue the dissection medially with diathermy and insert the bivalve speculum once the anal margin is reached.
- Continue to carefully separate the internal haemorrhoidal tissue from the white internal sphincter muscle fibres using diathermy.
- Achieve haemostasis with diathermy during this dissection.
- Divide mucosa at the apex of the haemorrhoid with diathermy or by transfixing with 2/0 Vicryl.
- Repeat the procedure to excise the haemorrhoids in other positions, taking care to keep skin bridges between excisions to avoid anal stenosis. During the operation repeatedly remove and reinsert the speculum to avoid overstretching the sphincter.
- At the completion of the procedure an anal pack is not required. Stool softeners may aid postoperative pain.

Perform digital rectal examination and proctoscopy 4–6 weeks after discharge.

The above description is of an open technique using diathermy. In the closed technique the skin edges and the mucosa are sutured together.

Postoperative complications
- Incontinence/major incontinence
- Acute urinary retention
- Recurrence/persistence
- Stenosis
- Bleeding/haematoma.

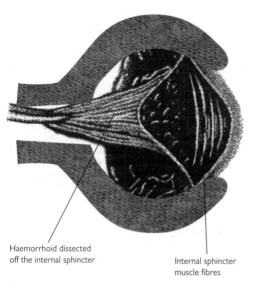

Haemorrhoid dissected
off the internal sphincter

Internal sphincter
muscle fibres

Fig. 7.6 Haemorrhoidectomy

Circular stapled haemorrhoidectomy (see also p366)

A new technique where a circular stapling device introduced per-anally is used to excise a rim of rectal mucosa above the haemorrhoids. The result is the prolapsed haemorrhoidal tissue is drawn back into a more physiological position and its blood supply is interrupted. The procedure claims to be less painful and allows rapid post operative recovery.

Perianal haematoma

Haematoma due to rupture of an anal venule. Surgery is indicated if the patient presents early with a painful lump. Incise the skin over the swelling and evacuate the clot. This can be done under local or general anaesthesia.

Thrombosed or strangulated haemorrhoids

Conservative treatment is usually successful. Immediate surgery, if undertaken, should be under antibiotic cover and carried out by an experienced surgeon.

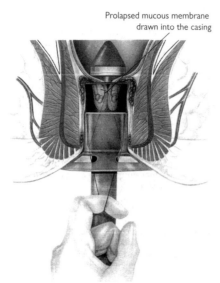

Prolapsed mucous membrane
drawn into the casing

Fig. 7.7 Circular stapled haemorrhoidectomy—insertion of stapling device

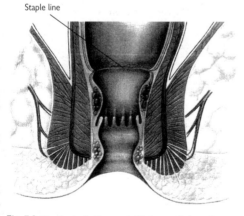

Staple line

Fig. 7.8 Circular stapled haemorrhoidectomy—final result

Fistula-in-ano

The majority of fistulas-in-ano arise from a diseased anal gland in the inter-sphincteric space. They are classified as crypto-glandular. Crohn's disease, infections, hydradenitis suppurativa, and malignancy may be associated with fistulas.

Preparation

Warn the patient of the possibility of further procedures if a complex or high fistula is encountered. A phosphate enema is administered one hour prior to the procedure.

Position

Lithotomy.

Procedure

Carried out under general anaesthetic usually as a day case procedure.

- Perform rigid procto-sigmoidoscopy.
- Identify the position of the external opening (or openings). Goodsall's rule is helpful in predicting the direction of tract. It states that a fistula where the external opening is situated behind the transverse anal line has a curved tract and opens in the posterior midline whereas anteriorly placed openings have straight tracts with an internal opening in the corresponding quadrant of the anal canal.
- Palpate the peri-anal skin carefully for induration. This helps to indicate the course of the fistulous tract.
- Perform a digital examination of the ano-rectum to feel for the internal opening and any supra-levator induration.
- Insert an Eisenhammer proctoscope and look for the internal opening.
- Gently insert a Lockhart–Mummery fistula probe in the external opening and ascertain the direction and depth of the tract. Look for secondary tracts. Allow the tip to exit through the internal opening. Bend the probe to bring the tip outside the anal orifice.

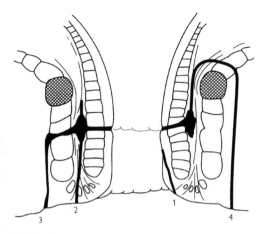

Fig. 7.9 Types of fistula-in-ano. 1) Superficial; 2) Inter-sphincteric;
3) Trans-sphincteric; 4) Supra-sphincteric

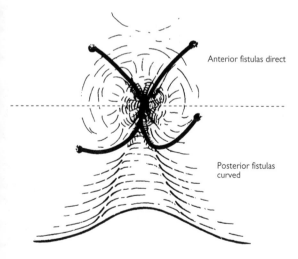

Anterior fistulas direct

Posterior fistulas
curved

Fig. 7.10 Goodsall's law

- Using diathermy cut onto the probe to lay open superficial, inter-sphincteric and low trans-sphincteric tracts. Use self-retaining retractors to expose the tract. Curette the granulation tissue away. Send tissue from the tract for histological examination. Cut away any overhanging skin edges. Lay open any secondary extensions.
- When the exact position and level of the tract in relation to the external sphincter is not clear insert a loose Setons such as a vascular sling or non-absorbable suture. Seton can similarly be used to drain acute infection secondary to a fistula-in-ano with definitive surgery being deferred until the acute inflammation settles.
- Lay open the tract outside the sphincters when you encounter a high trans-sphincteric or supra-sphincteric tract. Encircle the muscle with a Seton. Tighten it at two weekly intervals until it cuts through. This allows the gradual severance of the muscle followed by fibrosis.

Advancement flaps have been used as an alternative method of sphincter preservation in this situation. Emphasise proper care of open wounds to prevent superficial healing before healing has taken place from the depths outwards.

Postoperative complications
- Incontinence
- Recurrence/persistence
- Bleeding/haematoma.

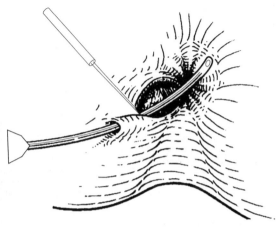

Fig. 7.11 Laying open of fistula tract

Pilonidal sinus

Pilonidal sinus occurs most commonly in the natal cleft. Enlargement of hair follicles with ingress of exogenous hairs results in the sinus, which may be asymptomatic. Treatment is only indicated when there is symptomatic disease. It may present acutely with cellulitis or as an abscess. The former may resolve with the use of antibiotics but an abscess requires drainage of pus, which can be done under local anaesthetic using a stab incision. The sinus is treated electively once the acute infection has settled.

Surgical options

Pilonidal sinus may also present as a result of chronic infection with discharge. The options are laying open of the tracts, wide excision with or without primary midline closure, asymmetric closure using Karydakis or Bascome's technique and Rhomboid flaps and Z-plasty. Low recurrence and high primary healing rates have been achieved by techniques which result in the main wound being placed away from the midline and which obliterate the natal cleft.

Bascome's cleft closure technique can be done under local anaesthetic as a day case procedure.

Position

Prone with table jack-knifed and the buttocks separated using tapes to expose the natal cleft.

Procedure

- Excise the affected skin in the midline and laterally.
- Lay open and curette the underlying sinus and chronically infected tissue.
- Suture the exposed fat together.
- Mobilise a flap of skin from the opposite side and suture it laterally over a suction drain.

Postoperative complications

- Recurrence
- Wound infection and dehiscence.

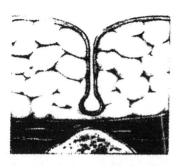

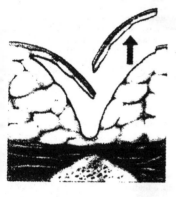

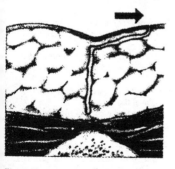

Fig. 7.12 Bascome's cleft closure technique

Rectal prolapse

Full thickness rectal prolapse can be treated by perineal and abdominal procedures.

Delorme's procedure
Position
Lithotomy.

Procedure
- Allow the rectum to prolapse to its full extent.
- Infiltrate saline containing 1 in 200 000 adrenalin in the sub-mucosal plane.
- Make a circumferential incision in the mucosa, 1cm proximal to the dentate line.
- Using diathermy carefully separate the mucosa circumferentially from muscle. Continue until the apex of the prolapse is reached.
- Plicate the muscle tube using 4–8 individual absorbable sutures.
- Divide the mucosal cylinder in stages and approximate the mucosal ends with interrupted absorbable sutures.

Postoperative complications
- Recurrence
- Bleeding, infection, obstruction.

Laparoscopic abdominal rectopexy
Position
Lloyd-Davies.

Procedure
Catheterise the patient.
- Make a vertical skin incision within the umbilicus. Expose the linea alba. Place two anchoring fascial sutures and incise linea alba between them.
- Open peritoneum and insert a Hassan cannula.
- Create pneumoperitoneum.
- Under laparoscopic vision insert a 5mm cannula in both iliac fossae. If necessary insert an additional 5mm suprapubic port to keep the sigmoid colon in left upper quadrant.
- Usually 30–40° of head down tilt is needed to keep small bowel out of the pelvis. Achieve this in stages to allow the anaesthetist to adjust ventilation.
- Insert two transcutaneous straight needled sutures to encircle Fallopian tubes to elevate uterus out of the way.
- Grasp the recto-sigmoid junction to tense the root of the mesocolon.
- Dissect with harmonic scalpel over the sacral promontory. Enter the bloodless plane behind the mesorectum.
- Divide the peritoneum on the right and dissect down to the pelvic floor. There is no need to divide the peritoneal reflection anteriorly, but complete mobilisation on the right and posteriorly.
- Swing the sigmoid colon to the right and divide the peritoneum on the left.

Mucosa separated circumferentially
and sutures in place to plicate muscle

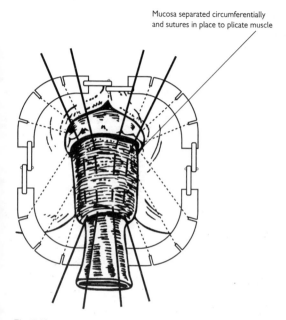

Fig. 7.13 Delorme's procedure

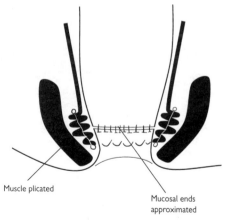

Muscle plicated

Mucosal ends
approximated

Fig. 7.14 Delorme's procedure

- Identify the ureter and dissect medial to it.
- Choose the points in the mesocolon for fixation to the sacral promontory. Place a suture through the mesorectum and sacral promontory on each side.
- Close the defect in the sigmoid mesocolon.
- Leave a drain in the pelvis.
- Remove uterine sutures.
- Remove carbon dioxide and withdraw cannula.
- Close fascia of 10mm port site.
- Use Steristrips to approximate skin.
- Infiltrate wounds with local anaesthetic.

Open abdominal rectopexy can similarly be carried out using sutures or mesh.

Postoperative complications
- Recurrence
- Bleeding, infection, obstruction, and inadvertent bowel injury.

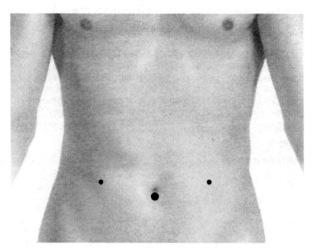

Fig. 7.15 Port placement for laparoscopic abdominal rectopexy (two 5mm and one infra umbilical 10mm port)

Acute anorectal infection (abscess)

Anorectal infection is usually linked to anal gland infection and is commonly associated with a fistula. Anorectal infection may also be seen in association with Crohn's disease, hydradenitis suppurative, and malignancy. Patients with perianal abscesses present with pain and a palpable tender lump at the anal margin. Those with an ischiorectal abscess have tenderness, induration, and fullness in the ischiorectal fossa. An inter-sphincteric or submucous abscess should be suspected in a patient with persistent anal pain and no obvious perianal abnormality. See Figs. 7.16–17.

Position

Lithotomy.

Procedure

The procedure is performed under general anaesthetic.
- Make a cruciate incision over the swelling and deepen it to the abscess cavity.
- Take a swab for bacteriology.
- Gently break down the fibrous septa in the ischiorectal fossa.
- Remove the corners of the incisions so that free drainage is provided and the final opening represents the entire floor of the abscess cavity.
- Loosely pack the cavity with an alginate dressing.
- Do not attempt to probe for a fistula tract or to lay it open.

Aftercare with loose packing and dressing ensures that healing occurs from deep to superficial and lessons risk of a further abscess.

Postoperative complications

- Development of fistula-in-ano
- Bleeding/haematoma.

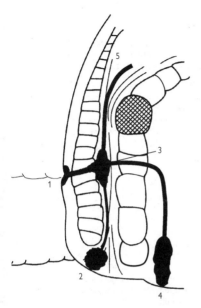

Fig. 7.16 Spread of infection from anal gland infection. 1) Submucous; 2) Perianal; 3) Inter-sphincteric; 4) Ischiorectal; 5) Pelvirectal

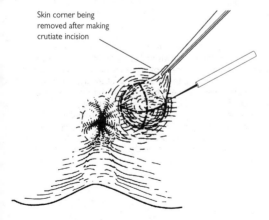

Skin corner being removed after making crutiate incision

Fig. 7.17 Incision and drainage of perianal abscess

Appendicectomy

Appendicitis is the most common major abdominal condition necessitating emergency operation. The exception to this is when an appendix mass is found without evidence of general peritonitis.

Preoperative preparation

- Give prophylactic metronidazole suppository or intravenously when the diagnosis is made. Prophylaxis with antiaerobic agent, such as a cephalosporin can be given IV at induction of anaesthesia.
- Commence IV fluids and naso-gastric aspiration if generalised peritonitis.

Open appendicectomy

Position
Supine.

Incision (Fig. 7.18)
Lanz.

Procedure (Fig. 7.18)
Palpate the abdomen again with the patient anaesthetised as it may help to locate the position of the appendix. If a circumscribed lump or a diffuse thickening is felt, plan the incision accordingly.

- Divide the aponeurosis of the external oblique in line with its fibres and split the internal oblique and transversus muscles. Retract the muscles to expose the peritoneum.
- Open the peritoneum between artery forceps. If wider access is required the internal oblique and transversus muscles can be divided in line with the fibres of the external oblique. Do this medially or laterally as required.
- Aspirate serous exudate or frank pus and send a sample for culture and sensitivity.
- Identify the caecum. Pick it up with fingers or Babcock's forceps applied to the tinea coli and slowly and carefully draw the caecum to the surface. If the appendix does not come into view pass an index finger along one of the tinea to their junction at the appendix base and then lift it out. If delivery of the appendix is difficult then create further access between forceps and ligate it to free under vision.
- Hold up the appendix with tissue forceps applied around it. Divide the mesoappendix with the appendicular artery between forceps and ligate it. Identify the base of the appendix, apply artery forceps to the base to crush it then apply again more distally. Ligate the crushed appendix area more proximally.

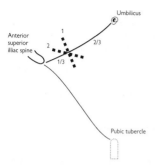

Fig. 7.18 Incisions for appendicectomy. 1) McBurney; 2) Lanz

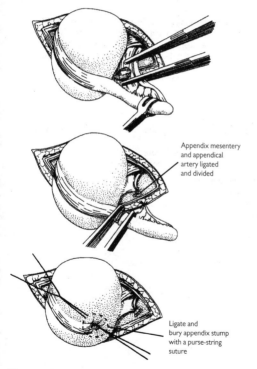

Appendix mesentery
and appendical
artery ligated
and divided

Ligate and
bury appendix stump
with a purse-string
suture

Fig. 7.19 Appendicectomy

- Pass a purse-string sero-muscular suture in the caecum about 1cm from the base of the appendix using a 3/0 Vicryl. Divide the appendix flush with the under surface of the artery forceps. Place the appendix and the instruments in a dirty dish taking care during and after division not to soil the wound or the peritoneum.
- Invaginate the stump and tie the purse-string suture. If the caecal wall is oedematous and friable, this is not necessary.

If the inflamed appendix is retro-caecal and cannot be delivered into the wound carry out a retrograde appendicectomy. Dividing the appendix first at its base, invaginating the stump and then dividing the meso-appendix in small segments. If the omentum is adherent to the inflamed appendix remove it with the appendix.

If a mass is encountered after opening the peritoneum, surround it with moist packs and gently explore the mass with the finger. Aspirate any pus, isolate the appendix and remove it in the usual way. If the appendix is divided at the site of the perforation take care to remove the entire appendix.

If the diagnosis of acute appendicitis was incorrect, most local abnormalities can be dealt with by extending the incision as described above.

- Make an appropriate vertical laparotomy incision if exposure is still inadequate or the abnormality lies outside the reach of the Lanz incision.
- If normal appendix is found search for an inflamed Meckel's diverticulum.

Closure

- Close the peritoneum with Vicryl.
- Allow the split muscles to fall together. Suture the external oblique aponeurosis with Vicryl.
- Close the skin incision with interrupted or subcuticular sutures. Drainage is not generally used after appendicectomy.

Postoperative complications

- Wound infection
- Pelvic or abdominal abscess
- Paralytic ileus
- Haemorrhage
- Incisional hernia.

Laparoscopic appendicectomy

Especially useful in women of child bearing age when the diagnosis of acute appendicitis is in doubt.

Position

Lithotomy.

Procedure

Empty bladder before commencing the operation.

- Make a vertical skin incision within the umbilicus. Expose the linea alba. Place two anchoring fascial sutures and incise the linea alba between them.
- Open peritoneum and insert Hassan cannula.
- Create pneumoperitoneum.
- Under laparoscopic vision place a 10mm and 5mm cannulae in the right and left iliac fossa respectively avoiding the inferior epigastric vessels.
- Table is tilted head down with left lateral position.
- Expose the appendix by displacing the ileum and caecum using atraumatic grasping forceps.
- Ligate or clip the mesoappendix and its artery.
- Apply two ligatures at the base of the appendix and transect the appendix between them. The appendix stump is not buried.
- Visualisation of the Fallopian tubes and ovaries is aided by manipulating the uterus with fingers placed in vaginal fornices.
- The appendix is removed through the 10mm cannula or by placing it in an endo bag, if bulky/friable.
- Lavage with normal saline.
- Remove carbon dioxide and withdraw cannula.
- Close fascia of 10mm port sites.
- Use Steristrips to approximate skin.
- Infiltrate wounds with local anaesthetic.

Postoperative complications

- Wound infection
- Pelvic or intra-abdominal abscess.

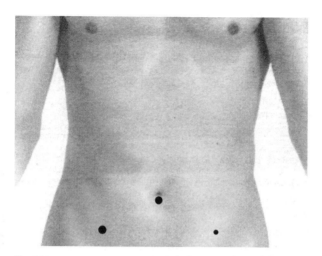

Fig. 7.20 Port sites for laparoscopic appendicectomy

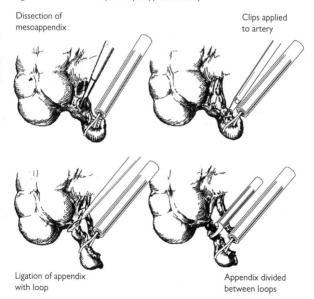

Dissection of
mesoappendix

Clips applied
to artery

Ligation of appendix
with loop

Appendix divided
between loops

Fig. 7.21 Laparoscopic appendicectomy

Excision of Meckel's diverticulum

Meckel's diverticulum is the persistence of a segment of vitello-intestinal duct on the anti-mesenteric border of the ileum. It is found in 2% of the population within two feet of the caecum (80cm) and is generally two inches long (5cm).

Indications

- Acute inflammation
- Bleeding from ectopic gastric mucosa
- Intestinal obstruction—volvulus around a persistent band or adhesion, intussusception
- An incidental finding at laparotomy. Consider excision of it because of the risk of associated pathology. A wide-mouthed, thin-walled unattached diverticulum in an adult patient may be left alone.

Position

Supine.

Procedure

The choice is between either diverticulectomy or excision of the segment of ileum carrying the diverticulum.

- Isolate the segment of ileum containing the diverticulum. Ligate any supplying vessels.
- Apply light occlusion clamps to the ileum and divide the diverticulum at its base and close the bowel wall transversely. The diverticulum can also be removed by a single firing of a transverse stapler.
- Resect the segment of ileum in patients with peptic ulceration or diverticulitis affecting the base.
- Restore intestinal continuity by a single or two layer anastomosis.

Postoperative complications

- Wound infection
- Pelvic or intra-abdominal abscess
- Ileus
- Incisional hernia
- Anastomotic leak.

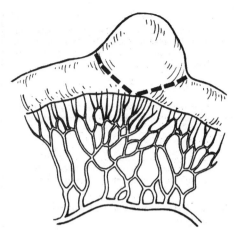

Fig. 7.22 Excision of Meckel's diverticulum—extent of excision

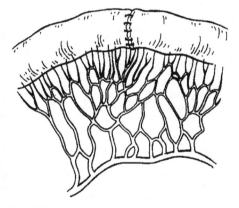

Fig. 7.23 Anastomosis following excision

Ileostomy

The terminal ileum is exteriorized as a spout in the right iliac fossa. Effluent is collected in a collecting bag (ileostomy bag). The ileostomy may be
formed as a loop of bowel to divert enteric contents temporarily or
more permanently as an end stoma.

End ileostomy

Indication

After proctocolectomy for inflammatory bowel disease, rarely for patients
with familial adenomatous polyposis and patients with synchronous colonic and rectal cancers.

Preparation

The ileostomy should be sited in the right iliac fossa clear of the umbilicus and anterior superior iliac spine and avoiding any scars or depressions. The optimal stoma site is identified and marked preoperatively.

Position

Supine or Lloyd-Davies position to allow a combined abdomino-perineal
procedure to be carried out.

Procedure

- In addition to laparotomy for the major procedure, make a trephine by
  excising a circular area of skin over the marked stoma site. Do this
  by picking up the skin with Littlewood forceps and excising a disc
  approximately 2cm in diameter. Alternatively make a cruciate incision
  and trim the edges using a cutting diathermy point.
- Excise a disc of sub-cutaneous fat to expose the anterior rectal sheath.
  Make a cruciate incision on the sheath.
- Use artery forceps to split the rectus abdominis muscle. Do this
  carefully to avoid injury to the inferior epigastric vessels.
- Expose the peritoneum by retracting the split muscle. Open the
  peritoneum between artery forceps. The trephine must admit the
  tips of two fingers to ensure there will be no obstruction to the
  blood supply of the bowel.
- Divide the ileum close to the ileo-caecal junction using a linear stapler.
- Divide the adjacent mesentery and partially remove the mesentery of
  about 5cm of terminal ileum.
- Deliver this length of ileum through the trephine onto the skin surface.
- The ileal mesentery should lie in a cephalad direction. Stitch the cut
  edge of the mesentery to the parietal peritoneum; it is not necessary
  to close the lateral gutter.
- Close and cover the abdominal incision.
- Excise the staple line.
- Insert eight 4/0 Vicryl sutures through the subcuticular skin edge, the
  adjacent sero-muscular wall of the ileum and full thickness of the open
  bowel end, avoiding the vessels of the mesentery.
- Clip the sutures long and tie them once all have been inserted. This
  everts the bowel end and results in a 2.5cm spout. This permits close
  application of the ileostomy bag with discharge of effluent away from
  the skin.

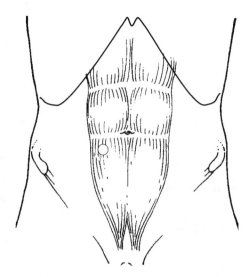

Fig. 7.24 Site of ileostomy

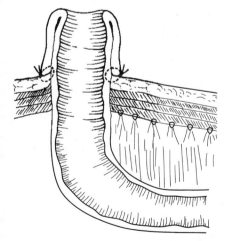

Fig. 7.25 End ileostomy

Postoperative complications
- Haemorrhage
- Parastomal herniation
- Prolapse
- Retraction
- Necrosis
- Stenosis.

Loop ileostomy

Indication
To divert faecal stream or protect large bowel anastomosis or ileal pouch anal anastomosis.

Preparation
As mentioned under end ileostomy.

Position
Lloyd–Davies position to allow stapling or suturing to be carried out peri-anally.

Procedure
- Select a loop of terminal ileum close to the ileo-caecal junction. This should be of sufficient length to be brought out without tension.
- Mark the distal limb with a suture.
- Make a mesenteric window adjacent to the wall of the ileum at the apex of the loop. Pass a Nylon tape through it.
- Using the tape deliver the loop through a trephine incision as described above.
- Remove the tape and insert a rod through the window in the mesentery used to pass the Nylon tape.
- Close and cover the abdominal incision.
- Make a transverse enterotomy in the distal limb at the junction with the skin using a diathermy point.
- Insert four to six 4/0 Vicryl sutures through the superior subcuticular skin edge, adjacent sero-muscular wall of the ileum and full thickness of the open proximal bowel end.
- On the distal limb open end insert a further four interrupted 4/0 Vicryl sutures through full thickness bowel and subcuticular skin so that the distal lumen is flush with the skin.
- Tie the sutures after all of them are in place. This forms a spout and avoids forceful grasping of the mucosa with forceps to evert the bowel.

Postoperative complications
- Haemorrhage
- Parastomal herniation
- Prolapse
- Retraction
- Necrosis.

Laparoscopic loop ileostomy
Indications and preparation as for open procedure
Position
Supine.

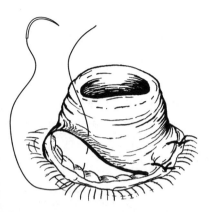

Fig. 7.26 End ileostomy

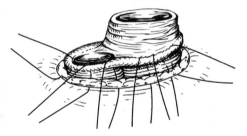

Fig. 7.27 Loop ileostomy

Procedure

Empty the bladder before commencing the operation.

- Make a vertical skin incision within the umbilicus and expose the linea alba.
- Place anchoring fascial sutures and incise the linea alba between them.
- Open the peritoneum and insert a Hassan cannula.
- Create pneumoperitoneum.
- A 5mm suprapubic working port is placed under vision.
- The table can be tilted head down and left lateral position to facilitate visualising the caecum.
- Identify the ileo-caecal junction and work proximally up the small bowel using atraumatic grasping forceps to identify a convenient loop of terminal ileum that will be able to be brought out easily and without tension. Orientate this loop carefully under vision so that the proximal bowel lies superiorly with the ileal mesentery lying in a cephalad direction.
- Make an open trephine by excising a circular area of skin over the marked stoma site. Ensure that the trephine admits two fingers to ensure there will be no obstruction to the blood supply of the bowel.
- Excise sub-cutaneous fat to expose the anterior rectal sheath. Make a cruciate incision on the sheath and use artery forceps to split the rectus abdominis muscle. Do this carefully to avoid injury to the inferior epigastric vessels.
- Expose the peritoneum by retracting the split muscle.
- Before opening the peritoneum grasp the loop of ileum laparoscopically and hold up to the surface just away form the trephine.
- Open the peritoneum between artery forceps and immediately grasp and deliver the ileal loop through the trephine incision with Babcock forceps.
- Remove carbon dioxide and withdraw the cannulas.
- Close fascia of 10mm port sites.
- Use Steristrips to approximate skin.
- Infiltrate wounds with local anaesthetic and dress the wounds.
- Continue with fashioning the loop ileostomy as for an open procedure.

Postoperative complications

- Development of parastomal hernia
- Prolapse
- Retraction
- Haemorrhage
- Necrosis
- Stenosis
- Inadvertent bowel injury.

Closure of loop ileostomy

Indication

When faecal stream diversion is no longer required. Check for anastomotic integrity and patency using contrast radiology or endoscopic examination prior to reversal.

Position
Supine.

Procedure
- Insert four muco-cutaneous stay sutures to help in mobilisation. Hold the long ends on an artery forceps.
- Using cutting diathermy to incise the skin circumferentially close to the mucocutaneous junction.
- Use sharp and blunt dissection to free the ileal loops from the parieties.
- Insert a finger in the peritoneal cavity and sweep it carefully around to separate adhesions and to allow withdrawal of sufficient length of small bowel for anastomosis.
- Separate the loops and divide the mesentery adjacent to the site chosen for anastomosis.
- Divide the ileum and carry out a single or two layered anastomosis or a stapled functional end to end anastomosis.
- Return the segment of bowel into the peritoneal cavity.
- Close with a single layer interrupted PDS sutures. Oppose the skin margins with interrupted non-absorbable sutures or skin staples.

Postoperative complications
- Acute obstruction
- Anastomotic leakage.

Colostomy

The colon may be exteriorized temporarily or permanently as an end or loop colostomy. Semi-solid faeces is collected in a collecting bag (colostomy bag).

End colostomy

Usually formed from the sigmoid or lower descending colon, which is brought to the surface through a trephine in the left side of the abdominal wall.

Indications
- After abdomino-perineal excision for distal rectal cancers and some anal cancers.
- After a Hartmann's procedure (potentially reversible).
- Irremediable faecal incontinence.

Preparation
The patient is counselled both in elective and emergency situations. The optimal site is identified and marked preoperatively. It is sited in the left iliac fossa clear of the umbilicus and anterior-superior iliac spine and avoiding any scars or depressions.

Procedure
- In addition to laparotomy for the major procedure, make a trephine by excising a circular area of skin over the marked stoma site. Do this picking up the skin with Littlewoods forceps and excising a disc of skin approximately 2cm in diameter. Alternatively make a cruciate incision and trim the edges using a cutting diathermy point.
- Excise a disc of sub-cutaneous fat exposing the anterior rectal sheath.
- Make a cruciate incision on the anterior rectal sheath to expose the rectus abdominis muscle.
- Split the rectus abdominus muscle using artery forceps muscle gently to avoid injury to the inferior epigastric vessels.
- Retract the muscle and open the peritoneum between artery forceps. The aperture should allow the tips of two fingers through it.
- The divided, proximal end of mobilised colon may be brought through the abdominal wall aperture using Babcock forceps and the lateral para-colic space closed with interrupted absorbable sutures or an extra-peritoneal tunnel may be dissected and the colon passed through this and out.
- Close and cover the main wound.
- Ask your assistant to retract the skin and sub-cutaneous tissue using two Langenbeck retractors. With your left index finger retract the colon.
- Insert four interrupted 3/0 Vicryl sutures into each quadrant to oppose the anterior rectus sheath to the colon taking sero-muscular bites.
- Excise the staple line and suture the skin edge to full thickness bowel end using interrupted 4/0 Vicryl sutures.

Postoperative complications
- Haemorrhage
- Stomal herniation
- Prolapse
- Retraction
- Necrosis
- Stenosis.

Loop colostomy

Is used to divert the faecal stream. The most commonly selected sites are the transverse and sigmoid colon. Should be avoided if an alternative as it is prone to so many complications.

Indications
- In patients with distal colonic obstruction as first part of a staged resection.
- As palliation for unresectable lesions.
- To defunction distal anastomosis.
- To protect anal operations for example anal fistula or sphincter repair.

Preparation

The patient is counselled regarding the stoma. The optimal site is identified and marked preoperatively.

Procedure

A formal laparotomy may not be needed.
- For a transverse colostomy make a horizontal incision midway between the umbilicus and the costal margin in the right upper quadrant.
- Incise all the layers of the abdominal wall. Divide the muscle fibres of the rectus abdominis.
- Mobilise the transverse colon from omental adhesions. Preserve the marginal vasculature.
- Make a window close to the bowel in the transverse meso-colon. Pass a Nylon tape through the window. Use this to bring the loop to the surface.
- Replace the tape with a rod. The latter supports the loop.
- Attach the bowel to the anterior rectus sheath with interrupted absorbable sutures.
- If a midline incision has been made close and cover it.
- Open the colon longitudinally. Suture the margin of the open colon to the adjacent skin edge with interrupted absorbable sutures.
- An appropriate sized hole is cut in the stoma bag to accommodate the rod and the looped colon.

For a sigmoid loop colostomy make a left grid iron incision. Carefully identify the sigmoid colon to make sure it is not small bowel. It has no omentum but has appendices epiploicae and taenia. Orient the loop to avoid rotation. The loop may be tethered with congenital adhesions which may need to be divided. The rest of the procedure is as described for a transverse colostomy.

Postoperative complications
- Haemorrhage
- Stomal herniation

- Prolapse
- Retraction
- Necrosis.

Closure of loop colostomy

Indication
- When faecal stream diversion is no longer required. Check for anastomotic integrity and patency using contrast radiology and endoscopic examination prior to reversal.
- Prepare proximal colon as for any colonic anastomosis.

Procedure
- Insert four muco-cutaneous stay sutures to help in mobilisation. Hold the long ends on an artery forceps.
- Using cutting diathermy incise the skin close to the muco-cutaneous junction.
- Use sharp and blunt dissection to free the colon loops from the parieties.
- Close the colostomy transversely using one layer interrupted sero-muscular extra-mucosal sutures.
- Replace the colon in the peritoneal cavity.
- Close the abdominal wall in one layer using interrupted PDS sutures. Close the skin with interrupted sutures or skin staples.

Postoperative complications
- Anastomotic leakage
- Wound infection.

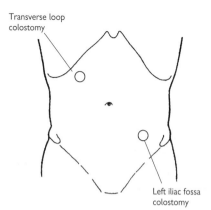

Transverse loop
colostomy

Left iliac fossa
colostomy

Fig. 7.28 Sites of colostomy

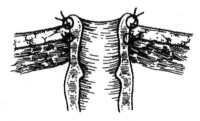

Fig. 7.29 End colostomy

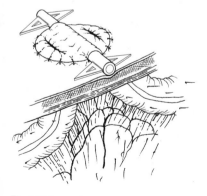

Fig. 7.30 Loop colostomy

Bowel resection and anastomosis

The essentials for any bowel anastomosis are:
- Tension free
- Adequate blood supply (pulsating mesenteric vessels)
- Accurate apposition using good surgical techniques
- Minimal local spillage.

Single layer interrupted seromuscular (extra-mucosal) technique

Mobile anastomosis (ileo-ileal, ileo-colic anastomosis)
- Line up the ends of the bowel.
- Ensure that the ends to be anastomosed are roughly equal in circumference. To achieve this make an incision on the anti-mesenteric aspect of the bowel or do an end-to-side anastomosis.
- Use non-crushing bowel clamps to prevent spillage.
- Isolate the operative field using moist packs.
- Use 3/0 absorbable suture material with an atraumatic round bodied needle.
- Insert stay sutures at the mesenteric and anti-mesenteric borders; do not ligate them but place them in haemostats.
- Starting from the mesenteric aspect, place interrupted sutures along the anterior wall of the bowel 0.5cm apart and tie as they are placed. Each suture should perforate the bowel from the serosal surface penetrating the muscle layer and sub-mucosa and emerging between the mucosa and sub-mucosa.
- Include the sub-mucosa as this is the strongest layer of the bowel wall.
- On completion, tie both stay sutures; do not cut but replace in haemostats.
- Use the stay sutures to reverse the bowel. The posterior wall will now lie anteriorly.
- Suture the new front wall in a similar manner. Ensure the angles are adequately sutured.
- On completion return the stay sutures to their original position and cut them.
- Close the mesenteric defect taking care not to damage the mesenteric vessels.

Immobile anastomosis (colorectal or ileo-rectal)
- Insert stay sutures at the lateral ends of the cut end of the bowel walls. Do not ligate them but place them in haemostats.
- Insert the posterior row of seromuscular sutures, hold suture ends in individual artery forceps. Thread the artery forceps to a forceps holder to avoid tangling. After insertion of the whole row 'parachute' the proximal bowel down to the rectum. Tie the knots; they will lie on the luminal side of the anastomosis. Cut the knot tails.
- Perform the anterior anastomosis in a similar fashion; the knots will lie on the serosal side of the anastomosis.

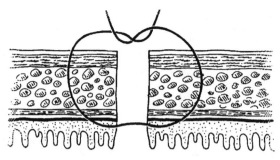

Fig. 7.31 Seromuscular suture

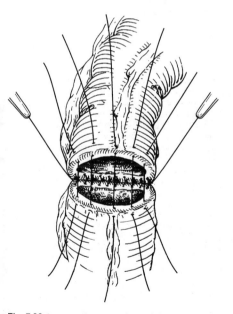

Fig. 7.32 Interrupted seromuscular single layer anastomosis

Two layer anastomosis

- Line up the ends of the bowel.
- Ensure that the ends to be anastomosed are roughly equal in circumference. To achieve this make an incision on the anti-mesenteric aspect of the bowel or do an end-to-side anastomosis.
- Use non-crushing bowel clamps to prevent spillage.
- Isolate the operative field using moist packs.
- Use 3/0 absorbable suture material with an atraumatic round bodied needle.
- Insert stay sutures at the mesenteric and anti-mesenteric borders; do not ligate them but place them in haemostats.
- Place a stitch between the adjacent cut edges of bowel in the middle of the posterior wall. Continue towards one corner with full thickness over-and-over stitches. The stitches should be less than 0.5cm apart and pick up about 0.5cm of bowel wall. To turn the corner pass the needle from the mucosa outwards on one corner to the serosa inwards on the other followed by the mucosa outwards on the same side to the serosa inwards on the other, thus forming a series of loops on the mucosal surface (Connell suture).
- Once around the corner, leave this stitch and return to the middle of the posterior wall. Using a new length of suture insert and tie a stitch close to the site of the previous ligature. Proceed towards the opposite corner and using the technique described above turn around the corner. Oppose the anterior walls using over-and-over stitches and tie off the ends of the suture in the middle. Remove the bowel clamps.
- Place a second layer of seromuscular continuous or interrupted sutures starting at one corner and going all the way round by rotating the bowel. The posterior layer of seromuscular sutures can be placed before the full thickness layer. The anterior seromuscular layer being completed subsequently.
- Close the mesenteric defect taking care not to damage the mesenteric vessels.

Anastomosis using staplers is described in chapters of right hemicolectomy and anterior resection.

Small bowel resection and anastomosis

Indications

- Obstruction leading to non-viable bowel
- Irreducible small bowel intussusception
- Mesenteric ischaemia
- Meckel's diverticulum
- Crohn's stricture
- Traumatic damage
- Tumours—primary or adherent small bowel loop to large bowel tumour.

Preparation

In cases of small bowel obstruction: naso-gastric aspiration, re-hydration with intravenous fluids, correction of electrolyte abnormality.

Position

Supine.

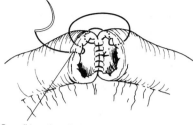

Connell inverting suture

Fig. 7.33 Two layer anastomosis

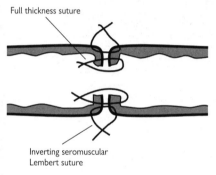

Full thickness suture

Inverting seromuscular
Lembert suture

Fig. 7.34 Two layer anastomosis

Incision

Midline, in case of strangulated external hernia make the appropriate incision.

Procedure

- Inspect the bowel requiring resection and also the remaining bowel. Choose the resection margins.
- Transilluminate the mesentery by shining a light from behind. This may not be helpful in Crohn's disease because of thickened mesentery.
- Between the margins of resection divide the mesentery using diathermy or scissors, leaving the vessels to be taken between artery forceps. Cut and ligate the vessels. Clear the mesentery up to the bowel wall. In malignant disease, take a V-shaped wedge of mesentery to remove the local lymphatic tissue which runs with the arteries. In benign disease keep close to the bowel wall.
- Apply crushing clamps to bowel immediately beyond the point of resection. Milk the bowel contents from the intervening section to reduce risk of spillage when bowel opened and apply non-crushing clamps proximal and distal to the crushing clamps.
- Divide bowel flush with the crushing clamp using a knife.
- Anastomose the two ends in one or two layers.
- Close the defect in the mesentery taking care not to damage the mesenteric vessels.

Closure

Single layer 1/0 PDS and subcuticular Monocryl.

Postoperative complications

- Anastomotic leak
- Bleeding

Large bowel resection and anastomosis

This is dealt with in the relevant chapters.

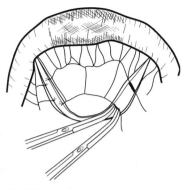

Fig. 7.35 Resection of small bowel

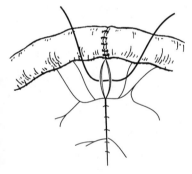

Fig. 7.36 Closure of mesentery after small bowel resection

Right hemicolectomy

Indications
- Malignant disease affecting the caecum, ascending colon, and hepatic flexure
- Inflammatory conditions such as Crohn's disease.

Preparation
- Thrombo-embolism prophylaxis
- Antibiotics administered after induction of anaesthesia
- Urethral catheter inserted after patient has been anaesthetised.

Position
Supine.

Incision
Midline with two-thirds of the incision above the umbilicus to ease mobilisation of hepatic flexure or transverse incision just above the umbilicus.

Procedure
- Carry out a full laparotomy to assess resectability and metastatic spread to the liver and peritoneum. Synchronous tumours should have been excluded by preoperative colonoscopy or barium enema. If not palpate the colon carefully.
- Cover the small bowel with wet packs and keep it away from the operative field by tilting the table to the patient's left.
- Stand on the left side of the table and retract the right colon.
- Using diathermy, divide the peritoneum on the right para-colic gutter from the caecum to the hepatic flexure and continue this dissection to develop the plane between the meso-colon and the posterior abdominal wall. In doing so the ureter and gonadal vessels will safely fall away.
- Carefully divide the vascular omental attachments of the hepatic flexure close to the colon.
- Identify the duodenum behind the right colon and gently dissect this away. Do not dissect medial to the duodenal loop to avoid injury to the small vessels around the pancreas.
- Enter the lesser sac distal to the hepatic flexure.
- Divide the greater omentum below the gastro-epiploic arcade to the junction between proximal third and distal two-thirds of the transverse colon.
- Now move to the right side of the table.
- Lift the terminal ileum and right colon.
- Transilluminate the mesentery and clamp, divide and ligate the ileo-colic and right colic vessels at their origin from the superior mesenteric. Clamp, divide, and ligate the right branch of the middle colic artery.
- Clear the bowel wall at the sites of transection and apply crushing clamps.
- Apply occlusion clamps on the proximal small bowel and distal large bowel.

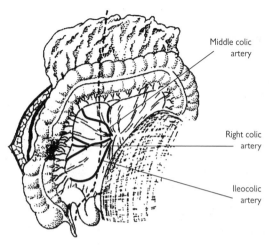

Middle colic
artery

Right colic
artery

Ileocolic
artery

Fig. 7.37 Right hemicolectomy

- Divide the bowel on the crushing clamps leaving them on the specimen.
- An end-to-end anastomosis is commonly performed but end-to-side with closure of the end of the colon is another option. Carry out the anastomosis either using a single layer of interrupted sero-muscular 3/0 Vicryl or PDS sutures or alternatively as a two layer suturing technique.

- *Alternatively* a stapled one stage functional end-to-end anastomosis and resection can be performed.
- Loop the portion of bowel to be resected and approximate the antimesenteric borders with stay sutures.
- Make a 1cm stab wound into the lumen of both the proximal and distal limbs and insert one fork of a GIA instrument into each lumen.
- Apply downward traction on the stay sutures to keep the mesentery out of the stapler.
- Close the instrument and fire the staples. Two double staggered rows of staples join the bowel; simultaneously, the knife blade cuts between the two staple lines creating a stoma.
- Inspect the anastomotic staple lines for completeness and haemostasis.
- Use a Babcock forceps to oppose the ends of the staple lines.
- Apply a GIA instrument across both limbs of bowel, distal to the Babcock forceps and fire the stapler to transect the bowel.
- Bury the transverse staple line using 3/0 PDS interrupted sutures.
- Close the mesenteric window, avoid taking the vessels in the bites.
- A drain maybe left in close proximity to the anastomosis.

Closure
- Single layer mass closure using 1/0 PDS
- Skin with subcuticular Monocryl or Prolene.

Postoperative complications
- Anastomotic dehiscence
- Postoperative paralytic ileus
- Wound infection
- Bleeding
- Incisional hernia.

Lesions of the transverse colon, splenic flexure, descending colon can be treated by extended right hemicolectomy.

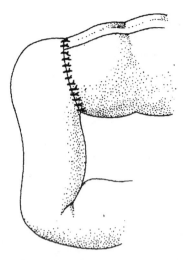

Fig. 7.38 End-to-end anastomosis

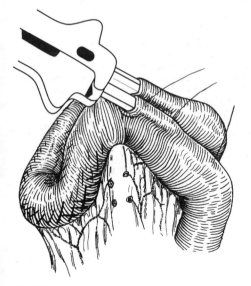

Fig. 7.39 Stapled anastomosis

Left hemicolectomy

Indications
- Neoplastic lesions involving distal transverse colon, descending colon or sigmoid colon.
- Complex, symptomatic diverticular disease.

Preparation
- Two units of blood are grouped and cross-matched
- Mechanical bowel preparation (usually with two sachets of Picolax)
- Thrombo-embolism prophylaxis
- Prophylactic antibiotics administered after induction of anaesthesia.
- Urethral catheter inserted after patient has been anaesthetised.

Position
Lloyd-Davies.

Incision
Midline.

Procedure
- Perform a full laparotomy to ascertain resectability of tumour, presence of liver metastases, peritoneal deposits and synchronous tumours.
- Cover the small bowel with wet packs and keep it away from operative field by tilting the table to the patient's right.
- Stand on the right side of the table and retract the sigmoid colon medially.
- Ask the assistant to retract the lower left abdominal wall.
- Divide the peritoneum lateral to the sigmoid and descending colon along the 'white line' of fusion using diathermy.
- Develop the plane between the mesentery and the retro-peritoneum. In the process the gonadal vessels and ureter are swept away. Identify and safeguard the hypo-gastric nerves.
- Lift the descending colon and its mesentery off the Gerota's fascia.
- Separate the greater omentum from the distal transverse colon. Continue the dissection laterally towards the flexure. For splenic flexure tumours the gastro-colic omentum is divided and the omentum removed with the specimen.
- Continue the incision along the left para-colic gutter upwards towards the splenic flexure.

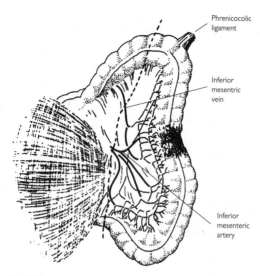

Fig. 7.40 Left hemicolectomy

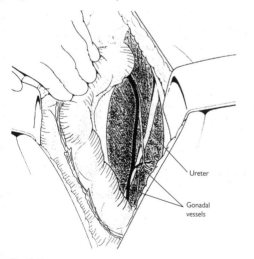

Fig. 7.41 Mobilisation of left colon

- Now grasp both limbs of the colon and under vision divide the peritoneum at the flexure. Bring the colon out of its splenic bed. Take care during the mobilisation of the splenic flexure that the tip of the retractor held by the assistant does not damage the spleen and avoid undue traction on the omentum during this manoeuvre as the splenic capsule can be torn.
- Lift up the sigmoid colon and divide the peritoneum on the right side from the origin of the inferior mesenteric artery down to the level of the sacral promontory.
- Pass a finger under the sigmoid colon and define the origin of the inferior mesenteric artery.
- Double clamp, divide and doubly ligate the inferior mesenteric artery.
- Then clamp, divide and ligate the inferior mesenteric vein below the inferior border of the pancreas taking care not to tear this vessel.
- Divide the transverse meso-colon at a convenient point. Isolate and ligate the marginal artery.
- Divide the transverse colon between occlusion and crushing clamps.
- Similarly divide the colon at the recto-sigmoid junction between Hayes clamps.
- Move to the left side of the table.
- Make sure there is no tension at the bowel ends and that it is adequately vascularised.
- Restore bowel continuity by using single layer of 3/0 PDS interrupted seromuscular sutures. (Fig 7.42)

- For a *stapled anastomosis* insert 2/0 Prolene purse-strings to both bowel ends. Make a colotomy through the anterior tinea and insert a circular stapler, placing the anvil in the distal segment. Tie the purse-strings and after approximation fire the stapler. (Fig 7.43) Alternatively a stapled anastomosis can be constructed introducing the stapler per-anally and placing the anvil in the proximal segment. (Fig 7.44)
- Check the donuts for completeness.
- Perform a leak test by insufflating air through a sigmoidoscope introduced per-anally and filling the peritoneal cavity with normal saline.
- Do a washout of the peritoneal cavity. Water is preferred for cytotoxic properties in cases of malignancy.
- Leave a tube drain in close proximity to the anastomosis.

Closure

In a single layer using number 1 loop PDS or Prolene and the skin with subcuticular Monocryl or Prolene.

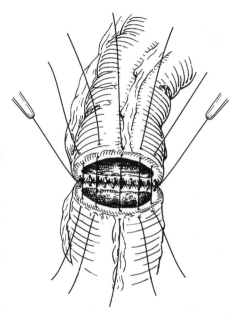

Fig. 7.42 Interrupted seromuscular single layer anastomosis

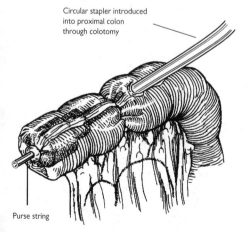

Circular stapler introduced
into proximal colon
through colotomy

Purse string

Fig. 7.43 Stapled anastomosis

Postoperative complications
- Anastomotic dehiscence
- Postoperative paralytic ileus
- Wound infection
- Bleeding
- Incisional hernia.

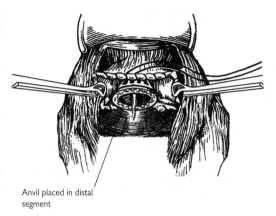

Anvil placed in distal
segment

Fig. 7.44 Stapled anastomosis

Transverse colectomy

Indications
Malignant tumour of the mid transverse colon.

Preparation
As for left hemicolectomy.

Position
Supine.

Incision
Midline.

Procedure
- Perform a full laparotomy to ascertain resectability of tumour, presence of liver metastases, peritoneal deposits, and synchronous tumours.
- Separate the omentum from the stomach below the gastro-epiploic vessels.
- Mobilise the hepatic and splenic flexures. The latter step may not be needed if there is a long transverse colon.
- A wedge resection based on the middle colic vessels is then undertaken with at least 5cm clearance from a malignant tumour.
- Clamp, divide, and ligate the middle colic artery at its origin.
- Clamp, divide, and ligate the meso-colon and marginal vessels up to the sites of bowel resection.
- Restore bowel continuity by using single layer of 3/0 PDS interrupted seromuscular sutures.
- Leave a drain in close proximity to the anastomosis.

Closure
Close the abdominal wall using single layer number 1 loop PDS, skin with subcuticular Monocryl (or Vicryl).

Postoperative complications
- Anastomotic dehiscence
- Postoperative paralytic ileus
- Wound infection
- Bleeding
- Incisional hernia.

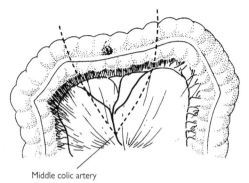

Middle colic artery

Fig. 7.45 Transverse colectomy

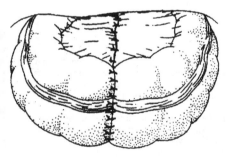

Fig. 7.46 Single layer interrupted anastomosis

Sigmoid colectomy

Indications
- To palliate a sigmoid tumour (left hemicolectomy is preferred for oncological reasons)
- Complicated diverticular disease
- Sigmoid volvulus
- As part of Hartmann's procedure.

Position
Lloyd-Davies.

Preparation
As for left hemicolectomy.

Incision
Midline.

Procedure
- Cover the small bowel with wet packs and keep it away from the operative field by tilting the table to the patient's right.
- Stand on the right side of the table.
- Retract the sigmoid colon medially.
- Ask the assistant to hold the lower left abdominal wall.
- Divide the peritoneum lateral to the sigmoid and descending colon along the 'white line' of fusion using diathermy.
- Develop the plane between the mesentery and retro-peritoneum. Identify and preserve the left ureter and gonadal vessels as they fall away in this dissection.
- The splenic flexure may need to be taken down for tension free anastomosis.
- Ligate the sigmoid arteries at their origin from the inferior mesenteric artery in malignant disease. In benign disease the mesocolon may be divided closer to the bowel wall.
- Apply crushing and occlusion clamps at the descending sigmoid colon junction and at the recto-sigmoid junction.
- Cut the bowel between the clamps.
- Carry out a sutured or stapled anastomosis.
- Perform a leak test.
- Leave a drain in close proximity to the anastomosis.

Closure
Single mass layer using number 1 loop PDS and subcuticular Monocryl.

Postoperative complications
- Anastomotic dehiscence
- Postoperative paralytic ileus
- Wound infection
- Bleeding
- Incisional hernia.

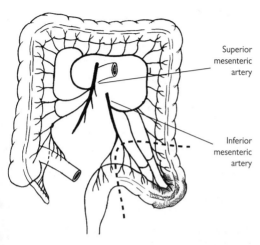

Fig. 7.47 Sigmoid colectomy

Total colectomy

Indications

- Inflammatory bowel disease—acute severe colitis failing to respond to medical treatment, toxic mega-colon, perforation, bleeding.
- Familial adenomatous polyposis.
- Left colonic obstruction with caecal perforation.
- Colonic inertia.

In the emergency setting for ulcerative colitis, colectomy with ileostomy and preservation of rectal stump is the operation of choice. Subsequent restorative proctocolectomy and avoidance of permanent ileostomy is a possibility.

Preparation

- Carry out adequate resuscitation when procedure done as an emergency
- Administer prophylactic antibiotics
- Thromboembolism prophylaxis
- Catheterise
- Counsel patient and have ileostomy site marked by stoma nurse
- Do not give bowel preparation when carrying out emergency colectomy.

Position

Lloyd-Davies.

Incision

Midline.

Procedure (Fig. 7.48)

- When carrying out emergency colectomy for inflammatory bowel disease, insert proctoscope to deflate bowel.
- Make the trephine for the ileostomy before opening the abdomen.
- Handle bowel with care to avoid perforation.
- Start with mobilising the right colon.
- Divide bowel at the ileo-caecal junction with a linear stapler.
- Continue mobilising the colon, transfixing relevant vessels.
- Leave a long recto-sigmoid stump which can be exteriorised to form a mucous fistula or closed depending on the state of the bowel.

Colectomy with ileo-rectal anastomosis can be carried out in selected cases of chronic inflammatory bowel disease (not Crohn's disease) and for familial adenomatous polyposis. Follow the steps for colectomy. Carry out a hand sutured or stapled ileo-rectal anastomosis.

Postoperative complications

- Bleeding
- Wound infection
- Anastomotic dehiscence
- Stoma complications
- Rectal stump suture line breakdown.

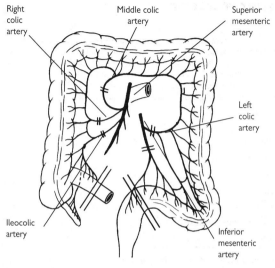

Fig. 7.48 Total colectomy

Anterior resection

Indication
Carcinoma of the rectum, where sphincter preservation is possible, high anterior resection is done for tumours of the upper third of the rectum. The anastomosis is made in the region of the junction of the mid and lower third of the rectum. Low anterior resection entails a total meso-rectal excision. The anastomosis is made at the level of the pelvic floor. For low anterior resections defunctioning stoma is made.

Preparation
As for left hemicolectomy. The stoma nurse marks the ileostomy site (for defunctioning).

Position
Lloyd-Davies.

Incision
Long midline.

High anterior resection
Procedure
- Stand on the right side of the table.
- Assess the position and resectability of the tumour. Assess liver and peritoneum for metastatic deposits and colon for synchronous tumours.
- Keep the small bowel away from operating field by tilting the patient to the right and covering the small bowel with moist packs.
- Retract the sigmoid colon to the midline and have the assistant to retract the lower left abdominal wall.
- Using diathermy divide the peritoneum along the 'white line'.
- Develop a plane between the mesentery and retro-peritoneum. In the process the gonadal vessels and ureter are swept away. Identifying and preserving these along with the hypogastric nerves.
- Lift the descending colon and its mesentery off the Gerota's fascia.
- Separate the greater omentum from the distal transverse colon and continue the dissection laterally towards the flexure.
- Extend the dissection along the left para-colic gutter towards the splenic flexure.
- Grasp both limbs of the colon and under vision divide the peritoneum at the flexure. The colon can now be brought out of its splenic bed. Take care during the mobilisation of the splenic flexure that the tip of the retractor held by the assistant does not damage the spleen and avoid undue traction on the omentum during this manoeuvre as the splenic capsule can be torn.
- Hold the sigmoid colon and descending colon up, divide the perito-neum on the right side from the origin of the inferior mesenteric artery to the level of the sacral promontory.
- Identify and preserve the right ureter.

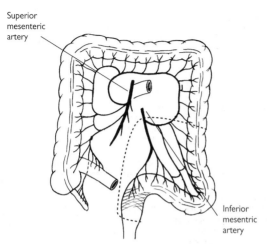

Superior
mesenteric
artery

Inferior
mesentric
artery

Fig. 7.49 Anterior resection

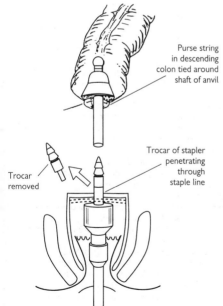

Purse string
in descending
colon tied around
shaft of anvil

Trocar of stapler
penetrating
through
staple line

Trocar
removed

Fig. 7.50 Stapled anastomosis: after anterior resection

- Pass a finger under the sigmoid colon and define the origin of the inferior mesenteric artery. Apply three artery forceps and divide the vessel between the two proximal forceps. This allows double ligation of the artery remnant.
- Clamp, divide and ligate the inferior mesenteric vein below the inferior border of the pancreas.
- Divide the meso-colon at the descending sigmoid colon junction ligating and dividing the marginal vessels.
- Transect the colon at this level using a side-to-side stapler.
- Now pack the small bowel and mobilised colon into the upper abdomen using two large moist packs. Place a Goligher's retractor to retract the wound edges using the central blade to hold the bowel in place.
- Remove the side tilt to the table and apply a head down tilt.
- Move to the patient's left side to carry out the pelvic dissection.
- When present the uterus can be hitched up by two sutures inserted through each broad ligament.
- Hold the sigmoid colon up and using diathermy develop the plane behind the superior haemorrhoidal vessels.
- Identify and preserve the pre-sacral nerves as they cross the pelvic brim medial to the ureters.
- Carry on the dissection in the avascular plane between the meso-rectum and the pre-sacral fascia posteriorly. Keeping in this plane dissect the lateral aspects of the meso-rectum.
- Having reached the level of the peritoneal reflection assess whether further mobilisation is needed.
- Aim for a 2cm clearance below the distal margin of the tumour and a 5cm clearance of the mesorectum.
- Then dissect anterior to Denonvillier's fascia, between the rectum and the bladder, seminal vesicles and prostate in men and the bladder and vagina in women.
- Divide mesorectum at the selected level. Do this by pinching the mesorectum between the index finger and the thumb off the rectum. Insert two right angled clamps through this window and cut between them. Transfix the meso-rectum held in the clamps.
- Then apply a right angled clamp across the rectum.
- Irrigate the rectum with Betadine or another tumouricidal aqueous antiseptic agent using a Foley's catheter introduced per-anally.
- Apply another right angled clamp below the previous one.
- Transect the rectum between the clamps.
- Remove the clamp on the rectal stump and apply Babcock's forceps to the cut edge. Suck any Betadine from the lumen.
- Place a purse-string suture using 2/0 Prolene, no more than 2.5mm from the cut edge to avoid tissue bunching.
- Remove the staple line on the colonic end and similarly place a purse-string. Insert the detached anvil of an end-to-end type circular stapler into the lumen and securely tie the purse-string around the shaft.
- Insert the stapler per-anally and unwind the stapler so the rod exits completely through the open rectal end. Secure the purse-string around the rod.

- Mate the central shaft of the anvil with the instrument shaft by pushing firmly until the shaft clicks into its fully seated position. Turn the wing nut clockwise to approximate the tissue and to close the space between the cartridge and anvil.
- Fire the stapler when close approximation is obtained (green colour appears on the window adhere to manufacturers instructions). Unwind and remove the stapler.
- Check to see the doughnuts are complete.
- Fill the pelvis with normal saline. Check for any leaks by insufflating air through a sigmoidoscope inserted into the rectum.
- Irrigate the peritoneal cavity.
- Leave a drain in close proximity to the anastomosis.

Alternatively a hand sewn anastomosis can be performed using interrupted sero-muscular extra mucosal 3/0 PDS sutures.

Closure

Close the abdomen in a single 'mass' layer using number 1 loop PDS, with subcuticular Monocryl for the skin.

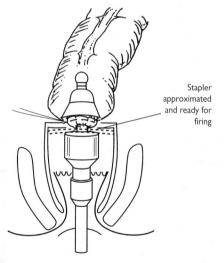

Stapler approximated and ready for firing

Fig. 7.51 Stapled anastomosis: after approximation of end-to-end stapler

Low anterior resection

Procedure

- Continue the rectal mobilisation to the pelvic floor performing a total meso-rectal excision.
- Cross-staple the rectum using a TA30 or 45.
- Carry out a Betadine washout of the rectum.
- Cross-staple the rectum below the previous staple line.
- Transact the rectum flush on the stapler.
- Open and remove the stapler.
- Insert the anvil of end-to-end stapler in the colon end as described above and secure its purse-string.
- Insert the end-to-end stapler with the sharpened point retracted into the rectal stump and bring it up to the staple line.
- Advance the spike so that it appears posterior to the staple line.
- Mate the central shaft of the anvil with the instrument shaft and approximate the two ends.
- Fire the stapler after the green spot appears in the window (check manufacturer's instructions).
- Check for completeness of the doughnuts.
- Perform a leak test as described above. A 5cm colonic pouch can be fashioned and a colo-pouch anal anastomosis made instead of the straight colo-anal anastomosis described. Instead of a stapled anastomosis, endo-anal colo-anal anastomosis can be performed.
- Leave a suction drain in the hollow of the pelvis.
- Washout the peritoneal cavity.
- Make a trephine in the marked site in the right iliac fossa and pull out a loop of terminal ileum to act as a defunctioning stoma.

Closure

Close the abdomen in a single mass layer using number 1 loop PDS, with subcuticular Monocryl for the skin. Make the ileostomy as described before.

Postoperative complications

- Anastomotic dehiscence
- Postoperative paralytic ileus
- Wound infection
- Bleeding
- Anastomotic stricture
- Urinary and sexual dysfunction
- Incisional hernia.

Proctocolectomy and ileostomy

Removal of the colon, rectum, and anus.

Indication
- Ulcerative colitis where medical treatment fails or there is malignant transformation, performed in patients where a sphincter saving procedure is not desirable or suitable.
- Colonic Crohn's disease.
- Synchronous colonic and rectal cancers.
- Familial adenomatous polyposis (for those with low rectal cancers).

Preparation
As for left hemicolectomy. Ileostomy site marked by stoma nurse.

Position
Lloyd-Davies with perineum protruding 5cm from lower edge of table.

Incision
Midline.

Procedure
- Make the trephine for the ileostomy before opening the abdomen.
- Start with mobilising the right colon.
- Divide the bowel at the ileo-caecal junction with a linear stapler.
- Follow the steps as described in relevant chapters when mobilising the colon. Preservation of the greater omentum is not necessary.
- When carcinoma or dysplasia is present perform wide clearance with high ligation of the lympho-vascular pedicle.
- Mobilize the rectum performing a total mesorectal excision, preserving the presacral nerves. In benign cases remove the rectum by close (peri-muscular) dissection.
- Do the perineal dissection by entering the inter-sphincteric plane.
- Follow the steps as mentioned in the chapter for formation of terminal ileostomy.

Postoperative complications
- Paralytic ileus
- Wound infection
- Bleeding
- Delayed healing of perineal wound
- Urinary or sexual dysfunction
- Ileostomy related complications.

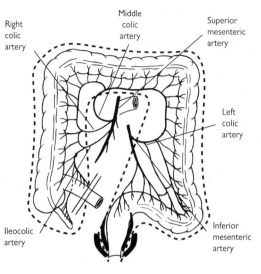

Fig. 7.52 Proctocolectomy and Ileostomy

Abdomino-perineal excision of rectum

Indications
- Low rectal carcinoma where adequate clearance will not be obtained by anterior resection. Other malignancies include those of the anal canal.
- Inflammatory bowel disease, such as severe Crohn's disease with multiple fistulae.
- As part of the procedure of proctocolectomy.

Preparation
As for left hemicolectomy. The stoma nurse marks the colostomy site in the left iliac fossa.

Position
Lloyd-Davies with the perineum projecting 5cm from the lower edge of the table.

Incision
Midline.

Procedure
Stand on the right side of the table.
- Assess the liver and peritoneum for metastatic deposits and the colon for synchronous tumours.
- Keep the small bowel away from operating field by tilting the patient to the right and covering the small bowel with moist packs.
- Retract the sigmoid colon to the midline and have the assistant retract the lower left abdominal wall.
- Using diathermy divide the peritoneum along the 'white line'. Develop a plane between the mesentery and the rectal peritoneum. In the process the gonadal vessels and ureter are swept away. Identify and preserve these along with the hypo-gastric nerves.
- Lift the descending colon and its mesentery off the Gerota's fascia.
- The splenic flexure may need to be mobilised.
- Hold the sigmoid colon and descending colon up. Divide the peritoneum on the right side from the origin of the inferior mesenteric artery to the level of the sacral promontory.
- Identify and preserve the right ureter.
- Pass a finger under the sigmoid colon and define the origin of the inferior mesenteric artery. Apply three artery forceps and divide the vessel between the two proximal forceps. This allows double ligation of the artery remnant.
- Clamp, divide, and ligate the inferior mesenteric vein.
- Divide the mesocolon at the descending sigmoid junction, ligating and dividing the marginal vessels.
- Transect the colon at this level using a side-to-side stapler.
- Now pack the small bowel and mobilised colon into the upper abdomen using two large moist packs.

- Place a Goligher's retractor to retract the wound edges, use the central blade to hold the bowel in place.
- Remove the side tilt to the table and apply a head down tilt.
- Move to the patient's left side to carry out pelvic dissection.
- When present the uterus can be hitched up by two stitches inserted through each broad ligament.
- Hold the sigmoid colon up and using diathermy develop the plane behind the superior haemorrhoidal vessels.
- Identify and preserve the pre-sacral nerves as they cross the pelvic brim medial to the ureters.
- Carry on the dissection in the avascular plane between the mesorectum and pre-sacral fascia posteriorly. Keeping in this plane dissect the lateral aspects of the mesorectum.
- Incise the peritoneal reflection anteriorly.
- Dissect anterior to the Denonvillier's fascia, between the rectum and the bladder, seminal vesicles and prostate in men and the bladder and vagina in women.
- Continue the rectal mobilisation to the pelvic floor, performing a total mesorectal excision.

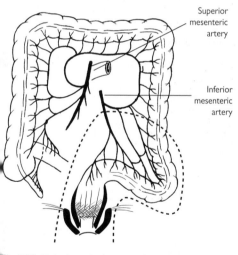

Superior mesenteric artery

Inferior mesenteric artery

Fig. 7.53 Abdominoperineal excision of rectum

The *perineal procedure* can be performed at the same time as the pelvic dissection from above, using a combined synchronous approach.

- Close the anal orifice with a 0 or 1 silk purse-string suture. Apply an artery forceps to the ends of the suture which is left long.
- Make an elliptical incision from the mid point of the perineal body, in the male or the posterior aspect of the vaginal introitus, in the female, to a point over the coccyx.
- Deepen the incision laterally into the ischio-rectal fossa. Control bleeding from the pudendal vessels.
- Use retractors to help dissect to the level of the levator ani.
- Carry the incision posteriorly to expose the anococcygeal ligament. Incise the ligament in front of the coccyx.
- Dissect behind the external sphincter to reach the levator muscles.
- Use the tip of the scissors to traverse the muscle, ask the abdominal operator to help to direct the scissors tip correctly. Avoid lifting the pre-sacral fascia from the sacrum and entering the pre-sacral venous plexus.
- Insert a finger into the pelvis and divide the levator muscles over it on either side.
- Continue the dissection anteriorly making a transverse incision in anterior decussating fibres of the external sphincter exposing the posterior fibres of the superficial and deep transverse perineal muscles. Deep to the latter identify the median raphe in the rectourethralis and puborectalis muscles. Follow the median raphe with blunt scissor dis-section into the pelvis with the abdominal operator guiding with his finger. Divide the remaining tissues to free the rectum and then remove it.
- Close the perineal wound in layers—approximating levator muscles and fibro-fatty tissue in the midline. Close the skin.
- Irrigate the pelvis and leave a suction drain. It is not essential to reperitonise the pelvis.
- Make a trephine at the marked site and deliver the colon end.
- Follow the steps as described for construction of colostomy.

Closure

In single mass layer using 1/0 PDS with subcuticular Monocryl for skin.

Postoperative complications

- Paralytic ileus
- Wound infection
- Bleeding
- Urinary or sexual dysfunction
- Colostomy related complications.

Restorative proctocolectomy

Proctocolectomy with ileal pouch—anal anastomosis.

Indications
- Chronic ulcerative colitis where medical therapy fails and patient wants to avoid permanent ileostomy.
- As a second procedure after colectomy in patients with acute severe ulcerative colitis.
- Familial adenomatous polyposis.

Patient should be highly motivated and have an adequate anal sphincter.

Preparation
As for left hemicolectomy. Ileostomy site marked by stoma nurse.

Position
Lloyd-Davies.

Incision
Midline.

Procedure
- Follow the steps as for conventional procto-colectomy.
- Mobilise the rectum to anorectal junction.
- For stapled anastomosis apply a transverse stapler at this level. For hand-sutured anastomosis divide the bowel to leave an open anal stump.
- Select the point on the ileum for ileo-anal anastomosis and attempt a trial descent to the anal canal level.
- Make a J or W ileal reservoir.
- Perform a stapled pouch-anal anastomosis or a hand sutured anastomosis after mucosectomy.
- Fashion a defunctioning ileostomy.

Postoperative complications
- Pelvic sepsis
- Stricture of the anastomosis
- Intestinal obstruction
- Pouch—vaginal, pouch—perineal fistula
- Excessive frequency of defecation
- Failure—need to remove the pouch and establish a permanent ileostomy
- Pouchitis.

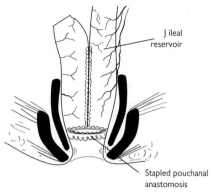

J ileal
reservoir

Stapled pouchanal
anastomosis

Fig. 7.54 Restorative proctocolectomy

Hartmann's procedure

Indications
A safe option when dealing with left-sided colonic emergencies (obstruction, perforation). The diseased colon is resected, divided colon is brought out as an end colostomy in the left lower quadrant, the rectal stump is closed or exteriorised. The procedure is performed when conditions are unfavourable for immediate anastomosis (faecal peritonitis, obstruction, unprepared bowel, unstable patient, inexperience of surgeon).

Preparation
- Ensure adequate resuscitation
- Prophylactic antibiotics
- Thrombo-embolism prophylaxis
- Cross-match blood
- Catheterise
- Forewarn the patient about colostomy and mark the site.

Position
Lloyd-Davies.

Incision
Midline.

Procedure
- As for sigmoid colectomy and colostomy.
- Close the rectal stump by cross stapling or suturing.
- Leave two long non-absorbable sutures at the lateral ends to help future identification of the rectal stump.

Postoperative complications
- Bleeding
- Wound infection
- Breakdown of rectal stump
- Colostomy complications.

Reversal of Hartmann's procedure
Usually considered six weeks after the initial surgery.

Position
Lloyd-Davies.

Preparation
As for left hemicolectomy.

Procedure

- Mobilise colostomy and re-open laparotomy incision.
- Mobilise adherent small bowel loops and identify the rectal stump. Introduce a rigid sigmoidoscope to aid identification if locating the stump is difficult.
- Mobilise proximal colon to bring it close to the rectum without tension. The splenic flexure may need to be brought down.
- Perform a stapled or a hand sewn anastomosis as described for anterior resection.

The operation can be performed laparoscopically assisted.

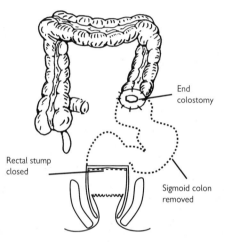

End colostomy

Rectal stump closed

Sigmoid colon removed

Fig. 7.55 Hartmann's procedure

Procedures for large bowel obstruction

Preparation
- Resuscitate the patient adequately.
- Perform a rigid sigmoidoscopy followed by water–soluable contrast enema to exclude pseudo-obstruction.
- Cross match two units of blood.
- Thrombo-embolism prophylaxis.
- Prophylactic antibiotics at induction.
- Catheterise patient.

Position
Lloyd-Davies.

Incision
Midline.

Procedures
- Consider decompression of gaseous large bowel distension. Insert a 14 or 16G needle through a tinea into the lumen of the bowel and attach to suction.
- If obstruction is due to a right-sided lesion consider a right hemicolectomy or for a fixed tumour an ileo-transverse anastomosis (hand-sutured single or two layered anastomosis or a stapled anastomosis).
- If obstruction is due to left sided lesion options are: three-stage approach (defunctioning loop colostomy → resection and anastomosis → closure of stoma); two-stage approach (Hartmann's procedure → reversal of Hartmann's); one-stage approach (sub-total colectomy with ileo-colic or ileo-rectal anastomosis or left hemicolectomy after an on-table colonic irrigation). Choice of operation depends on patient fitness, stage of disease if malignancy and local conditions for primary anastomosis.

On-table colonic irrigation
- Make a colotomy proximal to the lesion causing obstruction.
- Insert anaesthetic scavenging tubing and secure with heavy suture around the bowel. Connect tubing into a plastic bag and place this into a bucket.
- Insert a large Foley catheter into caecum via appendix stump or an enterotomy in the terminal ileum.
- Infuse 2–3 litres, or more, of warm saline into caecum and manipulate colonic contents into anaesthetic tubing. Mobilise colonic flexures if necessary to achieve this. Continue this until effluent is clear.
- Carry out a left hemicolectomy as described previously.

There are kits available on the market for carrying out on-table colonic irrigation.

Self-expanding metal stents are now being used in large bowel obstruction secondary to malignancy either for palliation or as a temporary bridge to surgery (stent decompression → elective resection).

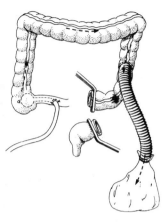

Fig. 7.56 On-table colonic lavage

Hepatobiliary surgery

R. Carter and C. W. Imrie

Introduction

As the morbidity and mortality associated with pancreatic surgery are amongst the highest in surgical practice, management of patients should take place within the context of multi-disciplinary team and they should be in optimal condition pre-operatively. They may be suffering from exocrine failure, altered glucose tolerance, or altered coagulation due to post-hepatic biliary obstruction. All these issues should be addressed. Most surgical procedures will require blood to be cross-matched.

Investigational procedures

Ultrasound

The first line investigation for most patients with pancreatico-biliary symptoms. Can detect:
- Cholelithiasis
- Hepatic abnormalities.

NB Image quality, especially of the pancreas, compromised by incomplete fasting or obesity.

Commonly performed procedures:
- Targeted biopsy
- Drainage
- FNA (Fine needle aspiration).

NB Fast patient for six hours to reduce bowel gas. If intervention is planned perform appropriate investigations (e.g. clotting screen) and exclude coagulopathy.

Endoscopic ultrasound

A mainstay of pancreatic investigation. Radial imaging used to:
- Assess venous invasion
- Locate islet cell tumours.

Linear array ultrasonography provides:
- Excellent images of the pancreatic parenchyma
- The opportunity for guided intervention, e.g. FNA, trucut biopsy of tumours, ultrasound guided drainage of cystic collections and celiac plexus blockade.

ERCP

Endoscopic retrograde cholangio-pancreatography (ERCP) is commonplace in surgical practice. The patient lies on an X-ray table in a semi-prone position with the head turned to the right. Venous access is via the right hand. Under conscious sedation, an endoscope is passed into the duodenum and catheters positioned within the bile or pancreatic duct for injection of contrast and imaging.

Therapeutic procedures:
- Sphincterotomy
- Stent insertion
- Biopsy
- Stone retrieval.

Major complications (commonly associated with therapeutic ERCP):
- Pancreatitis
- Duodenal perforation
- Post-sphincterotomy haemorrhage.

MRCP

Magnetic resonance cholangio-pancreatography. In many situations this is the preferred investigation. In 72 weighted images, static fluid is represented as a strong white signal. That within the common bile duct and pancreatic duct can be represented as an image resembling an ERCP, which can provide excellent diagnostic information of the biliary tree in particular (NB still inferior to direct radiology).

Contraindications and problems:
- Intracorporeal implants (pacemakers, intracranial vascular clips, metallic foreign bodies)
- Intensive care organ support
- Claustrophobia
- Lengthy image acquisition times.

Staging laparoscopy

Laparoscopy is commonly used to assess upper GI malignancies.

Position of patient
Supine.

Intraperitoneal access
This is achieved using a cut-down technique with the use of a Veress needle, but is associated with the risk of visceral or vascular injury.
- Insert a blunt port sub-umbilically
- Create a pneumo-peritoneum using carbon dioxide at a pressure of 10–13mmHg. Two further subcostal ports are then inserted under direct vision.

Procedure
- Inspect the peritoneum by starting to the left of the falciform ligament and working clockwise, examining the lower abdomen for trans-coelomic spread before returning to the right upper quadrant.
- Inspect the superior and under-surface of the liver, anterior aspect of the stomach and omentum for peritoneal metastasis.
- Lift the omentum allowing examination of the root of the mesentery for local invasion. The pancreatic head can then be assessed for mobility.
- Instil 500ml of saline for cytology and also to promote an acoustic window for laparoscopic ultrasound. Insert a laparoscopic ultrasound probe through the left upper quadrant port and placed along the right side of the falciform ligament, over segment four, to identify the hepatic veins for orientation. Then examine hepatic parenchyma in segmental fashion looking for metastasis. Then place the ultrasound probe along side the coeliac axis and superior mesenteric artery and follow the vessels proximally searching for significant lymphadenopathy The pancreas is usually easily identified and the pancreatic duct followed from the body towards the head of the gland.
- Identify the splenic veins and superior mesenteric confluents and assess them for venous involvement.
- Aspirate the fluid for cytology and remove the ports removed under vision to ensure there is no internal bleeding.

Pancreatic mobilisation

Elective pancreatic surgery is usually performed within specialised units. Approaching the pancreas in an unstructured manner can result in significant (particularly venous) haemorrhage. Most general surgeons operate on the pancreas during emergency trauma procedures. Nevertheless the principles of mobilisation apply to all pancreatic procedures and are designed to promote vascular control during procedures.

Position of the patient
Supine.

Incision
Transverse (rooftop) or midline incision.

Procedure
- Elevate the colon and omentum and dissect the omentum from the colon to allow entry to the lesser sac. Mobilise the hepatic flexure and retract inferiorly. Open the peritoneum parallel to the duodenum to allow entry to the plane between the inferior vena cava (IVC) and the duodenum.
- Extend the incision from the reflected colon up to the inferior aspect of the liver to develop the foramen of Winslow, encircling the hepato-duodenal ligament to permit, if necessary, the application of a Pringle manoeuvre. Roll the duodenum medially exposing the anterior aspect of the IVC, the left renal vein and the anterior aspect of the aorta. The duodenum and pancreatic head can then be held in the left hand between fingers and thumb, allowing pressure to be applied in an antero-posterior direction if significant venous bleeding is encountered.
- Follow the middle colic veins downwards, often dividing a branch of the uncinate process to expose the superior mesenteric vein as it descends beneath the pancreatic neck.
- Expose the anterior aspect of the head of the pancreas by dividing the gastro-epiploic vessels, which emerge from the pancreatic parenchyma close to the lower border of the pancreatic neck.
- Expose the portal vein as it emerges from the superior border of the pancreatic neck by ligating the gastro-duodenal artery, divide and retract it superiorly and medially to expose the vein.
- In the trauma situation, mobilise the pancreatic tail by bringing the tail and spleen forwards and medially from the posterior abdominal wall and open the lesser sac as described above and mobilize the splenic flexure and the colon and retract them inferiorly. The splenic artery can be ligated at its origin on the superior aspect of the pancreas in the midline. Divide the short gastric vessels between the stomach and spleen to expose the anterior aspect of the pancreatic tail and divide the lieno-renal ligament lateral to the spleen, rolling the spleen and pancreas medially in the plane behind the splenic vessels. This manoeuvre compresses the splenic vessels and as it is performed permits vascular control to be maintained during dissection.

Management of tumours

Pancreatic head resection—pancreatico-duodenectomy

Position of the patient

Supine.

Incision

Rooftop or midline.

Procedure

- Mobilise the head of the pancreas as described above. Divide the omentum up to the gastro-epiploic vessels preserving the gastro-epiploic arcade down to the level of the pylorus. Divide the lesser omentum at the level of the liver and mobilise it down to the pylorus taking care to preserve the right gastric arcade.
- Transect the duodenum approximately 2cm beyond the pylorus. Perform a retrograde cholecystectomy by exposing the anterior aspect of the common hepatic duct and dividing it approximately 1cm below the hilar plate. Skeletalise the right side of the hepatic artery and the portal vein down to the superior border of the pancreas.
- Lift the colon superiorly allowing release of the duodeno-jejunal flexure divide the jejunum at the level of the first arcade and divide the mesenteric vessels down toward the superior mesenteric artery and vein. Having freed the vascular supply to the proximal jejunum, pass it beneath the superior mesenteric vessels to lie in the right sub-hepatic space. Hold the uncinate process and proximal jejunum in the left hand and divide the pancreatic neck to expose the superior mesenteric vein (SMV)/portal vein. The inferior mesenteric vein (IMV) often joins the SMV rather than the splenic vein. Two further veins usually enter the SMV/portal vein from the pancreatic head.
- Dissect the remaining tissue from the lateral border of the superior mesenteric artery and remove the specimen.

Reconstruction

There are three common reconstruction techniques. The choice is usually determined by personal preference.

Pylorus preserving pancreatico-duodenectomy (PPPD)

- Bring the distal jejunal loop into the upper abdomen by the retro-colic route. As the initial anastomosis is usually end-to-side pancreatico-jejunal, an interrupted posterior layer of sutures is inserted and tied. Then perform a small enterotomy allowing a mucosa-to-mucosa pancreatico-jejunal anastomosis to be fashioned using interrupted sutures. This anastomosis can be facilitated by the use of a stent. Complete the anastomosis with an interrupted anterior layer.
- Perform an end-to-side biliary anastomosis.
- Place an anterior layer of interrupted sutures from the outside to the inside of the bile duct lumen. Then hold them in forceps for future use with the needles left in situ.
- Perform a small enterotomy.

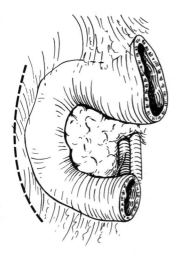

Fig. 8.1 Kocherization of duodenum

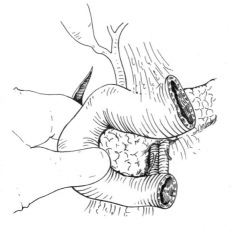

Fig. 8.2 Mobilisation of head of pancreas

- Place a posterior wall of interrupted sutures through both the jejunum and posterior bile duct.
- Then 'parachute' the duodenal loop down into position and tie the posterior row of sutures.
- Next place the anterior layer of sutures, already through the bile duct, through the jejunum and tie them to complete the anastomosis. Finally, fashion an end-to-side duodenal-jejunostomy with a continuous single layer technique. The exact position and order of these anastomoses can vary depending on the individual anatomical orientation.

Closure

Mass technique. Clips or sutures to skin. Suction drain to right upper quadrant.

Variations

- *Classical 'Whipple' operation.* Rather than preserving the antrum, pylorus and first 2cm of the duodenum, an antrectomy is performed by dividing the stomach from the incisura to the greater curve. Reconstruction is achieved by using either and end-to-side Billroth II type anastomosis in a continuous two layered technique or, if a roux loop has been fashioned, by a functional end-to-end anastomosis with continuous one or two layer sutures.
- *Pancreatico-gastrostomy.* The pancreas can be anastomosed to the posterior wall of the stomach rather than to the jejunum. This can be achieved using a 'dunking' technique with interrupted sutures to pancreas and stomach.

Standard distal pancreatectomy with splenectomy

Having mobilised the pancreatic tail, the splenic artery is dissected at its origin from the coeliac axis and doubly ligated. The neck of the pancreas is then divided to the medial aspect of the superior mesenteric vein to expose the splenic vein, which is also ligated and divided. The tail of the pancreas and spleen are then resected. The cut end of the pancreas is oversewn using interrupted sutures ensuring inclusion of the main pancreatic duct if possible and leaving a drain in situ.

Splenic preserving distal pancreatectomy

The anterior aspect of the pancreas is exposed and the superior and inferior aspects of the neck of the pancreas dissected to expose the superior mesenteric vein. The spleen is not mobilised. The pancreas is then divided and the dissection continued towards the tail. Small pancreatic tributaries from the splenic artery and vein are ligated and divided, resecting the pancreatic tail whilst leaving the vessels in situ. The cut edge of the pancreatic neck is then secured as above, and a drain left in situ.

Total pancreatectomy

This is a rarely performed operation due to its potential morbidity. The usual indications are IPMT with positive resection margins preventing a local resection or, in certain rare circumstances, chronic pancreatitis. This essentially involves a combination of 'Whipple' resection with a distal pancreatectomy.

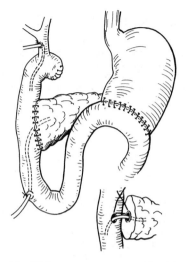

Fig. 8.3 Pancreaticoduodenectomy (Whipple's operation) showing three anastomoses

Enucleation of islet cell tumour

Some pancreatic endocrine tumours may be enucleated at open or laparoscopic surgery. The main complication with this technique is the development of a postoperative pancreatic fistula due to involvement of the ductal system in the resection margin. The extent to which the tumour is intraparenchymal is therefore important in the pre-operative choice of procedure as a distal pancreatectomy may be more appropriate for deeply sited lesions.

Pre-operative localisation

Use EUS, CT plus intra-operative ultrasound scanning to identify the lesion.

Procedure

This is the same whether via a rooftop incision or laparoscopy. Dissect the gastro-colic omentum from the colon to expose the anterior aspect of the pancreas. A superficially sited tumour may be shelled out from underlying pancreatic tissue, excision being confirmed by frozen section.

Closure

Mass, clips or sutures to skin. Leave a drain along the anterior aspect of the pancreas.

Management of pancreatic necrosis

Surgery is usually required for the management of complications rather than for the necrosis itself. The commonest procedure for infected pancreatic necrosis, or necrosis in a patient failing to respond to conservative treatment, is an open necrosectomy. This may be performed through an open anterior, a lateral retroperitoneal, an anterior laparoscopic or a percutaneous approach.

Open anterior approach

Position of patient
Supine.

Incision
Rooftop.

Procedure
- Perform a laparotomy. Open the lesser sac, as previously described, or by dividing the gastro-colic omentum.
- Mobilise both hepatic and splenic flexures to exposure the anterior aspect of the pancreatic abscess. Open the abscess through the lesser sac; use finger dissection to tease all necrotic material out. Avoid sharp resection as this may lead to haemorrhage which is difficult to control. Cholecystectomy and operative cholangiogram are usually performed and the cavity cleared of all necrotic tissue.

Closure
Close the abdomen over paired drains, usually 4–6 to allow postoperative lavage at a rate of 250ml/hour.

Complications
In the event of significant oozing, pack the abscess cavity with lubricated gauze swabs with a view to a re-laparotomy 48 hours later.

Lateral retroperitoneal approach

Position of patient
Right lateral.

Incision
Left flank.

Procedure
- Mobilise the colon medially allowing retroperitoneal access to the lesser sac.
- Remove the necrotic material by blunt finger dissection and manage the cavity by either drainage or packing, as described above.

Anterior laparoscopic approach

Position of patient
Supine.

Access

- Use a cut-down technique to insert a blunt port subumbilically. Insert a further 10mm and 5mm ports to provide both operative access and upward retraction of the colon to expose the transverse meso-colon.
- Enter the lesser sac by opening the transverse meso-colon and remove the abscess and necrotic material through this opening.
- Tube drainage postoperatively to control the necrosectomy cavity.

Percutaneous necrosectomy

This procedure has been developed in Glasgow and involves the dilatation of a drain tract to promote adequate drainage and lavage of an abscess cavity. It is most commonly used for infected necrosis.

Procedure

- Insert a percutaneous catheter into the abscess cavity under CT guidance.
- Insert a guidewire into the drain and dilate the tract to 34Fr. gauge using either a balloon dilatation system or graduated dilator. Then insert an Amplatz® sheath to maintain tract integrity. This permits the cavity to be explored using an operative nephroscope and any solid material can be removed under direct vision.
- Suture a tube drain with a parallel lavage catheter in place at the end of the procedure to permit continuous postoperative lavage at a rate of 250ml/hour.

Management of pseudocyst

Drainage of a pseudocyst may be either into a Roux loop or more commonly into the back of the stomach. It is particularly useful for post inflammatory cysts containing necrotic debris, which may prevent resolution if a minimally invasive technique of drainage is employed.

Cysto-gastrostomy
Position of patient
Supine.

Incision
Midline.

Procedure
- Identify the anterior aspect of the stomach and perform a longitudinal gastrostomy approximately 10–15cm in length.
- Confirm the site of the retroperitoneal pseudocyst by either intra-operative ultrasound or needle puncture. Then open the cyst with diathermy and over-sew its edge to prevent bleeding. The length of the cysto-enterostomy is usually 5–10cm. Remove any necrotic material within the cyst.
- Close the anterior wall of the stomach using continuous 3/0 PDS sutures.
- Identify the anterior aspect of the stomach and perform a longitudinal gastrostomy approximately 10–15cm in length.
- Confirm the site of the retroperitoneal pseudocyst by either intra-operative ultrasound or needle puncture. Then open the cyst with diathermy and over-sew its edge to prevent bleeding. The length of the cysto-enterostomy is usually 5–10cm. Remove any necrotic material within the cyst.
- Close the anterior wall of the stomach using continuous 3/0 PDS sutures.

Closure
Mass. Sutures or clips to skin. No drainage
NB Endoscopic cysto-gastrostomy (with or without EUS control) is becoming increasingly common and is the approach of choice where necrosis is minimal.

Cyst-enterostomy
Where the site of the cyst precludes drainage into the posterior aspect of the stomach, a Roux loop can be used as an alternative. The loop is brought up to lie adjacent to the pseudo-cyst and its position can, once again, be confirmed by intra-operative ultrasound or needle puncture. The cyst is then opened and a side-to-side anastomosis established using a continuous suture technique.

Management of chronic pancreatitis

Minimally invasive endoscopic procedures for the management of chronic pancreatitis are a viable alternative to surgical decompression in selected patients.

Frey procedure

Position of patient
Supine.
- Mobilise the head of the pancreas and identify the dilated pancreatic duct with either intra-operative ultrasound or needle aspiration.
- Excise the anterior pancreatic parenchyma to expose the posterior aspect of the pancreatic duct leaving a tadpole-shaped defect in the anterior aspect of the pancreas. The depth of the head dissection is determined by the size of the pancreatic head mass and the presence or absence of the significant extra-hepatic bile duct obstruction.
- Create a Roux loop after the resection is completed. Bring it through the transverse meso-colon to the retro-colic position.
- Anastomose this side-to-side to the pancreatic parenchyma using multiple interrupted sutures in with parachute technique to ensure correct placement. The amount of pancreatic tissue excised in the classical procedure is 5–6g.

Closure
Close the wound in layers with staples to skin and a drain is left within the lesser sac.

Beger procedure
A duodenum-preserving pancreatico-jejunostomy was initially described for the management of a pancreatic head mass in the presence of an essentially normal pancreatic tail. The procedure involved formal transection of the pancreas at the medial border of the superior mesenteric/portal vein, as in a 'Whipple' resection.
- Core the pancreatic head out leaving a small rim of pancreatic tissue around the internal circumference of the duodenal loop and the posterior wall of the pancreas to expose the common bile duct, which is on occasion opened.
- Perform an end-to-side pancreatico-jejunostomy as in the 'Whipple' procedure. The Roux loop is also anastomosed onto the exposed pancreatic head.
- This procedure has been modified extending the dissection into the pancreatic tail for those patients with tail involvement, and may be considered as a modification of a longitudinal pancreatico-jejunostomy. Approximately 20–40g of pancreatic tissue is removed. However, in practice, the amount removed is a function of the volume of the pancreatic head mass, if present, and the need to decompress the biliary system.

Minimally invasive thoracoscopic splanchnicectomy (MITS)
This procedure is used for relief of pancreatic pain in patients with either chronic pancreatitis or pancreatic carcinoma, and is an alternative to coeliac plexus block.

Position of patient
Prone.

Incision
Achieve intra-thoracic access using a cut-down technique similar to that described for the ATLS insertion of a chest drain, just below the inferior border of the scapula.

Procedure
- Open the pleura, with a finger inserted to ensure there are no significant adhesions. Then insert a blunt port at this site with a pneumothorax created using carbon dioxide at a pressure of 6mmHg.
- Insert a second 5mm port two rib spaces below this.
  The splanchnic nerves emerge from the sympathetic chain within the chest between T5 and T12 and converge to form the *greater, lesser* and *least splanchnic nerves*, which are easily visible using a 30° camera running beneath the pleura overlying the vertebral bodies.
- Divide the nerve branches using a nerve hook pressing against the vertebral body to avoid the intercostal vessels. Move the ports at the end of the procedure under vision and have the lung re-inflated. There is no need for long-term water-sealed drainage of the pleural cavity.
- Repeat the procedure on the opposite side, so that bilateral splanchnicectomy is performed.

Common pancreatic complications

General considerations

Pancreatic conditions are associated with considerable morbidity whether presenting with an acute illness or following elective surgery. Organ dysfunction is common and patients are usually managed in a high dependency environment. As with all surgical patients, chest infections, line sepsis and catheter related sepsis occur, and low molecular weight heparin and physiotherapy is considered standard care. Organ dysfunction may require support within an intensive care unit. However, some complications are specific to pancreatico-biliary conditions:

- *Bleeding.* Pressure bleeding from a surgical drain should be reported immediately to a senior colleague, particularly where sepsis has been present. An initial 'herald' bleed may be followed by an exanguinating bleed, so early recognition is essential. Although definite definitive surgical control may be required, management may be possible by angiographic embolisation.

- *Biliary fistula.* Leakage of bile following surgery can occur following a dislodged surgical tie, a leaking anastomosis or iatrogenic ductal injury. Management is largely determined by the post surgical anatomy, as access to the ampulla of Vater may allow endoscopic decompression. The principle of management is to gain control of infection by surgical, endoscopic or percutaneous drainage, maintaining nutritional support whilst resolution occurs.

- *Pancreatic fistula.* This most commonly occurs following surgery but can follow percutaneous drainage of a peri-pancreatic fluid collection. It many settle spontaneously but stenting of the pancreatic duct at ERCP can expedite resolution. Pancreatic resection may be required for persistent fistulas.

- *Post ERCP pancreatitis.* Abdominal pain is relatively common following ERCP due to gaseous distension. However, if this persists for more than a short period or increases in severity, peripancreatic or pancreatic inflammation should be suspected. Post ERCP pancreatitis may be confirmed by a two hour post procedure serum amylase being greater than three times normal. This is more common following interventional procedures, or following a pancreatogram. Duodenal perforation should be suspected if there are any signs of early infection or sepsis and can be confirmed by an urgent contrast CT scan.

- *Cholangitis.* This is life-threatening and usually secondary to biliary obstruction. The classical clinical syndrome with pain, fever, rigors and jaundice should be managed by urgent biliary decompression, usually by ERCP. Delay in treatment may result in the rapid development of multi-organ dysfunction syndrome.

Laparoscopic surgery

S. Rawat, L. Horgan, and
C. M. S. Royston

Laparoscopic staging for abdominal malignancies

Laparoscopy is an effective and useful tool for the diagnosis and staging of abdominal malignancies. Staging is of paramount importance in planning treatment for localized and advanced disease. It is imperative to accurately identify those patients with a potentially resectable, localized tumour and those patients with advanced disease or distant metastasis. Despite improvements in preoperative staging with dynamic computed tomography (CT) and endoscopic ultrasonography, unexpected liver or peritoneal metastases are found in 10–20% of patients with oesophageal, gastric and pancreatic cancer. The need for laparotomy can therefore be obviated in these patients.

Aim of laparoscopic staging
- Confirm the findings of preoperative investigations
- Assess spread—local and distant
- Biopsy of suspicious lesions
- Cytology of ascitic fluid/peritoneal washing.

Indications
- Oesophageal cancer
- Gastric cancer
- Pancreatic cancer
- Hepatobiliary tumours
- Lymphoma.

Contraindications
- Disseminated disease
- Unfit for general anaesthesia
- Open procedure is indicated for palliation
- Procedure unlikely to alter plan of care.

Technique
The procedure is performed under general anaesthesia.

Position of patient
Supine.

Procedure
- Create pneumoperitoneum.
- Introduce a 30° telescope through a midline periumbilical trocar. Place one or two additional trocars in each upper quadrant depending on area to be visualised.
- Perform a systematic four-quadrant visual inspection. Carefully inspect all peritoneal and omental surfaces for seedlings. Send ascitic fluid sample for cytology.
- Assess the primary tumour—size, location, local extent, fixation, extension to adjacent organs.

- Place the patient in a 20° reverse Trendelenburg position with 10° left lateral tilt. Visualize anterior, posterior and inferior surface of both lobes of liver. Inspect the hilum of the liver and biopsy any periportal nodes if suspected.
- Place the patient in a 10° Trendelenburg position without lateral tilt. Identify the omentum and retract it to the left upper quadrant. This allows identification of ligament of Treitz and inspection of mesocolon.
- Incise the gastrohepatic omentum to expose the caudate lobe of the liver, vena cava and the coeliac axis. Take care to preserve any anomalous left hepatic artery. Biopsy any suspicious enlarged lymph nodes in this region (coeliac, portal, or perigastric).

Laparoscopic ultrasonography (LUS)

Laparoscopic ultrasound has enhanced the sensitivity of staging as the direct contact of the probe with the organ of interest affords superior resolution especially in pancreatic tumours. Ultrasound probes use conventional B-mode and colour Doppler technology and permit identification of deep liver lesions, small peritoneal lesions, vascular invasion, and abnormal lymph nodes in the coeliac, gastric, portal, and peripancreatic regions. LUS may also accurately direct biopsy and assess proximity to surrounding structures.

Criteria for unresectability
- Metastasis: hepatic, serosal or peritoneal
- Involvement of the mesocolon
- Invasion or encasement of coeliac, hepatic, superior mesenteric artery or involvement of portal vein.

Complications
- Haemorrhage
- Bowel perforation
- Wound infection
- Port site herniation and recurrence.

Laparoscopic splenectomy

Since it was first described by Delaitre and colleagues in 1992, laparoscopic splenectomy has become the method of choice for elective splenectomy in patients with a splenic weight estimated to be <1.5kg. Massive splenomegaly (palpable clinically) still remains a technical challenge. Increasing operative experience and technical refinements have produced good results compared to open splenectomy in terms of wound infection, pulmonary complications, patient discomfort, outcome and length of hospital stay.

Indications
Essentially the same as for open splenectomy.
- Idiopathic thrombocytopenic purpura
- Hereditary spherocytosis
- Haemolytic anaemia
- Lymphoma
- Lymphocytic leukaemia.

Relative contraindications
- Massive splenomegaly
- Abscess
- Tumour
- Splenic artery aneurysm.

Preparation
- Preoperative immunization with pneumovax, Haemophilus influenza and meningococcal vaccines.
- Cross match packed red blood cells for all patients and platelets for thrombocytopenic patients (platelets count <50 × 10^9/l).
- Preoperative splenic artery embolization for large spleens to minimize bleeding has been suggested by some.
- Give steroid cover to patients with idiopathic thrombocytopenic purpura or patients on long-term corticosteroids.
- Take advice of haematologist regarding pre and postoperative care.
- Informed consent for both laparoscopic and open splenectomy.
- Prophylactic antibiotics (penicillin) at induction of general anaesthesia.
- Two operative techniques are described—the anterolateral and the posterior approach. The anterolateral approach is preferred as it is associated with better access, reduced operative time, postoperative stay and blood transfusion.

Position
Reverse Trendelenberg semi lateral tilt.

Technique
- Create pneumoperitoneum (via umbilical route). Introduce 30° angled telescope. Place three further cannulas, 10mm in epigastrium and two 5mm in left mid-clavicular and left anterior axillary lines.
- Exploratory laparoscopy looking especially for accessory spleens in the hilum, gastrosplenic ligament, splenocolic ligament, splenorenal ligament and greater omentum.

- Divide splenocolic ligament with harmonic scalpel.
- Dissect the short gastric vessels and divide them using clips, harmonic scalpel or bipolar diathermy.
- Retract the spleen medially, divide lienorenal ligament close to the splenic capsule using diathermy or harmonic scalpel.
- Clear any adhesions posteriorly to create a space for a laparoscopic stapling device to be placed across the hilum.
- Locate the hilar vessels. Transect it using an Endo GIA ensuring that fundus of the stomach or the tail of the pancreas is excluded. Other methods of ligation such as clips or ties may also be used.
- Insert Endocatch II instrument into 12mm cannula and place spleen in bag. Withdraw the bag and remove the spleen piecemeal after sectioning into smaller pieces with sponge-holding forceps or digital fracture technique.
- If spleen is required intact for histological examination or is too large to be placed in a retrieval bag, use a small Pfannenstiel incision for organ removal.
- The harmonic scalpel facilitates control of the short gastric vessels and splenic attachments and reduces the operative time.

Operative complications

- *Bleeding.* Correct any coagulation defect preoperatively. Control haemorrhage with cautery, clips, endoloops, Endo GIA Staplers or open conversion.
- *Injury to adjacent organs*—colon, stomach, small bowel, pancreas. Laparotomy may be required.
- *Subphrenic abscess.* Start antibiotics and drain percutaneously under CT guidance.
- *Pancreatitis and pancreatic fistula.* Percutaneous drainage for fistula.
- *Overwhelming postsplenectomy infection* (OPSI). Patients should receive preoperative vaccination at least 2 weeks before surgery. Give advice regarding immunization, foreign travel and prophylactic antibiotics.
- *Thrombocytosis.* Can lead to DVT and pulmonary embolus. Routinely use subcutaneous heparin and TED stockings.

Laparoscopic inguinal hernia repair

Laparoscopic hernia repair has the advantages of reduced discomfort after surgery, early return to full activity, low incidence of wound infection and chronic groin pain. Recurrence rates are comparable to Lichtenstein open mesh repair. In January 2001, the National Institute for Clinical Excellence (NICE) guidelines suggested that open mesh repair should be the preferred procedure for primary unilateral inguinal hernias, and the laparoscopic repair should be considered for recurrent or bilateral hernias. NICE has also expressed a preference for one of the two laparoscopic techniques available, the totally extraperitoneal (TEP) rather than the transabdominal preperitoneal (TAPP) method, even though there is no proven difference in outcome between the two techniques. These guidelines have been controversial and are widely debated.

Indications
- Recurrent inguinal hernia—universally accepted indication. Open surgery for recurrence is more difficult, with higher risk of damage to cord structures, including testicular vessels and higher risk of recurrence.
- Bilateral hernia—laparoscopic surgery permits repair in the same session with shorter convalescence time.
- The role of laparoscopic repair of primary unilateral hernia is debated and is not recommended by NICE.

Contraindications
- Patients unfit for general anaesthesia
- Active infectious or inflammatory process (mesh at risk)
- Strangulated/incarcerated hernia
- Previous retropubic open prostate surgery.

Preparation
- Obtain informed consent including conversion to open repair if necessary
- Consent for contralateral repair if unsuspected hernia identified at laparoscopy
- Mark the hernia side
- Empty the urinary bladder immediately before induction of anaesthesia
- Place the patient supine with the head end slightly lower (Trendelenburg position)—keep bowel away from operating site
- Place the monitor at the foot end of the table
- The surgeon stands on the side opposite the hernia.

Technique
Repair can be performed by either TAPP approach or TEP approach.

TAPP approach
- Create pneumoperitoneum.
- Position the cannulae; one at the umbilicus (12mm) and one on each side at the lateral border of the rectus muscle (both 5mm).

- Establish the anatomy from medial to lateral—bladder, medial umbilical ligament (obliterated umbilical artery), area of direct inguinal hernia, inferior epigastric vessels, internal ring, and anterior superior iliac spine.
- The internal ring is confirmed by looking for two divergent structures, which emerge from it; medially the vas deferens (round ligament of the uterus in females) beneath the peritoneum, and laterally a less distinct ridge caused by the gonadal vessels. Between the two is the 'triangle of doom'; deep to the peritoneum are the external iliac vessels.
- Identify whether the hernia is direct (medial to inferior epigastric vessels) or indirect (lateral to inferior epigastric vessels), unilateral or bilateral.
- Create a peritoneal flap from lateral to deep ring to medial umbilical ligament horizontally and well above and below the inguinal ring vertically. Inferiorly, strip the peritoneum off the gonadal vessels and vas for a few centimetres (beware not to damage them).
- Create an identical contralateral space for bilateral hernia.
- Retract the direct sac, or small indirect sac along with the peritoneal flap.
- Divide the large indirect sac at the level of the external ring and leave the distal part in situ.
- Introduce a 15 × 10cm mesh through the umbilical port and ensure it covers the entire posterior wall, extending behind the pubic bone to cover direct, indirect and femoral ring.
- Fix the mesh at Cooper's ligament and along the upper border with staples or sutures. Biologically compatible glues may be an inexpensive alternative to stapling or suturing.
- Do not apply staples below and lateral to the ileopubic tract to avoid injury to the lateral femoral cutaneous nerve. Never staple close to the 'triangle of doom'.
- Close the peritoneal flap by using staplers or by suturing (prevent gaping between the flaps).
- Ensure complete peritoneal coverage of the mesh to avoid small-bowel obstruction.
- Close the rectus sheath at the 10mm port site.

TEP approach

Without entering the peritoneal cavity, this approach reduces the risk of port site hernia and possibly bowel adhesions. Presence of a lower abdominal incision may make the TEP operation difficult or impossible because of adherence of the peritoneum to the muscles and tissues of the anterior abdominal wall. Complete withdrawal of a very large indirect hernial sac may also prove difficult by TEP.

Technique

- Make a transverse sub-umbilical incision to expose the anterior rectus sheath on the side of the inguinal hernia.
- Divide the anterior rectus sheath to expose the rectus muscle.
- Retract the muscle laterally.
- Create an extraperitoneal space behind the rectus abdominis muscle. A specially designed balloon or its substitutes can be used.

- Insufflate the extraperitoneal space with carbon dioxide to a pressure of 10mmHg.
- Expand the space by separating the peritoneum from the posterior abdominal wall to the anterior superior iliac spine laterally and well beyond the defect vertically in a manner similar to TAPP repair.
- Place 10mm trocar port at the midline, about 8cm from the pubis. Enlarge the preperitoneal space by blunt dissection.
- Insert an additional 5mm trocar either in the midline approximately 3cm caudal to the 10mm trocar or on the side of the hernia at the level of the anterior superior iliacspine (ASIS), along the anterior axillary line.
- Create and dissect extraperitoneal space by endo-scissors. Separate the peritoneum from the posterior abdominal wall up to the ASIS laterally and well beyond the defect vertically in a manner similar to TAPP repair.
- Dissect and reduce the hernial sac.
- Introduce a 15 × 10cm prolene mesh, similar to one used in TAPP. Anchor the upper border of it to the abdominal wall and fix the lower medial part to Cooper's ligament or pelvic bone with an endo-stapler.
- Desufflate at the end of the procedure. Ensure the mesh remains flat and does not roll.

Complications

- *Bladder injury:* avoid sharp instruments near bladder, avoid patients who may have had previous surgery in the area (previous retro pubic prostatectomy).
- *Bleeding:* avoid injury to iliac vessels and inferior epigastric artery by ensuring systematic identification of anatomical structures and avoiding dissection in triangle of doom. Take care when stripping the peritoneum from the gonadal vessels. Beware of accessory obturator artery (10% of cases).
- *Damage to vas.*
- *Seroma/hydrocele:* aspirate if large or causing concern.
- *Retention of urine:* usually resolves spontaneously or following a period of catheter drainage. Cover any urethral catheterisation with antibiotics in early post operative period. Take urological opinion to rule out latent prostate obstruction in elderly men.
- *Haematoma.*
- *Neuralgia:* due to injury to genitofemoral or lateral femoral cutaneous nerves.
- *Bowel obstruction:* due to adherence to mesh (disturbing complication occasionally reported with TAPP procedure).
- *Mesh infection.*
- *Recurrence:* the common cause is technical fault and use of a small mesh.

Laparoscopic Nissen fundoplication

Minimal access anti-reflux and hiatus hernia surgery is becoming increasingly established throughout the world.

Indications

- Failure of or side effects from medical therapy
- Healthy young patients who prefer surgery to lifelong medication
- Complications of gastrooesophageal reflux disease (GERD)—continued oesophagitis, Barrett's oesophagus, oesophageal stricture
- Complications of large hiatus hernia. (e.g. bleeding, dysphagia)
- Atypical symptoms of gastro-oesophageal reflux (hoarseness, cough, chest pain, nocturnal choking, recurrent aspiration pneumonia, loss of teeth enamel) with documented reflux on 24-hour pH monitoring.

Preparation

Investigate to confirm the diagnosis and select patients for surgery.

- *Endoscopy*—usually the first test to be performed. Assess hiatus hernia, oesophageal length, mucosal abnormalities, ulceration, stricture and Barrett's oesophagus. Biopsies of suspected Barrett's epithelium may show severe dysplasia or carcinoma. In such case, antireflux procedure alone would be inappropriate (resection or close endoscopic surveillance may be indicated).
- *24-hour pH monitor*—most specific and sensitive test for GERD. Quantifies the actual period of acid contact with the oesophageal mucosa and allows correlation with subjective feeling of heartburn. A normal 24-hour pH study rules out reflux disease and strongly suggests alternative diagnosis.
- *Oesophageal manometry*—tests for oesophageal motility, helps individualize the surgery. The lower oesophageal sphincter (LES) pressure in patients with reflux disease is usually $\leq$ 6mmHg and most patients require a 360° wrap. A partial wrap is indicated if LES pressure is high or if oesophageal motility is poor (diminished contraction amplitude, diminished peristalsis).
  Patients with aperistalsis may have achalasia and may require different therapy. Abnormal findings may also suggest significant risk of dysphagia following fundoplication (need to modify the procedure).
- *Barium swallow*—in cases of diagnostic or anatomic confusion.

Position

Lloyd-Davies position with knees slightly flexed and reverse Trendelenburg position. Surgeon between the legs using 2-handed technique.

Technique

- Create pneumoperitoneum by Veress needle or open Hassan entry.
- Angled 30° or 45° laparoscope is helpful for adequate visualization.
- Five ports are used: two 10mm, three 5mm. Place camera port in the midline at junction of upper 2/3 and lower 1/3 between umbilicus and xiphoid process. Introduce subsequent four ports under direct vision, angling them towards the hiatus. Operating ports are in the right

(5mm) and left (10mm) midclavicular lines. Place liver retractor through the subxiphoid port (5mm). This may be hand-held or attached to a mechanical holder secured to the table (Natensen's). Retract the stomach with a grasper or Babcock's forceps introduced through the port in left anterior axillary line (5mm). This manoeuvre opens up the gastro hepatic ligament.

- Open the avascular aspect of lesser sac; divide the gastro-hepatic ligament from about the level of the left gastric artery to the hiatus using diathermy forceps or harmonic scalpel.
- Extend the dissection to the right to allow identification of right crus. Adequate crural dissection reveals the oesophagus, which can then be separated from right and left crura with gentle dissection. Never grasp the oesophagus for retraction.
- Fully mobilise the angle of His from the left crus and free the medial part of greater curve from the diaphragm.
- Create a window posterior to the oesophagus, just below the left crus and above the posterior gastric fundus. Identify and preserve both vagus nerves. Insert a soft sling to retract the oesophagus.
- Divide the short gastric vessels only if necessary to create a loose floppy wrap without tension.
- Reconstruct the normal hiatus by closing the left and right crura with two or three interrupted 2/0 Ethibond sutures. Avoid injury to the posterior wall of the oesophagus. Maintain a distance of approximately 1cm between the highest suture and the oesophagus.
- Pass atraumatic forceps behind the oesophagus from right to left, grasp the greater curve of the stomach, pull it behind, forming the wrap. Use shoeshine manoeuvre in which surgeon alternately retracts the left and right portions for proper wrapping. Use three interrupted 2/0 Ethibond sutures to form a 2–3cm wrap for a standard Nissen fundoplication (360°). Place a full-thickness suture through the stomach but include only the muscular wall of the oesophagus to avoid the risk of post-operative oesophageal leakage. Some prefer fashioning a wrap over bougie (56F) to prevent tying too tightly but there is a small risk of oesophageal perforation by this. Do not pass a nasogastric tube unless you suspect injury to the stomach or oesophagus.

Difficulties

- *Large paraoesophageal hernia*—consider anterior repair with mesh reinforcement.
- *Laparoscopic partial fundoplication*—various techniques e.g. Toupet fundoplication. Consider in patients with compromised oesophageal motility, in order to decrease the risk of postoperative dysphagia.
- *Open conversion*—if dense adhesions, difficult exposure due to large left lobe of the liver, uncontrolled bleeding or repair perforations.

Postoperative care

- Encourage oral fluid intake after 6 hours.
- Start sloppy diet within 24 hrs.
- Soft diet for the next 2 weeks (eating slowly, chewing carefully and avoiding meat and bread). Most patients can be discharged within 48 hours.

Complications

- **Oesophageal perforation** (<1%)—more likely in severe oesophagitis or large hiatus hernia. Avoid forceful introduction of bougie (if used), dissect bluntly and gently around oesophagus and do not grasp the oesophagus for retraction.
- **Bleeding**—during dissection of short gastric vessels or from accidental injury to the spleen or liver.
- **Pneumothorax** (1–5%)—caused by dissection into the mediastinum and pleura.
- **Subcutaneous and mediastinal emphysema**—in extensive dissection of large hiatus hernia.
- **Dysphagia**—remains the most troublesome and frequent complication. Minimised by formation of loose floppy fundal wrap, use of Toupet partial fundoplication instead of Nissen complete fundoplication in patients with oesophageal dysmotility (weak or uncoordinated peristalsis). If dysphagia continues to be severe after three to four weeks postoperatively, dilatation is performed. Reoperation for dysphagia is seldom necessary.
- **Wrap migration and para-oesophageal herniation**—due to failure to repair the oesophageal hiatus and breach of the pleura. Always close crura, prevent vomiting with routine use of ondansetron. Surgical correction may be required.
- **Gas bloating, inability to belch and hyperflatulence**—occur occasionally, usually improve with time.
- **Delayed gastric emptying, dumping, and diarrhoea.**
- **Recurrent reflux symptoms**—consider suture line failure, slipped fundoplication, paraoesophageal hernia, dysphagia secondary to fundoplication.

Laparoscopic cholecystectomy

Indications

- Symptomatic cholelithiasis
- Acute calculous cholecystitis
- Acute acalculous cholecystitis
- Gallstone pancreatitis
- Symptomatic gallbladder polyp.

Contraindications

- Absolute: Cirrhosis with portal hypertension due to low peripheral resistance and increased risk of bleeding which is difficult to control.
- Relative contraindications include cirrhosis, coagulopathy, pregnancy (second trimester) and severe cardio respiratory insufficiency.

Preparation

- Confirm diagnosis on ultrasound, provides information about the stones, gallbladder wall thickness (chronic cholecystitis), pericholecystic fluid (acute cholecystitis), and the size of the common bile duct (CBD). FBC, U&E, liver function tests, and blood is obtained for group and save. Evaluate the overall surgical risk including cardiorespiratory assessment.
- MRCP/ERCP in patients with a history of jaundice, abnormal LFTs or dilated common duct on USS.
- Rule out other pathology e.g. gastritis, peptic ulcer disease, irritable bowel syndrome and pancreatitis in patients with atypical symptoms and presentation.
- Administer single dose of antibiotic for prophylaxis at the start of the operation. Give further two doses postoperatively doses if there is bile leak
  during the operation. Treat the patients with acute cholecystitis and cholangitis as their clinical course warrants.
- Institute thromboprophylaxis (subcutaneous heparin and TED stockings) because the reverse Trendelenburg position and pneumoperitoneum increases the risk for deep venous thrombosis.
- Use a radiolucent operating table which allows on table cholangiography.
- Obtain informed consent for laparoscopic cholecystectomy including discussion of possible conversion to an open procedure. Conversion rates vary with experience of the surgeon and are 2–5%. Conversion rate is higher with previous upper abdominal surgery, acute cholecystitis, or CBD stones. Consider conversion as good surgical judgement rather than failure.

Position

- Supine (classical)—UK and North America. Surgeon stands on left side of the patient.
- Leg abduction position (frog-legged)—French approach. Surgeon stands between the patient's legs.

Technique

- Perform under general anaesthesia with endotracheal tube and full abdominal relaxation.
- A urethral catheter is unnecessary provided patient empties his/her bladder before coming to the theatre. Insert NG tube only if the stomach is distended with gas to facilitate exposure.
- Access the abdominal cavity using an open (Hassan) or closed (Veress) technique. Surgeon's preference usually determines the choice of technique. Introduce 10mm umbilical port for the camera; achieve pneumoperitoneum and maintain intraabdominal pressure of 12mmHg.
- Place other ports under direct vision as demonstrated in Fig. 9.1 10mm with 5mm reducer in the epigastrium 2–5mm below the xiphisternum (working port); 5mm anterior axillary line (lateral port) to retract fundus of gall bladder; 5mm right upper quadrant port placed in right mid clavicular line to manipulate the neck of the gallbladder.
- Laparoscope the entire abdomen to exclude injury/bleeding during creation of pneumoperitoneum, and also to identify any gross additional disease.
- Place the patient in reverse Trendelenburg position with tilt to the left to allow the colon and omentum to fall inferiorly.
- Use most lateral grasper to grasp the fundus of the gallbladder and push it (laterally and anteriorly) over the anterior edge of the liver by progressive traction. Avoid this manoeuvre in patients with contracted gallbladder or fibrotic/cirrhotic liver. In these cases, push fundus gently against the liver with care not to penetrate the parenchyma of the liver.
- Dissect the adhesions off the gallbladder.
- Identify the Hartmann's pouch and grasp it with the lateral working grasper, pull it laterally exposing Calot's triangle, which includes the cystic duct and artery as well as the common bile duct. Constantly maintain this traction. Start the posterior dissection of Calot's triangle, divide the inferior peritoneal leaf.
- Start anterior dissection from Hartmann's pouch and move toward the cystic duct. This is particularly important in acute cases, when anatomical landmarks are difficult to find. Separate/divide peritoneum over the Calot's triangle as far back as the liver.
- Create a window posterior to cystic duct and cystic artery.
- Gently separate the cystic duct from the cystic artery by using dissector.
- Define junction of cystic duct with gall bladder, defining the junction with CBD is not necessary. In doubt, check with an intraoperative cholangiogram.
- Coagulation in Calot's triangle should be minimal and used with extreme caution.
- Apply two proximal and one distal titanium clips to the cystic duct and artery.
- Withdraw the applicator and introduce the scissors or endoshears instrument is inserted to cut them.

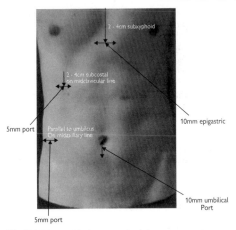

Fig. 9.1 Port sites for laparoscopic choleeystectancy

Retract the Hartmann's pouch upwards and place the tension on the surgical plane between the gallbladder and its liver bed. Begin dissection at the infundibulum of the gallbladder and proceed to the fundus with the aid of an electrosurgical hook or scissors, although more recently, the harmonic scalpel has been used. Facilitate by alternate anterolateral and anteromedial traction. Take care not to enter the gallbladder, which would release stones or the liver, which would cause bleeding.

- On reaching the fundus inspect the liver bed. Ensure haemostasis. Separate the gallbladder from its bed.
- Extract the gallbladder from the umbilical or epigastric port using claw shaped gallbladder extraction forceps (alligator forceps). Pull forceps, cannula and neck of the gallbladder out of the fascial opening.
- Use endobag to extract the gallbladder in cases of empyemas and iatrogenic perforations of gallbladder with spilled gallstones.
- Drainage is not always necessary. When in doubt, drain (bleeding or oozing from liver bed, bile leak).
- Perform final inspection of the abdomen.
- Deflate the abdomen and remove the trocars under direct vision.
- Close the muscle sheath of trocar size 10mm with 2/0 Vicryl or PDS on J needle to prevent herniation. Use subcutaneous Vicryl or Steristrips to close the skin.
- Infiltrate all port wounds with long-acting local anaesthetic.

Difficulty and cautions

- *Cystic artery*—beware of a short cystic artery arising from looped right hepatic artery. Early division of the cystic artery—risk of bleeding from the posterior branch if overlooked; other anomalous origin cystic artery of the hepatic or right hepatic artery from the superior mesenteric artery.

- *Cystic duct*—short cystic duct–risk of damage to common bile duct; Accessory cystic duct—postoperative bile leakage if unrecognised.
- *Perforation of gallbladder*—aspirate bile, locate and remove stones, place gall bladder and large stone in retrieval bag, thoroughly irrigate the cavity with normal saline.
- *Decompression*—initial decompression facilitates approach to tense gall bladder in acute cholecystitis (mucocele/empyema).
- *Wide cystic duct*—tie with a Roeder knot/Endoloop or apply Endo GIA staples.
- *Difficult extraction*—multiple or large stone. The neck is opened outside the abdomen, bile is sucked out and the stones can either be crushed or removed with Desjardin forceps to debulk the gallbladder. Thick walled gallbladders may be extracted by extending the fascial opening. Temptation of excessive traction should be avoided.
- *Porcelain gallbladder*—calcified rim, difficult grasping or decompression due to higher incidence of carcinoma; the specimen should be removed in a nonporous retrieval bag.
- *Large/floppy left lobe of the liver* can obstruct the view of Calot's triangle. Use a liver retractor placed through an additional 5mm port in the left upper quadrant.
- *Retrograde, fundus first* in difficult cholecystectomy (acute, inflamed, distortion of Calot's triangle).
- *Subtotal cholecystectomy*—very difficult. Chronic fibrotic, Calot's triangle obliterated—divide gallbladder at Hartmann's pouch, extract stones, ligate the pouch with endoloop/oversew.
- *Partial cholecystectomy*—if gallbladder very adherent to liver, diathermize mucosal surface of residual gall bladder (partial cholecystectomy).
- *Open conversion*—consider in technical difficulties, anatomic uncertainties or anomalies, uncontrollable bleeding, suspected common duct injury, visceral or major vessel damage.
- *Intraoperative cholangiogram*—liberal use is desirable to clarify difficult anatomy and to detect common bile duct stones. Some surgeons use it routinely for education and training and others pursue a policy of selective cholangiography based on a history of jaundice, pancreatitis, ultrasound evidence of a CBD stone, serum elevation of bilirubin, alkaline phosphatase, and intraoperative abnormal findings or difficulties. The cystic duct is occluded distally with a clip and a small proximal incision is made in the cystic duct anterosuperiorly with fine scissors. A catheter is guided into the duct and held there with a special instrument or a loosely applied titanium clip. The contrast medium is injected during screening. Evaluation of the CBD includes the size of the duct, filling defects, visualisation of major intrahepatic ducts, and flow of contrast into the duodenum. If the cholangiogram is normal, the catheter is removed and the cystic duct is secured just inferior to the ductotomy with two titanium clips and divided.
- *Co-existing ductal calculi*—the usual management consists of endoscopic tone extraction followed by laparoscopic cholecystectomy during the same hospital admission, if possible. The alternative, if local expertise is available, is single stage laparoscopic management with extraction of the ductal calculi through the transcystic approach, if small (<0.6mm), or by direct supraduodenal common bile duct exploration for large or occluding stones.

- *Carcinoma of the gallbladder*—high index of suspicion is important. Consider open conversion with excision of the gall bladder, regional lymphadenectomy and excision of trocar site.
- *Diathermy hazards*—risk of occult injury. Avoid high-power setting and use diathermy under direct vision only.

Postoperative care

- Remove NG tube (if inserted) at the end of operation.
- Postoperative antibiotics are not required for elective cases.
- Start clear fluids when the patient is fully awake and proceed to normal diet as tolerated.
- Remove the drain, if inserted, the following day provided the drainage is minimal.
- Encourage early ambulation. Most patients are ready for discharge within 24 hours. Increasing trend towards day-case laparoscopic cholecystectomy in some centres.
- Patient is generally able to return to normal activity within 2 weeks.

Complications

- *Bleeding*—during the operation from the cystic artery or the liver bed. It is usually easily controlled by electrocautery, clips, and or suture ligatures. If haemostasis is not achieved using these methods, the procedure should be converted to an open procedure. Major vascular damage (aorta, iliac vessels, and vena cava) can occur during introduction of cannula is rare but reported. It must be remembered that the distance between the anterior abdominal wall and the aorta and its bifurcation into the iliac vessels averages only 2.0cm in thin patients. Significant bleeding with hypotension requires immediate laparotomy.
- *Major bile duct injuries*—occur when the common bile duct is mistaken for the cystic duct and divided (complete transection). Other mechanisms of injury include indiscriminate clipping or cautery to hastily control bleeding, clipping of the cystic duct with the tips of the clip, and occluding the common bile duct. Major bile duct injuries should be referred to and are best treated in specialised unit for ERCP stenting, for example.
- *Visceral injury*—rare but well documented. Can occur with introduction of a cannula, insertion of an instrument without visualisation or careless use of electrocautery.
- *Gallbladder perforation*—visible stones should be retrieved to prevent complications related to lost gallstones (Intraabdominal abscess and fistula).
- *Postoperative bile leak*—0.02–2.7%. Patients may present with symptoms of shoulder pain, abdominal pain, and fever. Bile leak may occur from the gallbladder bed, cystic duct (dislodged clips), or as a result of injury to the common bile duct. Most bile leaks resolve spontaneously if adequately drained (ultrasound or CT scan guided), and there is no distal bile duct obstruction. MRCP/ERCP is recommended if no intraoperative cholangiogram was obtained in order to rule out a major ductal injury. ERCP should be performed if bile leak persists beyond 1 week after drainage. If a retained common bile duct stone is found, it is removed. A sphincterotomy and/or stent placement decompresses the biliary system, thus helping resolution of the leak.

- *Wound infection*—may occurs when bile is spilled during extraction of gallbladder or when there is direct contact between an infected gallbladder and the incision. Avoid seeding when removing an infected specimen through a tight trocar site. Use extraction bag.
- *Incisional hernia through port sites*—most commonly occurs in 10mm port sites. Patient usually presents with pain and small bowel obstruction three to 5 days post-operatively.
- *Deep vein thrombosis*—risk related to duration of surgery, reverse Trendelenburg position and the pressure of insufflation. Use DVT prophylaxis such as LMWH and TED stockings.
- *Post-cholecystectomy syndrome*—this is the persistence of symptoms despite surgery. Some of these patients may have a retained stone in the bile duct—MRCP or ERCP may be needed. The gallbladder may not have been responsible for the pain in the first place—the pain may have been due to peptic ulcer, irritable bowel syndrome or to disease of the liver or pancreas.
- *Death*—occurs in 0.1–0.5% of cases (1–5 per 1000 operations). The risk increases with age.

Laparoscopic appendicectomy

It has been demonstrated to be safe and efficacious. However, its superiority to the traditional open technique continues to be debated. Decision of laparoscopic versus open appendicectomy is based on many factors including patient's wishes, surgeon's experience, equipment availability and time of day.

Advantages (demonstrated by several prospective clinical trials): ability to explore the peritoneal cavity, reduced postoperative pain, decreased rate of wound infection, less postoperative adhesions, shorter hospital stay, more rapid return to normal activity, and better cosmesis. Make a definite diagnosis in females.

Disadvantages: higher total cost, increased operating time, need for experienced surgeon/theatre staff and appropriate equipment. It is not yet the gold standard for the management of appendicitis but may become the standard approach in future.

Indication
Acute/suspected appendicitis.

Preferred in
- Premenopausal women with uncertain diagnosis
- Obese patients (large incision otherwise required)
- Athletes and others who need rapid return to full activities
- Patients concerned about cosmesis.

Preparation
- Informed consent for both laparoscopic and open procedure
- DVT prophylaxis
- Prophylactic antibiotics
- General anaesthesia with endotracheal intubation and muscle relaxation
- Catheterisation to reduce risk of bladder injury and aid pelvic examination.

Position
- Patient in supine position.
- Surgeon and assistant standing on patients left side, nurse on the right and monitor at the foot of the table towards the right.

Technique
- Re-examine the abdomen when patient is anaesthetised—appendicular mass.
- Induce pneumoperitoneum using either Veress needle or open technique.
- Perform quick diagnostic laparoscopy first, through 10mm umbilical port.
- Place second 5mm suprapubic (lower midline, above symphysis pubis) and third 10mm trocar either in the right lower or right upper quadrant. Upper quadrant placement preferred because it allows better caecal retraction.

- Trendelenburg with left sided tilt facilitates inspection of the right lower quadrant and appendix.
- Complete the diagnostic laparoscopy to exclude ovarian cyst, pelvic inflammatory disease, cholecystitis, perforated ulcer, Meckel's diverticulum, colonic diverticulitis, Crohn's disease and ischaemic bowel.
- Identify the appendix. Signs of appendicitis include omental adherence, caecal inflammation, presence of turbid fluid in the region of the appendix, increased vascular injection of the serosa and wall thickening, perforation and gangrene.
- Grasp and elevate the tip of the appendix. If tip is not visible, identify the base and then follow this using two atraumatic graspers until you see the tip.
- Free the appendix off the surrounding adhesions to define its entire length.
- Divide the mesoappendix with clips, bipolar cautery or linear stapling device or tie.
- Identify the base of the appendix (convergence of taenia), and secure it with a pretied suture ligature/endoloop or a linear stapling device.
- Divide the appendix between two pre-tied endoloop ligatures.
- No need to bury the stump of the appendix.
- Place the purulent appendix into retrieval bag and remove the specimen.
- Irrigate the peritoneal cavity.
- Place suction drain into the pelvis if localized collection.
- Remove trocars under direct vision.
- Remove the Foley catheter in theatre at the end of the procedure.

Retrograde appendicectomy—useful in severe inflammation or gangrene. Begins with dissection, ligation, and division of the appendicular base, which is then retracted to complete the dissection.

Appendicular abscess—if surrounding tissue is too inflamed and friable to allow safe appendicectomy, perform laparoscopic drainage and irrigation. Place a closed suction drain in the abscess cavity and bring it out through the right trocar site. Perform interval appendicectomy, either laparoscopic or open, at a later date.

Perforated appendix—occlude its lumen using an endoloop proximal to the perforation to prevent spread of its content in the peritoneal cavity.

Open conversion—in cases with difficult dissection, uncontrollable bleeding or suspected visceral damage.

Normal looking appendix and no other pathology identified—remove the appendix (early appendicitis cannot be confirmed until histological examination is undertaken). Failure to remove the appendix may result in confusion if the patient continues to have right iliac fossa pain.

Postoperative care

- Continue antibiotics as treatment if there is peritonitis or gross faecal spillage.
- Encourage early ambulation.
- Start oral diet usually after 8–12 hours post operative.
- Patients can be discharged as early as 24 hours after surgery and are advised to resume normal activities as tolerated.

Complications

- *Bleeding*—sources include the inferior epigastric artery, appendicular artery and the staple line. Avoid injury to inferior epigastric vessels by placing the cannula lateral to the rectus abdominis muscle. Do not hesitate to convert if bleeding is uncontrollable.
- *Bowel perforation*—by inadvertent injury by diathermy or the trocar.
- *Bladder injury*—avoid by catheterisation and introduction of the suprapubic cannula under direct vision.
- *Wound infection*—avoid contact between the wound edges and the appendix. Use an Endobag.
- *Intra-abdominal and pelvic abscess*—higher incidence in patients with appendicular perforation. Careful dissection and lavage are key factors in avoiding it.
- *Recurrent appendicitis*—due to incomplete appendicectomy. Avoid by removing the entire appendix.
- *Incisional hernia*—may develop if fascial site of 10mm port is not closed.
- *Deep venous thrombosis and pulmonary embolism*—avoid by heparin prophylaxis and TED stockings.

Obesity surgery

Laparoscopic surgery is ideally suited to bariatric surgery. The absence of large wounds and related complications is especially advantageous in this group of patients and obesity in itself poses less of a problem for the laparoscopic surgeon than for the open surgeon. All types of bariatric procedure can be performed laparoscopically and with increasing experience in similar operating times as for open surgery.

Indications
- Morbid obesity uncorrected by dieting and non-operative interventions.
- BMI (body mass index) >40kg/m^2.
- BMI >35kg/m^2 with an obesity related comorbidity (diabetes, hypertension, sleep apnoea etc.).

Contraindications
- Previous gastrooesophageal surgery.
- Multiple previous laparotomies.
- Co-morbidities precluding general anaesthesia.

Three types of operation are commonly performed

1. Purely restrictive procedures: laparoscopically placed adjustable silicone gastric bands (LASGB)

A variety of bands are now available and involve passing an adjustable band around the stomach just distal to the gastro-oesophageal junction, above the lesser sac posteriorly giving a 'proximal' gastric pouch of between 25–30ml. The channel/stoma between proximal and distal pouches is adjusted postoperatively in the outpatient clinic by injecting fluid into the inner balloon via a subcutaneously placed port.

Technique
- General anaesthesia.
- Patient in Lloyd-Davies and reverse Trendelenberg's position on the operating table.
- Creation of pneumoperitoneum (Veress needle preferable).
- Primary 10mm laparoscope trocar in midline 4 inches beneath xiphoid.
- 30° laparoscope.
- Insertion of Nathenson retractor to retract left lobe of liver cephalad under direct vision via sub xiphoid route.
- 5mm left hand working cannula midclavicular line.
- 15mm right hand working port midclavicular line.
- 5mm retractor cannula to right of 15mm port anterior axillary line.
- Assess for presence of hiatus hernia and (optional) repair of crura.
- Dissect angle of his from left crus.
- Create retrogastric tunnel via pars lucida passing left hand instrument behind gastrooesophagel junction to emerge between left crus and angle of His.
- Insert band with attached tubing into abdomen through 15mm port and draw through retrogastric tunnel to place band around gastro-oesophageal junction posteriorly.

- Place 25ml balloon into stomach transorally and withdraw to gastro-oesophageal junction (GOJ) to assess size of proximal gastric pouch.
- Close band locking mechanism anteriorly below level of intragastric balloon to create pouch.
- 3–4 anterior gastro-gastric sutures to cover the pouch anteriorly and prevent later band slippage.

Complications
- Bleeding
- Gastric perforation
- Damage to band during gastro-gastric suturing.

2. Combined restrictive/malabsorptive procedures: Laparoscopic roux-en-Y gastric bypass
Technique
- General anaesthesia.
- Patient in Reverse Trendelenberg's position on the OR table with modified Lloyd-Davies positioning.
- Creation of pneumoperitoneum (Veress needle preferable).
- Primary 10mm laparoscope trocar in midline 4 inches beneath xiphoid.
- 30° laparoscope.
- Insertion of Nathenson retractor to retract left lobe of liver cephalad under direct vision via sub xipoid route.
- 12mm left hand working cannula midclavicular line.
- 12mm right hand working port midclavicular line.
- 5mm retractor cannula to right of 15mm port anterior axillary line.
- Dissection begins at lesser curve 2cm below GOJ at level of left gastric vein exposing lesser sac.
- First (blue cartridge) gastric staple layer placed transversely separating stomach. Repeated progressive stapling (3–4 firings in total) directed to angle of Hiss to complete transection of the stomach leaving 30ml proximal stomach.
- Identify duodeno-jejunal (DJ) flexure in retrocolic compartment and identify suitable site of small bowel for gastrojejunal anastomosis. This loop of jejunum may be divided before or after gastro-jejunal (GJ) an-astomosis and must by brought to the gastric pouch either ante-colic and ante-gastrically (in which case omental division aids passage) or retrocolic, retrogastric (in which case passage must be made through the transverse mesocolon).
- The GJ anastomosis may be sutured or stapled with either a linear stapler or circular stapler.
- The jejunojejunal anastomosis is then fashioned at a point 100cm distal to the GJ (sometimes 150cm in the super-obese patients).

3. Malabsorptive procedures: Biliopancreatic diversion (Scopinaro technique)
This technique relies predominantly on malabsorption to maintain weight loss by ensuring a 'common alimentary channel' (ileum) of no greater than 100cm preventing nutrient absorption. Metabolic and mineral deficiencies are more common with this technique than with either of the above methods but sustained weight loss may be better. Two variants are

described. The classical approach involves a distal gastrectomy (Fig. 9.2); a more recent modification especially used by laparoscopic surgeons involves a 'sleeve' gastrectomy with duodenal switch (Fig. 9.3) either as a single or as a staged procedure.

Sleeve gastrectomy with duodenal switch

Stage 1: Sleeve gastrectomy.
The harmonic scalpel is used to free the greater curve of the stomach from the gastrocolic omentum. Sequential firings of linear staples from the antrum to the angle of His then create a gastric tube 1.5cm in diameter based on the line of the lesser curve. Bleeding from the staple line and perforation/staple line disruption (especially at the gastrooesophageal junction) are the major operative complications.

Stage 2: Biliopancreatic diversion.
The duodenum is freed at the junction of D1 and D2 and transected with a linear stapler. A point on the small bowel 250cm from the ileocaecal valve is divided and the distal cut end anastomosed to the duodenum with a hand suturing technique. The proximal end is then anastomosed into the side of this alimentary channel with either sutures or staples 50–100cm from the ileocaecal valve. The shorter the common channel the more pronounced is the malabsorptive effect and steattorrhoea is frequent with common channels shorter than 75cm.

Distal gastrectomy with biliopancreatic diversion (single stage operation)

A distal gastrectomy is performed with a proximal stomach remnant of approximately 150–200ml. The biliopancreatic diversion is performed as above to restore intestinal continuity. This technique removes the pylorus and the dumping syndrome which results may aid carbohydrate malabsorption.

All the above techniques are in common use and it is currently unclear which will emerge as the 'best' overall technique for long-term weight loss when balanced with their complications and side effects. In general the greater the degree of obesity the more likely a malabsorptive or bypass approach will be preferred particularly when the patient has a 'sweet tooth' in which case purely restrictive approaches are less likely to be effective.

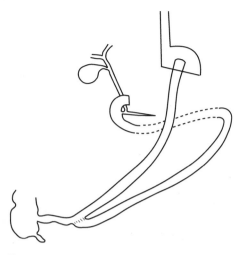

Fig. 9.2 Scopinaro biliopancreatic diversion

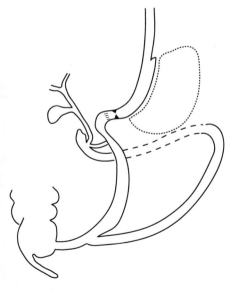

Fig. 9.3 Sleeve gastrectomy with duodenal switch (pylorus preserving)

Stapling in surgery

V. J. Kurup, A. Gillian and David J. Leaper

Introduction

The first linear stapler used successfully in surgery was described by Professor Humer Hultl in Hungary in 1908. This large instrument weighed 5kg and took 2 hours to load. He used the instrument to close the stomach during gastrectomies. In 1921 Aladar von Petz, another Hungarian, described a much lighter, easier to use instrument. These early instruments inserted a double row of staples giving a B-closure to achieve haemostasis without necrosis of the suture line. Modern instruments are disposable and some have a multiple-fire facility allowing them to be used several times without the need to re-open a basic unit. The range of staplers consists of four categories (circular, linear, linear cutting, and skin staplers), along with recent variations that lend themselves to minimally invasive surgery. Within each category, several commercial models are available, many of which have their own unique features modified by the manufacturer. Some of these instruments have different staple heights, which can be adapted for use in different thicknesses of tissue.

Staple or sew?

Staplers facilitate gastrointestinal surgery by rapidly closing or anastomosing bowel. Some anastomoses (e.g., choledochojejunostomy) are best done by hand but in others, such as joining colon to a rectal remnant after a low anterior resection, stapling is easier and faster as it creates a more consistent anastomosis in an inaccessible location. For most procedures, however, the choice is up to the surgeon. Stapling has the advantage of speed and also facilitation of access but has the disadvantage of increased cost. Mechanical failure is now rare and malfunction is generally due to operator error. Complications related to the stapling technique are uncommon, although anastomotic stricture may be more frequent than when handsewn anastomoses are performed. Stapled anastomoses cannot be expected to succeed under conditions that would make construction of a sutured anastomosis dangerous. There is no evidence that staples are safer than sutures, for instance, in the presence of advanced peritonitis or poor tissue perfusion. Modern gastrointestinal staplers are designed to preserve the viability of the tissues distal to the staple line. This is analogous to the 'approximate but do not strangulate' principle used when a bowel anastomosis is handsewn. However, it should be stressed that these are an adjunct to, and not a substitute for, meticulous surgical technique.

Circular stapler

This stapler applies a double row of staples in circular fashion while transecting the tissue within the circle, and is used for creating visceral end-to-end or end-to-side anastomosis. Some of the instruments are curved with a detachable or rotatory anvil which allows much greater adaptability, particularly when transecting oesophageal varices or carrying out transabdomino-oesophagojejunal anastomosis or a low anterior resection. There are varied diameters between 21–33mm to accommodate the bowel lumen being anastomosed. Circular staplers are not reloadable.

Linear stapler

This inserts two parallel staple lines. The lengths vary from 30–90mm, with the shorter ones being used for closing a small bowel enterotomy, the intermediate ones for closing the duodenal stump after a partial gastrectomy, and the longer ones for creating a new lesser curve after distal gastrectomy. Two standard staple sizes are available for the standard linear stapler. The 3.5mm staple is 3.5mm in leg length and 4.0mm wide across the base. The 4.8mm staple is 4.8mm in leg length but also 4.0mm wide across the base. The 3.5mm stapler achieves a closed size of 1.5mm, and the 4.8mm stapler closes to 2mm. Smaller (3.5mm) cartridge is blue and the larger (4.8mm) cartridge is green; mnemonic 'little boy blue and the jolly green giant'. The 3.5mm cartridge is appropriate for most tasks. The 4.8mm cartridge is used for thicker tissues, such as stomach.

Linear cutter

Here four parallel staple lines are inserted with a cutting blade between. The tissue is stapled before knife activation so staples are completely formed before the knife cuts the tissue. The lengths vary from 50–90mm permitting side-to-side anastomosis or making terminal closures. The Linear cutter may be reloaded during a single procedure. This is particularly useful if speed is important or in less accessible operations. These instruments can also be used for laparoscopic work, allowing bowel anastomosis through 10mm ports.

Accessories are available, for example the tissue-measuring (sizers) and purse-string-inserting devices. Some operations are made easier or carried out more quickly with staples, and this justifies their cost in many cases.

Skin staplers

They are designed for fast skin closure with good cosmetic results. They are applied with force just sufficient to achieve approximation without producing cross-hatching of the skin. The wound edges must be everted during approximation. Staples are delivered one by one and are placed 5–10mm apart depending on the thickness of the skin and underlying structures.

Metal clips

Metal clips offer a secure and quick method for obtaining haemostasis provided the entire circumference of the vessel is visible. Furthermore, ligating clips can be used to mark internal structures as they can be clearly identified on X-ray. There is a wide range of clip applicators with different sizes for both open and laparoscopic surgery. Multiple clip applicators are also available. They have a ratchet mechanism, which prevents accidental fall of clips from the jaw, and also have an integrated mechanism that reloads the instrument enabling comfortable, efficient and fast ligation.

Stapling technique in anterior resection

Advantages

- Permits a low anastomosis with greater ease and safety
- Is time-saving and permits optimal sterility of the operative field
- Has lower risk of neoplastic spillage
- Eliminates technical problems such as the preparation of the distal purse-string suture and the inequality between the two intestinal stumps to be anastomosed.

Preparation, anaesthetic, and incision are as for hand-sewn anterior resection. The table should be in Lloyd-Davies position to allow per annum access.

Procedure

(Also see Figs.7.44, 7.50, and 7.51)

- Proceed exactly as hand-sewn until the ends of the bowel have been prepared for anastomosis.
- Be certain that the proximal colon reaches the pelvis easily and mobilize the splenic flexure if not. Additional mobility may be gained by ligating the inferior mesenteric vein just below the inferior margin of the pancreas.
- 'Single stapled' anastomosis (proximal and a distal purse-string suture) or a 'double stapling' technique (the rectum being closed with a straight/transverse stapled suture and a circular anastomosis made through the stapled suture row of the closed rectum) can be used.
- Remember that the stapler removes an extra 8mm of rectum and this is included when distal clearance is estimated below the tumour.
- Place a purse-string suture in the proximal colonic resection line using a disposable purse-string device, a modified Furness clamp, or by hand. Use 2/0 Prolene on a round-bodied needle. Start extraluminally on the anterior aspect and then continuously over and over, in and out, to invert the bowel edge. Prolene sutures must include both muscular and mucosal layers and must be placed close to the cut edge so as to ensure a snug approximation of the entire bowel wall around the stapling instrument when it is tied.
- Place distal purse string on the rectal stump, which can be performed by hand (single staple) or staple (double stapling technique). Transverse or adjustable-angle linear stapler (roticulator) is used to staple the rectum below the tumour.
- Metal sizers used to assess which size of stapler to use can be traumatic, and simple measurement with a ruler is safer. However, when a sizer is introduced through the anus it can lift a very low anterior rectal stump into the pelvis, making the insertion of the purse-string easier (single staple).
- Choose the largest stapler that can safely be introduced into the two bowel lumens. A curved instrument usually makes this easier. If the pelvis is narrow, use an instrument with a head that can be revolved (roticulator).

- Introduce the stapling device through the anus with its safety catch on. Open the instrument to separate the firing end from the distal anvil.
- Tie the purse-string sutures over the separated ends (single staple) or allow the spike of the gun to pass through the posterior aspect of the stapled rectal stump in the middle and just behind the staple line (double stapling).
- Manipulate the end of the descending colon over the top of the anvil and tie the purse-string.
- Connect the anvil and secured descending colon into the cartridge.
- Close the instrument and ensure that no extraneous tissues enter it.
- Remove the safety catch and fire the instrument.
- Open the gun to separate the anvil from cartridge, two to three turns and rotates the stapler through 360°, which should be easy.
- Remove the stapler through the anastomosis carefully as if undoing a button from a buttonhole, but keeping your left hand around the anastomosis.
- Remove the stapler, detach the anvil and remove the two colon ends. Both should be complete 'doughnuts', confirming a complete anastomosis, which is secure. If these are not complete, it may be necessary to redo the anastomosis or repair the defect.
- Send the doughnuts for histological examination.
- Some surgeons test the anastomotic integrity by filling the pelvis with saline containing a weak antiseptic and looking for air leaks with air insufflation through the sigmoidoscope. The presence of air bubbles confirms the presence of a leak that must be repaired by interrupted sutures.
- Consider a temporary ileostomy or colostomy when there is any doubt concerning the security of the final anastomosis.

Stapling technique in oesophagojejunostomy (Roux loop) after transabdominal total gastrectomy

Preparation, anaesthetic, position, and incision are the same as in abdominal total gastrectomy.

Procedure

- After the oesophagus has been transected and the specimen removed, prevent proximal retraction of the oesophagus by applying stay sutures in each of the four quadrants of the oesophagus, going through all layers.
- Attach a hemostat to each suture.
- Place a 2/0 Prolene purse-string suture as for a stapled anterior resection ensuring that the ends are outside the lumen. Include full thickness no more than 3–4cm proximal to the cut edge of the oesophagus.
- Attach a haemostat to the completed purse-string suture.
- Measure the oesophageal size with a calibrated sizing instrument. Some prefer to dilate the end of the oesophagus by inserting a Foley catheter (size 16Fr) into the lower oesophagus and injecting approximately 7–10ml of saline, which gently dilates the end of the oesophagus for the easier introduction of the anvil of the stapler. This may permit the introduction of a larger stapler.
- Be gentle as vigorous attempts to dilate the oesophagus will result in mucosal tear.
- Fashion a Roux loop of jejunum, either retrocolic or antecolic. This can be done quickly using a multifire side-to-side stapler.
- Leave the end of the proximal jejunum open, ensuring that it can reach the oesophagus below the hiatus.
- Insert an appropriately sized circular end-to-end stapler with the anvil removed through the open end of the jejunal loop.
- Ensure that the safety catch is on, that the stapler is the largest you can safely use, and that you have checked staple heights and tissue thickness.
- Push the spindle spike through the jejunum 4–5cm from the bowel end on the antimesenteric side. A curved stapler with a detachable roticulating head makes this easier. Some use a jejunal purse string, which is securely tied.
- Tie the purse string in the oesophageal resection line over the anvil and join the stapler.
- Close the stapler and fire it after removing the safety catch.
- Open the stapler two to three turns and then remove it, holding the anastomosis with your left hand and using the buttonhole technique.
- Confirm that there are two intact fragments (doughnuts) of oesophagus and jejunum on the spindle. If necessary reinforce it partially or completely with sutures.

- If the oesophagus is very thick, dissect back the muscular coat as a cuff. Do not include this in the stapler. After stapling, unite the oesophageal muscle to the jejunum with a continuous ring of sutures. Feel the anastomosis through the open jejunum and ensure that it is intact and that the efferent long loop is open.
- Close the open jejunum with a linear stapler or by hand using two layers of Vicryl or PDS.

Stapling technique for transection of bleeding oesophageal varices

Indication

Consider transection when varices continue to bleed despite medical therapy, resuscitation, and insertion of Sengstaken tube.

Preparation, anaesthetic, position on the table, and incision are the same as for other variceal procedures.

Procedure

- Divide the phreno-oesophageal ligament and dissect free the lower oesophagus.
- Place an atraumatic sling around it, taking care not to damage the vagal nerves.
- Pass 2/0 silk or an atraumatic sling around the cleared oesophagus before the insertion of the stapling device; otherwise it is technically more difficult and there is risk of damage to the oesophageal wall when the rigid gun is in position.
- Make a small gastrostomy in a relatively avascular part of the high anterior surface of the stomach.
- Pass the sizer into the oesophagus to determine the largest size of gun head that can be slipped into the oesophagus without risk of damage.
- Select the correct size circular end-to-end stapler with adjustments calculated for staple height and tissue thickness.
- Insert the complete stapler (closed gun) into the oesophagus with the safety catch on making sure that neither the sling nor the encircling ligature around the oesophagus impedes the passage of the gun up the lumen.
- Advance the gun into the oesophagus for 5–6cm; open the stapler three or four turns so that there is a gap between the anvil and the firing end (3–4cm).
- Tie encircling 2/0 silk or other easily tied braided suture into the gap, thereby inverting the whole circumference of the oesophagus into the gun. It takes time to ensure that the ligature is firmly tied.
- Close and then fire the gun with a protective hand around the site of anastomosis. Open the gun two or three turns and rotate it through before removing it with the buttonhole technique.
- Check the doughnuts and the anastomosis which should be 2–3cm above the oesophagogastric junction.
- Close the gastrostomy with a linear stapler or with two layers of Vicryl or PDS.

Stapling technique for transection of duodenum

Linear staple closure of the bowel is safe, haemostatic, and quick to perform. Closure of the duodenum by this method applies equally well to closure of other bowel segment.

Preparation, anaesthetic, position on the table, and incision are as for gastrectomy.

Procedure

- Mobilize the stomach during total or Polya gastrectomy.
- Prepare the duodenum for transection.
- Place a linear stapler (30 or 60mm long) just distal to the proposed transection line.
- Ensure that the catch is on and that the correct staple heights have been taken into account.
- Place a crushing clamp (Parker-Kerr or Payrs) adjacent and proximal to the linear stapler.
- Remove the safety catch and fire the staple.
- Divide the duodenum between the stapler and clamp-using knife.
- Remove the specimen or displace it medially.
- Open the jaws of the stapler and remove it.
- Check the staple line for bleeding. If there is a bleeding vessel, under run it with 2/0 Vicryl.
- Drainage to cover the risk of blowout is no more necessary than after hand-sewn closure.

A new lesser curve to the stomach during distal gastrectomy can be fashioned similarly using the longer 90mm linear stapler. Continuity can be re-established with a gastroenterostomy using a side-to-side stapler (Polya) or an end-to-end stapler to the duodenum (Bilroth I).

Stapling technique for gastroenterostomy

Stapled gastroenterostomy using a side-to-side technique is easy and rapid to perform in distal gastric resection or palliative proximal bypass for unresectable antral cancer.

Procedure

- After resecting the distal stomach or realizing that the antral cancer cannot be resected, bring up a loop of jejunum ante or retrocolically so that it reaches the stomach without tension.
- In palliative surgery exclude the distal stomach (the 90mm linear stapler is ideal for this).
- Position the jejunal loop with the afferent loop to the lesser curve so that the proposed stoma lies in the most dependent part of the stomach.
- Plan the position of the stomach and jejunal loop for stapling to ensure that vessels in the gastric arcade and jejunal mesentery are not embarrassed.
- Hold the proposed suture lines adjacent with four Babcock's forceps. Make two enterotomies opposite each other in the duodenum and stomach with diathermy.
- These should admit the jaws of a side-to-side stapler and be approximately 1cm across. Insert the open jaws of the stapler fully into each viscus and approximate the proximal end first.
- Ensure that the vessels and other structures are not incorporated and fire the stapler. Open the stapler and remove it.
- The anastomosis can be inspected for completeness and bleeding through the now single enterotomy.
- Close the enterotomy with two layers of continuous 2/0 Vicryl or with a linear stapler.
- It is not necessary to reinforce the staple line, but a Vicryl suture placed seromuscularly at each end of the anastomosis may take the strain off it.

Stapling technique for bowel resection and functional end-to-end anastomosis

After bowel resection, e.g. right hemicolectomy, an end-to-end anastomosis can be fashioned quickly using the side-to-side stapler.

Preparation, anaesthetic, position on the table, and incision are the same as conventional hand-sewn anastomosis.

Procedure
- After right hemicolectomy line up the distal ileum and transverse colon with their open lumina adjacent using Babcock's tissue forceps.
- Ensure that the mesentery of each viscus is as far away from the proposed anastomosis as possible. Ideally the staple line should run along the antimesenteric border.
- Insert the open jaws of the stapler down each bowel limb, close and fire.
- Open and remove the stapler and inspect the long side-to-side join.
- Close the open ends of the ileum and colon with two layers of continuous 2/0 Vicryl or by using a linear stapler.
- A similar palliative gastroenterostomy bypass can be fashioned quickly for an unresectable cancer by lining up two loops of bowel as in gastroenterostomy.

Stapling can be justified when operative procedures can be undertaken more quickly and easily. Stapling further facilitates other more complex operations. Such operations include small bowel pelvic pouches and Koch reservoir ileostomy, vertical banded gastroplasty (for obesity) and reverse gastric tubes. Oesophageal replacement using stomach, colon, or small bowel is also quicker using stapling techniques.

Stapling technique for prolapse and haemorrhoids

This operation involves excision, pulling up and anchoring of excess rectal mucosa using a circular stapler. The technique has been shown in several randomised trials to shorten anaesthetic time and in-patient stay, reduce pain scores and analgesic requirements allowing more rapid return to normal activities. Symptom control and functional outcome are comparable at 3 months follow up.

Position

Prone. Jackknife that allows good visibility and access.

Equipment

33mm haemorrhoidal circular stapler, suture threader, circular anal dilator, purse-string anoscope.

Procedure

- Insert the circular anal dilator and remove the obturator. This device allows easy introduction of the instruments and protects the internal sphincter.
- Suture the dilator to the anoderm.
- Identify the dentate line. Some surgeons infiltrate marcaine with adrenaline 0.5% into submucosa to contribute to analgesia and haemostasis.
- Introduce the purse-string suture anoscope through the anal dilator. Place 2/0 Prolene/Monocryl purse-string suture containing only rectal mucosa.
- Rotate the purse-string suture anoscope to allow the placement of purse-string suture around the entire circumference. Apply the suture at least 5cm above the dentate line. Pull the end gently to confirm mobility of the mucous membrane and to ensure no muscle bites have been taken.
- Apply KY Jelly® to head of gun to allow easy insertion through purse-string.
- Open the circular stapler fully and position its head proximal to the purse-string. Tie with one throw loose enough to allow tissue to slip down the shaft when traction is applied.
- Pull the ends of the suture through the lateral holes of the stapler and tie the knot externally. Introduce the cartridge housing of the stapler in the anal canal and confirm that the upper rim of staples is at least 2cm above the dentate line using cm marking.
- With moderate traction on the purse-string draw the prolapsed mucous membrane into the casing.
- Close the stapler tight enough to optimize haemostasis before firing. Open the circular stapler and extract the head. Examine the staple line using the purse-string suture anoscope.
- Apply any additional stitches if needed.
- Diclofenac (100 mg) and/or paracetamol (1g) suppositories can be inserted post-procedure and topical GTN 0.2% cream applied to ano-derm, to reduce iatrogenic anal fissures and sphincter spasm.
- Bleeding has been observed in approximately 20% of patients on stapler extraction: in 10% of cases haemostasis occurs spontaneously (within 5min), the remainder of patients will require the insertion of a 2/0 Vicryl suture to the bleeding point.

Hernias

F. Di Franco, G. R. McLatchie,
David J. Leaper

Inguinal hernia

Indications
- Elective: all symptomatic hernias need operation, particularly if indirect.
- Emergency: irreducible or strangulated hernias.

Preoperative preparation
- Elective: can be performed as a day case in patients fulfilling the criteria. Antibiotic prophylaxis if planning to perform a mesh repair.
- Emergency: IV fluids, antibiotic prophylaxis, and NG suction are required. Emergency situations associated with intestinal obstruction.

Position of patient
Supine.

Incision
- Make a curved inguinal incision in skin crease approximately 2cm above the medial two-thirds of the inguinal ligament.
- Incise fat and Scarpa's fascia, ligating the superficial epigastric veins which cross the line of incision.

Procedure
- Identify the external ring. Divide the external oblique aponeurosis along the line of its fibres over the inguinal canal. Open the external ring.
- Pay attention to the ilioinguinal nerve, which exits the external ring and the iliohypogastric nerve, which is superior.
- Apply artery forceps to the edges of the external oblique. Turn back the edges and identify the internal oblique and the conjoint tendon above the cord and inguinal ligament below. In the Shouldice repair divide the cremasteric muscle and open the fascia transversalis.

Indirect hernias
- Identify the sac after picking up the cord at its medial end. Split its investing fibres in the line of the cord and dissect the sac to its origin, avoiding injury to the vas deferens. Transfix the sac at its base and excise it, except when there is a sliding hernia in which case the sac should be reduced.
- Repair the transversalis fascia margins of the internal ring and repair the posterior wall of the inguinal canal with non-absorbable sutures.

Direct hernias
Push the sac inwards and repair the posterior wall. If the sac is very large divide the sac near its origin and leave the distal portion open.

Lichtenstein 'mesh' repair (see Fig.11.1)
This is now a popular procedure.
- Tailor the mesh as shown (made of Prolone or Marlex).
- Place the mesh over the conjoint tendon/internal oblique with the two limbs around the cord. It should overlap the pubic tubercle and the conjoint tendon and be adjacent to the inguinal ligament.

- By using monofilament stitches, suture the mesh to the inner surface of the inguinal ligament and conjoint tendon.
- Suture the tail ends of the mesh to one another around the cord.
- The mesh allows reinforcing the posterior wall of the inguinal canal in a 'tension free' fashion.

Shouldice repair (see Fig.11.2)

- Suture the lateral flap of the fascia transversalis to the under-surface of the medial flap.
- Suture the medial flap of the fascia transversalis to the anterior surface of the lateral flap.
- Suture the conjoint tendon to the inguinal ligament.
- The external oblique is closed anterior to the cord.
- Use non-absorbable monofilament sutures for the repair.

Bassini repair (see Fig.11.2)

This is no longer recommended because of the high risk of recurrence.
- It is performed by suturing the conjoint tendon to the inguinal ligament using a non-absorbable suture.

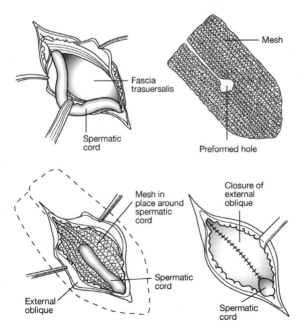

Fig. 11.1 Lichtenstein mesh repair

Closure

- Approximate the external oblique with an absorbable suture.
- Close the wound in layers with clips or a subcuticular suture to skin.
- Inject local anaesthetic at wound site and apply adhesive strips.

Complications

- Acute urinary retention
- Haematoma
- Wound infection
- Infection of the mesh
- Exacerbation of prostatic symptoms
- Chronic pain (trapping of the ilioinguinal nerve)
- Recurrence.

Bassini repair

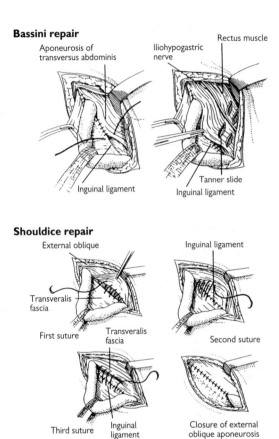

Aponeurosis of transversus abdominis

Inguinal ligament

Rectus muscle

Iliohypogastric nerve

Tanner slide

Inguinal ligament

Shouldice repair

External oblique

Transveralis fascia

First suture

Inguinal ligament

Second suture

Transveralis fascia

Third suture   Inguinal ligament

Closure of external oblique aponeurosis

Fig. 11.2 Inguinal hernia

Repair of femoral hernia (see Fig.11.3)

There are several approaches to the repair of femoral hernia which are all safe, but the operator must witness all of them and decide which procedure suits his/her needs most.

Position of patient

Supine, regardless the approach used.

McEvedy approach

Incision

Oblique vertical or transverse over the femoral canal with the lower part of the incision over the sac.

Procedure

- First isolate the sac by a preperitoneal approach through the external oblique aponeurosis and conjoint tendon.
- Open the transversalis fascia and dissect between it and the peritoneum to the neck of the sac. The inferior epigastric vessels may have to be divided in this plane.
- Reduce the sac by manipulating it from above and below. Then isolate and open it, ensure that it is empty, and transfix, ligate and divide it.
- Carry out the repair of the hernia by uniting the inguinal and pectineal ligaments for a distance of 0.5–1cm laterally without constricting the femoral vein. Use monofilament Nylon.
- Retract the vein laterally with an index finger, insert the stitch into the inguinal ligament, have your assistant retract the ligament upwards; take a large bite of the pectineal ligament. A single stitch may be all that is required. If not, insert a further stitch.

High approach

Incision

Inguinal incision about 1cm above the medial two-thirds of the inguinal ligament.

Procedure

- Identify the external oblique aponeurosis. Split it as for the approach to an inguinal hernia repair and then displace the cord or round ligament upwards.
- Incise the transversalis fascia in line with the incision to identify the neck of the sac and the external iliac vein.
- Gently isolate the sac, open it, and empty it. Then transfix, ligate, and divide it.
- Affect this by placing non-absorbable sutures between the pectineal ligament and the inguinal ligament, not constricting the femoral vein.

Low approach (not recommended for strangulation)

Incision

5–10cm long in the line of the groin crease, centred between the anterior superior iliac spine and the symphysis pubis.

Procedure
- Deepen the incision to identify the hernial sac. Ligate veins as necessary.
- Clean the sac, open and empty its contents, transfix, ligate and divide it, then carry out the repair as above.

Closure
Close the skin wounds with subcuticular sutures to the skin.

High approach

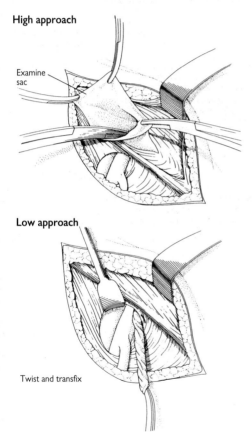

Examine sac

Low approach

Twist and transfix

Fig. 11.3 Repair of femoral hernia

Adult umbilical hernia (Mayo's 'vest over pants' repair)

Position of patient
Supine.

Incision
Horizontal elliptical (with excision of stretched skin).

Procedure
- Deepen the incision to reach the rectus sheath. Expose the neck of the sac. Open it in proximity of its neck. Return any protruding bowel to the peritoneal cavity.
- Any protruding omentum may be excised to reduce the volume of contents to be reduced. Remove the whole sac.
- Use non-absorbable mattress stitches.
- Suture the lower edge of the rectus behind the upper flap.
- Carry the upper flap down to overlap the lower flap.

Closure
Close the skin either with clips or a subcuticular suture.

Complications
- Rise in the intra-abdominal pressure due to the return of mesentery, bowel and omentum into the abdominal cavity.
- This may affect venous return and diaphragmatic movements leading to both circulatory and respiratory problems.
- Recurrence. Mesh repair is preferable in large umbilical hernias.

Epigastric hernia

Indications
- Symptomatic
- >2cm in diameter

Position of patient
Supine.

Incision
Vertical midline.

Procedure
- Deepen the incision around the margin of the hernia until healthy linea alba is identified.
- Then dissect towards the free edges of the sac. Excise the sac and repair the defect in the linea alba with non-absorbable sutures.

Closure
Close the skin either with clips or a subcuticular suture.

Incisional hernia

Aim
- To close the abdominal wall defect and prevent recurrence.
- Carry out either a side-to-side suture of healthy aponeurosis, overlap of the defect edges, or interposition of a prosthetic patch or mesh.

Position of patient
- Supine. Most hernias are midline.

Procedure
- Excise the old scar and deepen the incision around the margins of the hernia until healthy aponeurosis is identified.
- Dissect towards the free edges of the defect.
- Return the sac, intact if possible, to the peritoneal cavity and suture its margins together.
- Clean the edges of the defect so that they are easily approximated.

Options
1. If the defect edges come together easily, suture them with continuous (mass type closure) or interrupted Nylon sutures.
2. Create a two-layer closure by incising along the edges of the muscular defect. Suture the opposing sides together in two layers.
3. Overlap the edges of the defect in two layers of sutures. Do this only if no tension is created.
4. The 'keel' repair involves inversion of the sac with suture of its margins followed by several layers of sutures to invert the edges of the defect.
5. If the defect is large or if there is only tension caused by approximation, use a mesh (Marlex or Prolene) or a patch (Teflon) to close the defect. Suture the prosthesis all the way round the palpable margins of the defect.

Closure
- Close the skin with clips, or interrupted, or subcuticular Nylon sutures.
- Bring a suction drain through a separate stab wound. When using a prosthesis give prophylactic antibiotics.
- Large defects can be closed with 2 layers of mesh, inlay and onlay, to the musculofascial margins of the defect.

Peripheral vascular surgery

A. E. Clason

Arterial anastomosis

Aim

The aim of arterial anastomosis is to achieve a watertight closure/join between the conduits concerned without tension and without compromise of the lumen. This is facilitated by first excising the adventitia. The intimal surface should be protected from damage. Gentleness at all times is mandatory and it is a vital principle of all anastomoses that the edges should always be everted to allow apposition of the intima of the artery with the graft lining.

Materials

Vascular sutures are usually produced with a needle at each end and polypropylene (Prolene) of various gauges is the commonest used. In general 3/0 Prolene is used for the aorta, whilst 4/0, 5/0, or 6/0 are used for smaller vessels. 8/0 to 10/0 sutures may be used in the formation of micro vascular anastomoses. Taper cut needles allow easier penetration of atheromatous vessels.

Arteriotomy

This is best fashioned longitudinally for several reasons:
- Longitudinal easier to close than transverse
- Easier to extend if necessary
- Transverse more difficult as intima tends to retract away from the edges.

Incise the artery wall with a 15 blade knife and extend the arteriotomy incision with Potts scissors taking care not to create any intimal flaps.

Techniques

Anastomosis may be end-to-end or end-to-side. Insert the sutures from inside to outside the artery and from outside to inside the graft. This avoids displacement of the intima and creation of intimal flaps that may occlude the vessel.

End-to-end (see Fig. 12.1A)

- Insert one of the double-ended needles from inside to outside the proximal end of the artery at the centre point of the back wall and the other similarly from inside to outside of the distal end, tying the knot on the outside.
- Take each needle and suture round the circumference of the vessel with an over-and-over stitch till you reach the centre of the front wall and tie both ends of the suture together on the outside of the artery. Avoid tension on the anastomosis and intimal damage. A continuous suture is appropriate in large vessels but interrupted (either simple or everting mattress) may be more suitable for smaller vessels.
- When it is possible to rotate the vessel the anastomosis may be facilitated by dividing the circumference into three with stay sutures and rotating the vessel by gentle traction on the stay sutures.

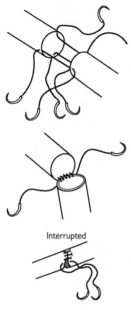

Interrupted

Fig. 12.1A End-to-end arterial anastomosis

- In the case of end-to-end suture of a graft to a large vessel, use a polypropylene suture and place the first four or five sutures before pulling down the graft, thus facilitating careful placement of sutures in the back wall (see Parachute technique). It is not necessary to cut the vessel completely across but approximately halfway or two thirds, so that it is opened like the leaves of a book. It is important to take an adequate bite of the posterior wall of the artery and pull it up. Then snug the graft down by pulling both ends of the suture at right angles to the artery wall and complete the suture line by a continuous over-and-over stitch till the sutures meet tying the knot externally.
- Wherever smaller vessels are to be anastomosed, cut the vessel ends obliquely. This increases the length of the suture line and reduces tension and the risk of stenosis.
- Pass two double-ended polypropylene sutures through the opposing ends of the vessel. Tie one end and hold the other in a rubber-shod mosquito forceps. Use one end of the tied suture to sew over and over to the other corner. On completion of one side rotate the vessel and
complete the second side similarly.

End-to-side (see Fig. 12.1B)
This is the standard form of anastomosis used for bypass procedures.
- Use a double ended vascular suture and pass the needles from outside—in on the graft side—out on the artery.
- Fashion an arteriotomy as above and cut the graft obliquely tailoring the length of the oblique cut to match the arteriotomy and spatulating the end by an 'S' shaped cut to form a 'cobra head'.
- Place a double-ended stitch from outside to inside in the heel of the graft and then pass both needles from inside to out at the proximal apex of the arteriotomy and tie the knot on the outside. Either anchor the toe of the graft to the distal apex of the arteriotomy with a separate double ended suture or leave it free (the latter allows clearer view of the inside of the anastomosis). Run the suture down each side of the anastomosis to beyond the mid point and retain the ends in rubber shod forceps.
- Now either take one suture around the lowermost part of the anastomosis to meet the second or alternatively insert a further stitch in the toe of the graft at the lower apex and complete either side, tying the knots on the outside of the artery.

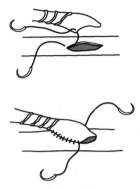

Fig. 12.1B End-to-end arterial anastomosis

Variation: parachute technique (see Fig. 12.1C)

With the graft and the recipient artery separated, place a number of running stitches from outside the graft to inside the apex of the arteriotomy at the heel, beginning from the mid point of the faraway wall and continuing around the heel without tying the knot (ensure no snagging). Then gently pull the suture ends at right angles to the artery wall as the vessels are approximated. Then complete the suture line as above.

Patch angioplasty (see Fig. 12.1D)

If the vessel being opened is <4mm in diameter or if it is desired to widen the lumen of a stenosed vessel (see Profundaplasty) then achieve closure of the vessel by patch angioplasty.

- Use a patch of autologous vein for small vessels (never sacrifice the proximal end of the long saphenous vein but rather harvest the vein patch from the ankle or a tributary). For larger vessels use a patch of Dacron or PTFE.
- Shape the patch to match the arteriotomy/defect and fix either end with a double ended stitch passing both needles from outside the patch to inside and inside to outside of the artery wall at the apex. Complete the suture line with a running stitch but do not finish at the apex, rather go round either side to the middle.

(C) Parachute technique

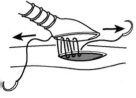

(D) Vein patch

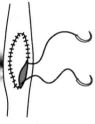

Fig. 12.1C and **D** Arterial anastomosis techniques

Exposure of major blood vessels

Carotid (see Fig. 12.2A)

Position
Supine with the neck extended (place a pad between shoulder blades and support the head in rubber ring). Turn the head to the contralateral side.

Incision
Along the anterior border of sternomastoid extending from 2cm below the angle of the jaw to just above the clavicle.

Procedure
- Divide the platysma and incise the deep fascia, divide the common facial vein and retract the internal jugular vein posteriorly.
- Mobilise the common carotid, superior thyroid, external and internal carotid arteries and control them with slings. The ansa cervicalis lies anterior to the vessels and leads superiorly to the hypoglossal nerve whilst the vagus nerve lies lateral to and posterior to the vessels. The carotid sinus nerves lie in the bifurcation above the artery.
- Divide the stylohyoid and digastric muscles if greater access to the internal carotid is required, as in the case of high bifurcation of the vessels.

Vertebral (see Fig. 12.2A)

Position
As for carotid.

Procedure
- Make an oblique incision lateral to sternomastoid, expose the internal jugular vein and retracted laterally to expose the vagus nerve.
- Dissect out the carotid artery and retract it medially and continue dissection in the angle between the artery and vein to expose the vertebral artery and vein crossed by the cervical sympathetic chain. Expose the lower part of the vertebral artery and the origin of the subclavian by downward dissection dividing the sympathetic chain and the vertebral vein.

Subclavian (see Fig. 12.2B)

Position
As for carotid.

Procedure
- Make a 10cm incision above medial half of clavicle and lateral to the insertion of sternomastoid muscle. Deepen the incision by dividing clavicular head of sternomastoid, platysma and deep fascia to expose omohyoid and fat pad with lymph node which is displaced superiorly.
- Identify the phrenic nerve lying in the anterior aspect of scalenus anterior and passing downward and medially, and protect it. Identify the brachial plexus and protect it laterally.
- Divide scalenus anterior over a blunt instrument to reveal the subclavian artery and the suprascapular and internal mammary branches.

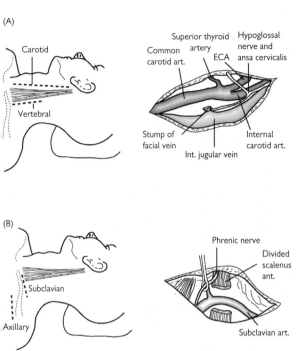

Fig. 12.2 Exposure of carotid and subclavian arteries

Distal subclavian/axillary artery (see Fig. 12.2B)
Position
As for Carotid.

Procedure
- Expose the distal subclavian artery as for Subclavian extending the incision over the clavicle, divide the clavicle if necessary.
- Approach the proximal axillary artery via a 10cm incision below the middle third of the clavicle.
- Incise the skin and deep fascia to expose the fibres of pectoralis major, split them and insert a self retaining retractor. Define the axillary artery in the depth of the wound. Exposure of the vessel may be aided by division or detachment of pectoralis minor from the coracoid process, the acromioclaviclar branches, if necessary, to allow full mobilization.

Brachial artery (see Fig. 12.2C)
Position
Supine with the arm on table and the hand isolated in a sterile translucent bag.

Procedure
- In the upper arm by an incision placed along the medial border, just behind biceps muscle. Divide skin and deep fascia and retract biceps anteriorly and triceps posteriorly. The median nerve lies anterior and superior to the artery.
- Achieve exposure of the brachial artery at the elbow by an S-shaped incision in the anticubital fossa. Expose the bicipital aponeurosis and divide it to expose the brachial artery and its bifurcation to radial and ulnar arteries, passing between brachioradialis and the flexor muscles. The median nerve and basilic vein are posteromedial to the artery.

Radial artery (see Fig. 12.2C)
Procedure
- Expose the radial artery via a vertical incision in the anterior aspect of the forearm.
- Expose it proximally by dissection between brachioradialis medially and flexor carpi radialis.
- Expose it at the wrist by a vertical incision beginning at the radial styloid. The cephalic vein lies above the deep fascia and the radial artery below it.
- Incise the deep fascia to expose the artery and its accompanying veins.

Ulnar artery (see Fig. 12.2C)
- Expose the ulnar artery likewise via vertical forearm incisions.
- Expose it proximally by dissection of pronator teres and the brachioradialis laterally and the flexor digitorum. The artery is found between them.
- For exposure at the wrist make a similar vertical incision medial to flexor digitorum and the ulnar styloid. The ulnar artery lies slightly deeper than its radial counterpart, expose it as it passes below the flexor retinaculum.

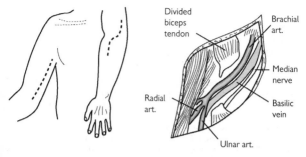

Fig. 12.2C Exposure of brachial artery

Exposure of the abdominal aorta (see Fig. 12.2D)

Position

Supine.

Incision

Long midline skirting umbilicus, transverse, or retroperitoneal.

Procedure

- Place self retaining retractors (Balfour, Finochetti, Omnitract) in the wound. Lift the transverse colon out of the wound or pack it under the upper abdomen/lower thorax. Displace the small bowel to the right and wrap it in moist packs in a gut bag.
- Expose the *coeliac axis* after opening the lesser omentum to identify the diaphragmatic crura. Divide them to reveal the aorta and origin of the coeliac axis. Supracoeliac approach can be used to gain rapid control of the aorta in the case of aortic rupture.
- Expose the *splenic artery* by dividing the greater omentum along the lower border of the stomach. Retract the stomach proximally to expose the upper margin of the pancreas and the splenic vessels.
- Expose the *superior mesenteric artery* by careful caudal dissection along the aorta utilising the supracoeliac approach as described above. An alternative and quicker approach to the SMA is via the root of the small bowel mesentery. Displace the transverse colon upwards and, with the small bowel to the right, expose the SMA in the small bowel mesentery using the point at which the middle colic artery ascends in the transverse mesocolon as a guide.
- To expose *the infrarenal aorta, renal arteries, and the aortic bifurcation* identify the peritoneum overlying the aorta and divide it over the bifurcation upwards to the right of the inferior mesenteric artery, mobilizing the duodenum to the right (you may need to divide the inferior mesenteric vein to gain access). Identify the left renal vein and carefully mobilise it passing a sling around it. The vein can be lifted or divided to expose the renal vessels.
- To expose each common iliac, lift the overlying peritoneum and divide it taking care to preserve the ureters and iliac veins (often adherent to the artery) and continue the exposure to the iliac bifurcation and origin of the internal iliac.

Common/external iliac artery (see Fig. 12.2E)

Incision

Oblique incision in iliac fossa lateral to edge of rectus sheath.

Procedure

- Deepen the incision and divide the abdominal wall muscles to expose the peritoneum which is displaced medially identifying the ureter and the iliac vessels.
- Insert deep self-retaining retractors to allow access. Expose the internal iliac by encircling the common and external iliac arteries with slings and pulling the vessel laterally to allow exposure of the origin of the internal iliac.

(D) Abdominal aorta

(E) Iliac vessels

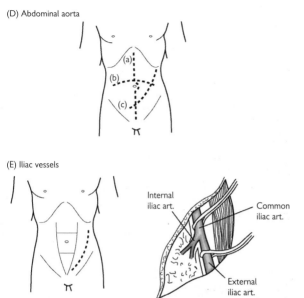

Fig. 12.2 Exposure of (D) abdominal aorta and (E) iliac arteries

Common femoral/profunda femoris arteries
(see Fig. 12.2F)

Incision

The surface marking for the common femoral artery is the mid inguinal point, halfway between the anterior superior iliac spine and the pubic tubercle.

Make 10–12cm vertical incision two fingerbreadths lateral to pubic tubercle extending one third above and two thirds below the inguinal ligament or over the palpable femoral pulse. Feel for the pulsation with your fingers. If exposure of the long saphenous vein is required use a lazy S incision curving medially over the vein.

Procedure

- Incise the fat and fascia and insert a Travers retractor. Do not cut across lymph nodes and ligate lymphatics. Feel for the pulse and expose the femoral sheath and incise longitudinally.
- Mobilise the artery using sharp dissection, ligating and dividing any small veins to allow exposure of the *common femoral* and the *superficial femoral* arteries. Pass a Lahey clamp under each vessel and draw a sling around each.
- Expose the *profunda* by gentle traction on the slings around the above vessels and pass a sling around it. Expose the profunda further. Divide the small vein which crosses it a short distance from its origin, this reveals the first bifurcation and the profunda vein. Ligate it and divide it to allow dissection to proceed distally.

Above knee popliteal artery (see Fig. 12.2G)

Incision

Longitudinal. Along the medial aspect of the lower thigh along the anterior border of Sartorius or over the previously marked long saphenous vein if a vein graft is contemplated.

Procedure

- Deepen the incision through the subcutaneous fat to expose the Sartorius and retract it posteriorly to reveal the neurovascular bundle and popliteal fat pad. The artery lies close to the bone and the nerve is some way away with the vein in-between.
- Gently mobilise sufficient artery to gain proximal and distal control with plastic slings passed around it using a Lahey clamp.

Below knee popliteal artery (see Fig. 12.2H)

Incision

Longitudinal over the medial aspect of the calf along the border of gastrocnemius 2cm below medial border of tibia.

Procedure

- With the knee flexed, deepen the incision and incise the deep fascia, sweep the fat pad and gastrocnemius away and retract it posteriorly.

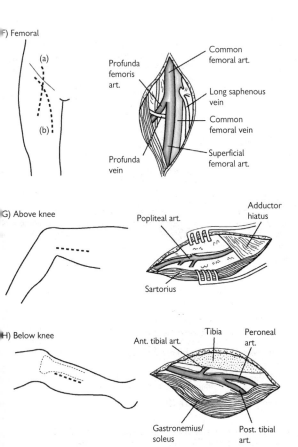

Fig. 12.2 Exposure of (F) femoral, (G) above knee, and (H) below knee arteries

- Continue dissection between the medial head of gastrocnemius and the tibia to expose the neurovascular bundle. Expose the vein first, carefully lifting it away to allow access to the artery. Mobilize a sufficient length for anastomosis passing slings proximally and distally. Proximal exposure of the artery is improved by dividing the tendons o sartorius, semimembranous, and gracilis.
- Divide soleal arch and detaching it from the medial border of the tibia dissection distally will expose the origin of the *anterior tibial artery and* allow access to the *tibioperoneal trunk*.

Crural vessels

Anterior tibial artery (see Fig. 12.2I)

Incision

Over the anterior tibial muscles on the lateral aspect of the calf, latera to the anterior tibial border.

Procedure

Dissect between the muscles in the line of their fibres to expose th artery lying deep on the interosseus membrane with the venae comm tantes. Dissect and mobilize the artery. This is aided by good retractio with a self retainer.

Posterior tibial artery

Incision

Longitudinal on the medial aspect of the distal calf centred over the junction of gastrocnemius and the Achilles tendon.

Procedure

- Deepen the incision and divide the deep fascia, develop the plane between gastrocnemius and soleus muscles to reveal the posterior tibial vessels and nerve on the surface of soleus, separate the artery by careful dissection.
- Alternatively find the artery more superficially by incising the deep fascia and retinaculum behind the medial malleolus.

Peroneal artery (see Fig. 12.2J)

Incision

- Longitudinal over lateral aspect of distal leg, expose the fibula and remove a segment. The artery lies behind the fibula.
- Alternatively approach as for the posterior tibial artery, split the latera fibres of soleus/flexor hallucis longus to reveal the peroneal artery.

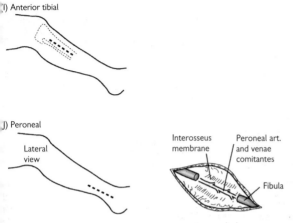

Fig. 12.2 Exposure of (I) anterior tibial and (J) peroneal arteries

Profundaplasty

The profunda femoris is part of an extensive vertical collateral network from the internal iliac to the tibial vessels and remains relatively free of disease when the other lower limb arteries are affected by atherosclerotic occlusion.

Indications
- Significant stenosis or occlusion of the origin or proximal portion of the deep femoral artery.
- Lower limb ischaemia with no possibility of femoropopliteal reconstruction.
- Adjunct to inflow procedure in multisegment disease (aorto-femoral/axillofemoral or femorofemoral graft).
- Limb salvage procedure in failed distal bypass.
- To aid healing of below knee amputation if profunda diseased.

Position of patient
Supine.

Procedure (see Fig. 12.3)
- Make a vertical incision over the common femoral artery, 5cm above the inguinal crease extending distally depending upon the length of the profunda to be exposed.
- Expose and mobilise the common femoral, profunda femoris and superficial femoral arteries and pass slings around them (the superficial femoral should be mobilised a variable distance as the outer wall of the vessel may be used as a patch). Dissect the profunda downwards dividing the small vein which crosses the primary stem to expose the first bifurcation and the profunda vein which should also be divided. Continue dissection along the artery can be continued until a satisfactory length of the vessel is exposed, and identify a soft portion for arteriotomy, controlling any muscular branches with slings.
- Give the patient 5000 IU heparin and apply vascular clamps to the common femoral and profunda vessels.
- Make an arteriotomy in a soft portion of the common femoral artery and extend it into the profunda. If there is occlusive atheroma proximally perform a local endarterectomy securing the distal flap with tacking sutures of 6/0 Prolene. Check for forward and backward bleeding and close the arteriotomy with a patch (vein, Dacron, PTFE, tongue of graft or adjacent SFA wall).
- Approach the mid portion of the profunda through an anterior thigh incision along edge of sartorius; retract it laterally to expose the superficial femoral artery. Retract the superficial femoral artery medially and incise the fascia deep to the vessel to expose the profunda deep to the 2nd and 3rd perforator branches.

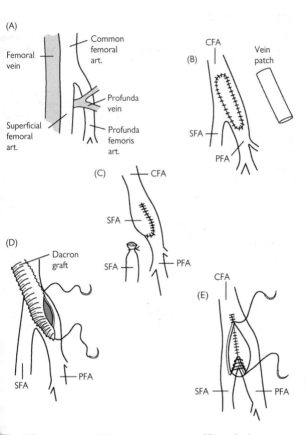

Fig. 12.3 Profundaplasty. CFA, common femoral artery; PFA, profunda artery; SFA, superficial femoral artery

Endarterectomy

Most frequently utilised in the internal carotid artery. It basically consists of removing the core of atheromatous and/or thrombotic material causing occlusion or stenosis of the vessel.

Indications

Restoration of blood flow in an artery with either a short occlusion or stenosis and in which the vessel is otherwise normal above and below the lesion. Heavily calcified vessels may not be suitable due to the risk of repeated vessel fracture and uncontrollable haemorrhage on application of clamps, but may be feasible using balloon occlusion catheters to gain control proximally and distally.

Procedure

• Expose the diseased artery and gain proximal and distal control of the vessel with slings.
• Apply arterial clamps above and below the lesion following systemic anticoagulation and the artery opened by a longitudinal incision along the length of the stenosed segment.
• Identify the plane of cleavage between the diseased and non-diseased zones of the arterial wall in the media and using a Watson-Cheyne dissector carefully separate the atheroma from the vessel wall. Then loosen the atheromatous core above and below being extra vigilant distally not to leave a loose flap. Secure the distal intimal division point by tacking sutures of a fine monofilament suture placed in through the endarterectomised artery and out through the non-endarterectomised wall, anchoring the flap. Close moderate sized arteries with a continuous or interrupted Prolene suture. Use a patch angioplasty for smaller arteries or if there is a risk of vessel stenosis.

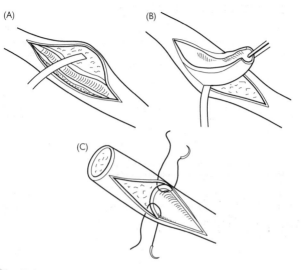

Fig. 12.4 Endarterectomy

Carotid endarterectomy

Aims
- Prevention of stroke by removal of the source of embolic material.
- Improvement in cerebral function by the removal of atheromatous occlusive material from the carotid bifurcation and origin of the internal carotid artery.

Indications
Symptomatic carotid occlusive disease with:
- Transient ischaemic attack
- Stroke with good functional recovery
- Reversible ischaemic neurological deficit (RIND)
- Amaurosis fugax
- >70% symptomatic stenosis—clear indication
  40–70% stenosis—if failed medical treatment.

Position
Supine with the neck extended and head supported on a ring, pad placed longitudinally between the shoulder blades and head turned toward the opposite side

Anaesthesia
General or local anaesthesia.
- Local anaesthesia allows evaluation of tolerance to cerebral clamping with/without the aid of transcranial Doppler assessment but disadvantage is restlessness/agitation of patient and patient/surgeon anxiety.
- General anaesthesia gives better control and the duration is unlimited.

Incision
- Vertical parallel to the anterior border of sternomastoid, the length is dependent on the location of bifurcation (X-ray, MRA).
- Oblique skin crease incision.

Procedure (see Fig. 12.5)
- Have all instruments (clamps and shunt) ready and available before the start. There are various shunts (Pruitt (balloon) Javid (clamps)) and snugging devices (Rummel).
- Divide the platysma and incise the fascia.
- Expose and divide the common facial vein and any anterior venous tributaries (facial vein is a useful marker of level of bifurcation).
- Enter the carotid sheath and carefully mobilise the common carotid artery passing a sling around it, keeping manipulation of the bifurcation to a minimum to avoid embolisation. If bradycardia ensues inject 1–2ml of 1% lignocaine into the tissues between the internal and external carotid vessels.
- Mobilize the hypoglossal nerve and protect it with a sling.
- Mobilize the internal carotid above the visible plaque and pass a sling. If there is a high bifurcation or access to the internal carotid is difficult, it can be improved by division of the posterior belly of the digastric muscle.

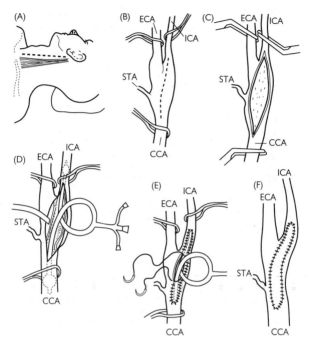

Fig. 12.5 Carotid endarterectomy. CCA, common carotid artery; ECA, external carotid artery; ICA, internal carotid artery; STA, superior thyroid artery

- Treat the external carotid and superior thyroid vessels similarly.
- Ask the anaesthetist to give the patient 4000–5000IU heparin intravenously, wait a suitable time for circulation before applying the vascular clamps, cross-clamping the internal carotid first to prevent debris entering it, followed by the common carotid and external carotid.
- Make an incision in the common carotid and extend it proximally to the palpable and visible limit of the diseased segment of the internal carotid revealing healthy intima.
- Insert the shunt with great care (it is the authors' practice to routinely shunt), beyond the diseased segment of the internal carotid and backbleed whilst releasing the internal carotid clamp and insert the backbleeding proximal end of the shunt into the common carotid artery and secure it ensuring a haemostatic fit at both ends of the shunt. Now perform careful endarterectomy in the appropriate plane using a Watson-Cheyne dissector. Transect the atheromatous core proximally and distally with iris scissors before completing the endarterectomy by avulsion of the core from the external carotid origin. Separation of the upper end of the core may result in feathering of the intima with no need for securing tacking sutures. It may, however, also create a step in the intima. Secure this with 3–4 tacking sutures of 6/0 Prolene. Carry out meticulous removal of any fragments of intima from the endarterectomy site and close the endarterectomy with a patch angioplasty (Dacron/Bovine pericardium/PTFE) with 6/0 Prolene.
- Before closing the anastomosis, remove the shunt, reapply the vascular clamps and flush the anastomotic site with heparinised saline. Release the clamps on completion of the anastomosis in the following order: external carotid, common carotid and internal carotid.
- Insert a suction drain and repair the carotid sheath and platysma with an absorbable suture, using staples or a subcuticular suture for the skin.

Prophylaxis

Give a single dose of antibiotic intravenously preoperatively. Postoperatively give aspirin 75mg/day and/or clopidogrel 75mg/day.

Complications

- Stroke
- Haematoma
- Haemorrhage
- Cranial nerve Injury.

Endovascular carotid stent

This technique is presently experimental and largely performed by or in conjunction with a vascular radiologist.

Patient selection

- Symptomatic high grade stenosis
- Surgical restenosis
- Hostile neck (burns/radiotherapy/high bifurcation)
- Possibly patients for CABG with concomitant carotid disease.

Preparation

Commence on clopidogrel 75mg/day prior to stent procedure.

Procedure

- Prepare the groin as for arteriography and gain arterial access to the common femoral artery percutaneously via the groin.
- Administer 5000IU heparin via the arteriography sheath. Introduce a stiff guide wire (0.035) and advance it with care into the external carotid artery to allow placement of a long sheath/catheter in the common carotid artery. Given the patient atropine and size the internal carotid artery using a catheter sheath or externally placed coin for reference.
- Pass a 0.014 wire across the stenotic segment in the internal carotid artery and pass a cerebral protection device along the wire and deployed to catch any debris.
- Pass a low profile balloon catheter of the appropriate size across the lesion with a 15 second inflation time, then exchange it along the wire for a self expanding stent deployed to abolish the stenosis.
- Obtain post deployment angiograms and remove the cerebral protection device and guide wires.

Excision of carotid body tumour

Carotid body tumours are rare and may be extremely vascular. Their excision may rarely involve excision of the carotid bifurcation or sacrifice of the external carotid artery. Handling of the tumour may result in significant haemodynamic upset and an experienced anaesthesia is essential. Dissection should proceed with great care.

Preoperative preparation

- Accurate localisation and diagnosis of the tumour by CT or MRI imaging.
- Vascular anaesthetic pre-assessment.

Position

Supine with the head of the table slightly raised, the head supported on a ring and extended to the opposite side away from the incision. A pad placed longitudinally between the shoulder blades.

Incision

Along the anterior border of the sternomastoid, from 2–3cm above its insertion to two fingerbreadths below the angle of the jaw.

Procedure (see Fig. 12.6)

- Expose the carotid bifurcation, preserve the greater auricular nerve. Dissect the internal jugular vein from the artery dividing the facial vein and anterior tributaries and retract the muscle with a Travers retractor. Dissect the internal jugular vein from the artery carefully preserving the vagus nerve in the groove between the artery and vein.
- Preserve the ansa cervicalis if possible and expose the common carotid proximally and the external and internal carotids distally passing slings around them.
- Identify and preserve the hypoglossal nerve which crosses the internal and external carotid vessels above the bifurcation.
- Begin with the external carotid side of the tumour and divide the plane between the tumour and the vessel wall. Numerous tiny vessels from the tumour to the vessel wall often make this dissection bloody. Secure them with bipolar diathermy. As dissection proceeds proximally, split the tumour along its midline. If the tumour completely surrounds the vessels divide it with diathermy to identify the plane, again on the external carotid side. It may be necessary to divide the external carotid to remove the tumour completely.
- Rarely when the tumour cannot be safely removed, as above, it may be necessary to resect the carotid bifurcation and re-establish vascular continuity to the internal carotid by insertion of a vein/prosthetic graft (see Resection of aneurysmal internal carotid artery).

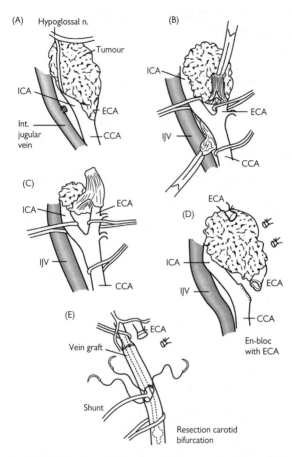

Fig. 12.6 Excision of carotid body tumour. CCA, common carotid artery; ECA, external carotid artery; ICA, internal carotid artery; STA, superior thyroid artery

Aneurysmal internal carotid artery repair

Aims
- To restore normal circulation
- To prevent risk of rupture, embolus and/or thrombosis associated with aneurysmal disease of the vessel.

Indications
Established aneurysmal disease of the extracranial internal carotid artery in a patient fit for surgery.

Preparation
- Vascular anaesthetic preassessment.
- MRA or CT angiographic assessment of the extracranial vessels and the Circle of Willis.

Position
Supine with the head extended, supported on a ring and turned away from the side to be operated upon with a pad placed between the shoulder blades.

Incision
Along the anterior border of the sternomastoid from two fingerbreadths below the angle of the jaw to just above the muscle insertion.

Procedure (see Fig. 12.7)
- Expose the carotid vessels as in carotid endarterectomy. Handle the aneurysm as little as possible to minimise the risk of dislodgement of any clot and subsequent embolisation. Control the vessels proximally and distally first, passing slings around them. Either ligate the external carotid artery or suture closed from within the opened aneurysm sac.
- Ask the anaesthetist to give 4000–5000IU heparin intravenously and apply vascular clamps to the carotid vessels. Open the aneurysm longitudinally; the neck of the aneurysm is usually clearly defined.
- Insert a Javid shunt into the internal carotid and pass the shunt through an appropriate length of a synthetic graft (woven Dacron/PTFE), backbleed the internal carotid through the shunt and insert the backbleeding shunt into the common carotid artery, applying ring clamps and/or snuggers to keep it in place and secure haemostasis at either end of the shunt.
- Suture the graft end-to-end starting with the internal carotid and beginning the suture in the middle of the posterior wall, working around each side to the front wall. Complete a continuous suture line to the posterior wall of the common carotid artery leaving a small gap on the anterior wall incomplete.
- Clamp the common and internal carotid arteries and remove the shunt, flushing the graft with heparinised saline to remove clots and debris and complete the anastomosis on the anterior wall of the common carotid.

- Release the clamps on the common carotid followed by the internal carotid securing haemostasis at the anastomotic lines as necessary.
- Plicate the opened aneurysm sac around the synthetic graft using an absorbable suture, insert a suction drain and close the wound in layers with either staples or a subcuticular suture for the skin.

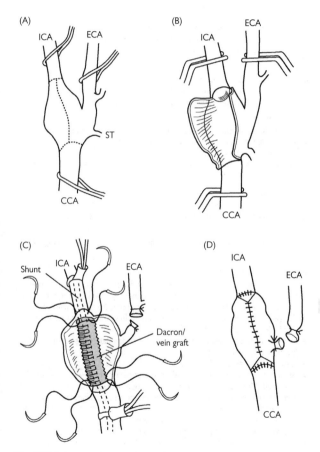

Fig. 12.7 Aneurysmal internal carotid artery repair. CCA, common carotid artery; ECA, external carotid artery; ICA, internal carotid artery; STA, superior thyroid artery

Sympathectomy

Thoracic sympathectomy

Aims

- To achieve permanent sympathetic blockade in the upper limb.
- No objective evidence for its use in pain syndromes or Raynaud's disease
- Primary indication is hyperhidrosis
- Also used in facial flushing/blushing(nerves of Kuntz)
- Less commonly—upper limb Ischaemia/post traumatic pain/rare cardiac arrhythmias (long QT syndrome)

Options

- Endoscopic—preferred option
- Open—transcervical/supraclavicular/transaxillary—when endoscopic not feasible (pleural adhesions, previous thoracic surgery).

Endoscopic

- 2nd and 3rd thoracic ganglia for supply to arteries and hands
- 4th thoracic ganglion for eccrine axillary glands
- Possible to do bilateral.

Take care to avoid azygos vein and tributaries on right and subclavian and aortic arch on the left.

Anaesthetic

General anaesthesia with either a single or double lumen tube, the latter facilitating collapse of ipsilateral lung to improve access to the chain.

Position

Supine with the arm(s) abducted to 90°, chest and axilla prepared and draped.

Procedure (see Fig. 12.8)

- Make a 10mm stab incision in the skin and subcutaneous tissues over the 4th intercostal interspace in the mid axillary line. Feel for the rib and ask the anaesthetist to deflate the appropriate lung if using a double lumen tube, insert a Verres needle into the pleural cavity and instil 700cc of carbon dioxide.
- Insert a 10mm laparoscopic port via the midaxillary incision and introduce the video camera.
- Orient the anatomical structures.
- Now make a 5mm stab incision on the anterior chest wall over the 3rd intercostal interspace and insert a 23 gauge hypodermic needle under direct vision to act as a guide for the insertion of a 5mm laparoscopic port through which a diathermy hook is inserted. Using the hook and video telescope displace the lung posteriorly to identify the thoracic sympathetic chain running below the pleura over the necks of the ribs.
- Open the pleura over the 2nd rib (the subclavian artery courses over the top of the 1st rib), elevate the chain and divide it using diathermy. Repeat the process over the 3rd and 4th ribs.

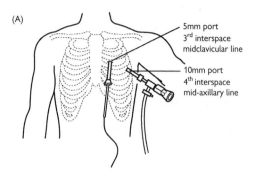

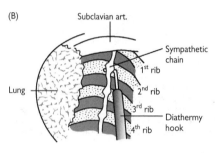

Fig. 12.8 Endoscopic thoracic sympathectomy

- To ensure obliteration of the nerves of Kuntz, if dealing with facial flushing or blushing, apply diathermy to the periosteum of the dissected rib necks on either side of the divided chain.
- Verify haemostasis and evacuate the carbon dioxide asking the anaesthetist to hand re-inflate the lung whilst re-expansion is confirmed on the video monitor.
- Remove the ports and close the wounds with absorbable sutures and steristrips to the skin

Open supraclavicular approach

Position
Supine on the operating table under general anaesthesia, with feet down tilt and the head turned to the opposite side.

Incision
Make a short 10cm long incision above the medial one third of the clavicle.

Procedure
- Deepen the incision and divide the clavicular head of sternomastoid.
- Identify the phrenic nerve running downwards from lateral to medial on the surface of scalenus anterior and mobilise it passing a sling around it. Elevate the nerve and divide scalenus anterior to expose the subclavian artery which is retracted inferiorly. Palpate the first rib and expose Sibson's fascia. Divide the fascia and expose the pleura which is pushed inferiorly and anteriorly to reveal the neck of the 1st rib and the stellate ganglion with the sympathetic chain palpable as a cord. Use good light and deep retractors to visualise the ganglion and the chain. Divide the stellate ganglion in its lower third to avoid a Horner's syndrome, elevate the chain and dissect it as far inferiorly as is safe below the third ganglion.
- Ensure haemostasis and check for pneumothorax by asking the anaesthetist to inflate the lungs before inserting a suction drain and closing the wound in layers with a subcuticular stitch for the skin

Complications
- Horner's Syndrome
- Pneumothorax
- Neuralgia.

Axillary transthoracic
Avoid in patients with apical pleural adhesions. Better access to the chain below the stellate ganglion than afforded by supraclavicular approach but first thoracic ganglion is not easily accessible.

Position
Lateral position with the arm supported to avoid brachial plexus traction.

Incision
Transverse incision in the axilla below the hair bearing zone in the line of the 3rd rib and approximately 15cm long.

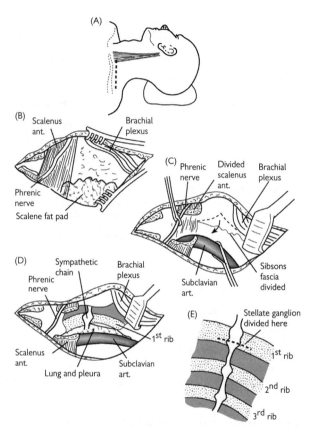

Fig. 12.9 Open supraclavicular cervical sympathectomy

Procedure
- Deepen incision through the fat of the axilla preserving the intercosto-brachial nerve, identify and retract the long thoracic nerve (beware of injury to this if the wound is extended).
- Enter the thorax via the 2nd interspace or by excision of a portion of the 3rd rib inserting rib retractors to provide access.
- Displace the lung downwards and retract it to expose the sympathetic chain lying below the posterior pleura.
- Incise the pleura over the chain, elevate the chain and excise it to the desired level.
- Ensure haemostasis, insert a chest drain and allow the lung to re-inflate, approximate the ribs and close the periosteum and muscle with a Nylon suture and the skin with a subcuticular absorbable suture.
- Perform a post operative chest X-ray to ensure no persistent pneumothorax and remove the chest drain at 24hrs.

Lumbar sympathectomy
- Relatively minor role in the management of vascular disease
- Maximal effects on blood flow in cutaneous arteriovenous anastomoses with small increase in tissue perfusion
- Results in alteration in extremity blood flow distribution and in pain impulse transmission

Indications
- Causalgia—if trial of LA blockade beneficial
- Ischaemic rest pain > ulcers—ABPI >0.3/absent neuropathy/limited tissue loss
- Small shallow ulcers/single digit gangrene—ABPI >0.3.

Techniques
- Phenol block/chemical sympathectomy
- Open surgical sympathectomy.

Phenol block
Useful in elderly/unfit patients and performed under image intensifier control.

Position
The patient lies on side with the side for injection uppermost.

Procedure
- Prepare the area between the 12th rib and the iliac crest with antiseptic solution. Infiltrate two sites corresponding to the position of the 2nd and 3rd lumbar vertebrae with local anaesthetic a few centimetres apart at the upper edge of quadratus lumborum and insert a spinal needle via the skin bleb and direct towards the vertebral column.
- When this is felt the needle is carefully marched forward tangentially and eased forward to penetrate the edge of the psoas sheath. Perform aspiration to ensure a blood vessel has not been penetrated and inject a few ml of dilute contrast medium slowly to ensure correct positioning of the needle. This is revealed by a satisfactory spread of contrast along the psoas sheath.

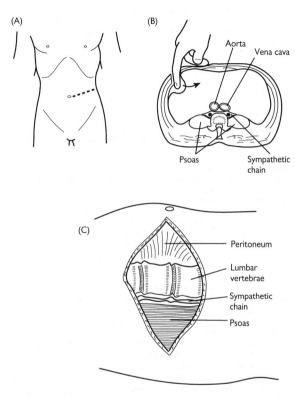

Fig. 12.10 Lumbar sympathectomy

- If satisfactory spread is observed slowly inject 3–5ml of 6% phenol in water into the space stopping after each millilitre for a minute or so, checking that the patient is comfortable. Repeat the process at the second site.

Complications
Neuralgia of upper thigh and groin.

Surgical sympathectomy (see Fig 12.10)

Position
The anaesthetised patient lies supine with a sandbag/padded rolls placed under the hip and thorax of the side to be operated on so that the interval between costal margin and iliac crest is opened and the table broken to 15°.

Incision
Oblique/transverse incision from the edge of the rectus sheath to approximately the anterior axillary line, halfway between the anterior superior iliac spine and the 12th rib.

Procedure
- Divide the musculofascial layers (external/internal oblique/ transversalis) or split them in the line of their fibres.
- Develop the lateral plane between transversalis and the peritoneum with the fingers and sweep the peritoneum towards the vertebral column. The ureter and gonadal vessels are left attached to the posterior peritoneum. Identify the anterolateral edge of psoas.
- Insert two deep retractors and feel for the sympathetic chain medial to psoas, lying over the transverse processes in the groove between the muscle and the vertebral column (take care to avoid the more lateral genitofemoral nerve).
- On the left the chain lies adjacent to the aorta and on the right just beneath the edge of the vena cava (take care!) Pick up the chain with a nerve hook and remove at least 2–3 ganglia placing ligaclips on the rami communicantes and diminish any bleeding with diathermy.
- Insert a suction drain and close the wound in layers with an absorbable suture to the muscle layers and subcuticular suture to the skin.

Repair of abdominal aortic aneurysm

Most abdominal aortic aneurysms are asymptomatic and less than 5% are suprarenal. Data from the UK small aneurysm trial suggests that at least in males surgical intervention is not required until the maximum transverse diameter of the aneurysm exceeds 5.5cm. Operative mortality for elective surgery is in the order of 3–5% but that for ruptured aneurysms is in excess of 40%. Screening for aneurysm disease has been associated with a reduced mortality rate for rupture (MASS Trial)

Preoperative preparation
- Accurate imaging and diagnosis—B mode ultrasound/CT scan/MRI
- Preoperative blockade reduces left ventricular workload.

Perioperative management
- Good intravenous access/intra-arterial pressure recording/urinary catheter/central venous line or Swan Ganz
- Haematological status/biochemistry
- Cross match 4–6 units of blood for elective surgery and 10 units for rupture.

Position
Supine with the arms abducted to 90° with a warming blanket appropriately applied.

Approaches/incision
Transperitoneal
- Midline xiphisternum to pubis
- Transverse mid-abdominal.

Retroperitoneal
- Left side usually (easier to mobilise the spleen)
- Hostile abdomen/stoma/horseshoe kidney
- May be difficult to access right iliac.

Endovascular
- Access by exposure of the groin arteries.

Transperitoneal
- Enter the peritoneal cavity and perform a thorough laparotomy to exclude concomitant pathology. Displace the transverse colon superiorly, divide the ligament of Treitz and displace the small bowel to the right between moist packs in a gut bag. ('Onion peel' the duodenum if an inflammatory aneurysm).
- Insert a fixed self-retaining retractor (Omnitract). Identify and retract/divide the inferior mesenteric vein. Incise the posterior peritoneum from lower border of pancreas to iliac arteries and identify the neck of the aneurysm (usually just below the left renal vein).
- Avoid incising the autonomic nerves (avoids sexual dysfunction in men) pass a sling around the left renal vein and lift it superiorly (take care—beware of the tributaries to the lumbar veins). Dissect the neck of the aneurysm and the iliac arteries.

- Apply a supracoeliac clamp if aneurysm neck is juxtarenal. Heparinise the patient with 5000IU heparin intravenously and apply arterial clamps to the iliac arteries and to the aorta.
- Open the aneurysm sac longitudinally away from the inferior mesenteric artery (IMA). Incise the proximal aorta transversely at the proposed anastomotic site. Remove the thrombus/atheroma and oversew any backbleeding lumbar arteries with 3/0 Prolene. Control the IMA temporarily with a bulldog clamp if it is patent. There is often a distinct ring at the proximal neck. If the bifurcation is healthy it may be suitable for a tube graft, if not, use a bifurcated graft.
- Select a suitable graft (if a bifurcation graft ensure it is long enough for the limbs to reach the groins) and suture it in position proximally end to end with 2/0 or 3/0 Prolene sutures taking good bites of the aortic wall. If the aortic wall is friable pledgelets of Dacron (from the redundant graft) can be incorporated in the anastomotic line.
- After completion of the anastomosis, clamp the graft and slowly release the proximal aortic clamp and check for suture line bleeding. Transfer the aortic clamp to the graft below and close to the anastomotic line and the flush graft with heparinised saline. Now complete the lower anastomosis similarly (if a tube graft) or if a bifurcation graft to either the iliac bifurcation (after opening iliac aneurysm) or to the junction of the common femoral arteries with the profunda and superficial femoral arteries (via retroperitoneal tunnels) after tying off the common iliac arteries. Complete the anastomosis to the iliac or femoral vessels with a 4/0 or 5/0 Prolene suture. Restore blood flow with slow release of the aortic clamps (warn the anaesthetist in advance to avoid declamping shock).
- Next assess the adequacy of lower limb perfusion by visual inspection of the feet/palpation of pulses. When adequacy of gut/limb perfusion and haemostasis has been secured plicate the aneurysm sac over the graft with an absorbable suture to prevent the formation of an aortoduodenal fistula and repair the peritoneum with Vicryl.
- Close the abdomen in layers or with a mass suture using non-absorbable suture material.

Retroperitoneal
Position
The left shoulder is elevated to 45° with the pelvis flat.

Incision
Make an incision centred on the 11th/12th rib, beginning at the lateral edge of the rectus sheath and curved laterally to the tip of the 12th rib.

Procedure
- Divide the underlying abdominal muscles and expose the peritoneum.
- Develop the retroperitoneal plane either anterior/posterior to the left kidney (anterior for most infrarenal aneurysms). For juxtarenal/suprarenal aneurysms mobilise the kidney anteriorly to allow an approach to the aorta behind the left renal artery.

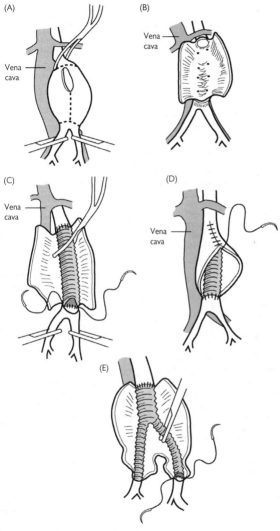

Fig. 12.11 Bifurcation graft

- Divide the inferior mesenteric artery to allow more complete access.
- If access to the right iliac artery is required extend the wound with division of the rectus muscle and/or make a separate right iliac fossa incision.
- Repair of the aneurysm and insert the graft as described above.

Endovascular

Preoperative assessment

Same intervention criteria as for open repair (maximum diameter >5.5cm).

- Maximum transverse diameter >5.5cm
- Proximal neck diameter 16–30mm diameter(no thrombus/plaque/calcification)
- Minimal iliac diameter 6–8mm
- Neck configuration not reversed cone and >15mm long
- Neck angulation <60°
- Evaluation of aneurysm by spiral CT scan, calibrated aortography
- Full anaesthetic preoperative assessment.

Position

Supine on an X-ray table/endovascular operating table under general epidural anaesthesia and with a radio-opaque ruler placed below the back to allow accurate assessment of deployment.

Incisions

Bilateral groin incisions either vertically or in the skin crease to expose and mobilize the femoral vessels (common femoral, profunda and superficial femoral) passing slings for control.

Procedure ('TALENT' device)

- Exposed the groin vessels. Give 5000IU heparin intravenously and apply arterial clamps to the profunda and superficial femoral arteries bilaterally. Make bilateral arterial punctures in the common femoral artery using an angiography needle and pass a soft guide wire into the aorta via a 6F sheath placed in each common femoral artery.
- Insert a 5F pigtail catheter via the left common femoral into the suprarenal aorta to allow peri-procedure imaging. Exchange the soft guide wire in the right femoral for a stiff Backup Meier wire and perform pre-deployment angiography to identify the renal artery origins whose position is marked on the X-ray monitor screen.
- Insert the main part of the modular bifurcated device is inserted over the Backup Meier and carefully advanced into the suprarenal aorta having ensured correct alignment of the contralateral limb markers. Begin the deployment of the device slowly and carefully to expose the suprarenal fixating bare stent and check the position of the renal arteries again by angiography.
- Now slowly drag the stent caudally until the upper fabric markers lie just below the origins of the renal arteries and continue deployment opening the stent into the right iliac system and deploying the short contralateral limb. Carry out moulding of the deployed stent rings using the included balloon.

- Now replace the left pigtail catheter with a stiff guide wire passed through the short limb of the stent graft (position checked by lateral views) and deploy the second modular component of the stent graft system within the short limb with a satisfactory overlap of the fabric markers. Mould the stent rings as before and iliac extensions if necessary.
- Carry out post implantation angiography to ensure no endoleaks.
- Repair the femoral artery insertion sites with 5/0 Prolene and close the wounds in layers.

Postoperative follow-up

Spiral CT scans and plain abdominal X-ray initially 3 monthly then annually to check for integrity/displacement or stent fracture.

Embolectomy

Aim to restore the circulation to the pre-occlusive state. It is often currently required in patients with advanced arteriosclerosis and underlying or medical comorbidity. It may be difficult to distinguish between embolus and thrombosis so preoperative angiography, although not always possible is the ideal and identifies the site, multiplicity and associated vascular disease allowing planning of any necessary reconstruction. Embolectomy using a Fogarty catheter is not without its complications and injurious effects and care must be exercised in performing this procedure.

Indications
- Loss of circulation due to embolus.
- Most are due to myocardial disease particularly atrial fibrillation and myocardial infarction but they may originate from in situ atheroma or thrombus (peripheral/aortic aneurysm).

Anaesthesia
Most embolectomies can be performed using local anaesthesia with intravenous sedation but GA may be occasionally required.

Basic principles
- Expose an adequate length of artery to gain proximal and distal control of the vessel(s) and pass slings around them.
- Next administer 4000–5000IU heparin systemically and apply arterial clamps.
- Open the artery through a longitudinal incision and check the artery lumen for visible embolic material. Check the balloon inflation/ deflation and introduce the uninflated balloon catheter into the artery, advancing it with care as far as it will proceed without resistance. Gentle retrieval of the inflated balloon is then performed partially deflating the balloon on resistance to adjust for calibre (plaque or narrowing). Remove the retrieved thrombus/embolus and flush the vessels with heparinised saline via a Tibbs cannula before closing the arteriotomy with either a continuous Prolene suture or patch angioplasty if there is a risk of narrowing.
- Use a single lumen/irrigating Fogarty catheter with a compliant balloon. Normally a size 3F will be suitable for the axillary/brachial artery, 4F for the common/superficial femoral artery and 5F for the aortic bifurcation.

Brachial embolectomy
Position
Supine with the affected arm extended on a board and the hand in a sterile/translucent bag.

Incision
Lazy S incision crossing the elbow joint to give access to the brachial artery and its trifurcation.

Procedure (see Fig. 12.12)
- Deepen the incision to expose the artery dividing the biceps tendon if necessary. The median nerve may be in the vicinity so care should be exercised as it sometimes lies superficial to the artery.
- Mobilise the artery and the trifurcation vessels passing slings around them for control.
- Make a vertical arteriotomy just above the trifurcation and proceed as above passing a 3F Fogarty catheter down each of the vessels distally, ensuring that there is backbleeding by releasing the tension on the slings. Ensure there is also forceful forward flow by releasing the proximal clamp. If insufficient flow, pass the catheter proximally to retrieve clot and restore flow.
- Flush the vessels, reapply the clamps and close the arteriotomy with 6/0 Prolene.

Femoral embolectomy

Position
Supine with both groins prepared and draped in case a crossover graft is required and with the foot in a sterile translucent bag.

Incision
Vertical groin incision over the femoral artery.

Procedure
- Expose and mobilise the groin vessels, passing slings around them for control. Give systemic heparin and clamp the arteries.
- Fashion a vertical arteriotomy and remove obvious clot with forceps. Pass a 3F/4F Fogarty catheter distally in the SFA and profunda, as described above, to retrieve propagated clot and ensure good backflow on withdrawal of the inflated balloon, making several passes to ensure that all clot is removed. (You may require two catheters, the first will likely enter the tibioperoneal trunk and the second will be guided into the anterior tibial.)
- Flush the vessels with heparinised saline and reapply the clamps. Pass a 4F/5F Fogarty catheter into the aorta until forceful downflow is re-established, flushing the vessel with heparinised saline.
- Before closure of the arteriotomy perform on table angiography to assess the distal vessels. If there is significant residual clot, instil 5mg of rTPA (Anteplase) and wait for 10min before reassessing and closing the arteriotomy with 5/0 or 6/0 Prolene.

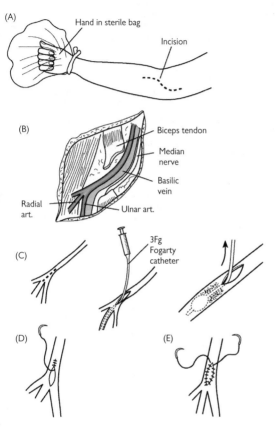

Fig. 12.12 Brachial embolectomy

In the case of a Saddle embolus, fashion bilateral groin incisions and expose and control the femoral vessels as above. Make an arteriotomy in the common femoral artery just above the bifurcation and proceed as above to remove the propagated clot from the distal vessels and proximal inflow.

Popliteal embolectomy

Position
Supine as for exposure of the infragenicular popliteal vessels.

Procedure
- Expose and mobilise the popliteal artery and tibioperoneal trunk, controlling the vessels with slings.
- Make an arteriotomy in the popliteal artery opposite the origin of the anterior tibial and proceed as described above using a 3F Fogarty catheter for the distal vessels and a 3F/4F catheter proximally.

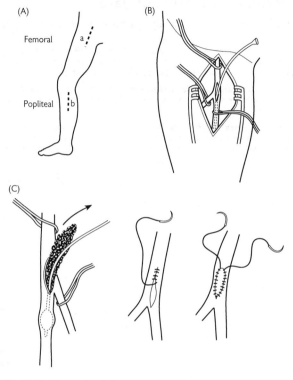

Fig. 12.13 Infrainguinal embolectomy

Aortoiliac occlusive disease

The *therapeutic options* for treatment of aortoiliac disease include:

Catheter based endovascular treatment by angioplasty with/without intravascular stent placement has largely replaced operative treatment in localised iliac disease but patient selection is of paramount importance and it is not appropriate in diffuse iliac disease.

Extra-anatomic reconstruction may be the treatment of choice in high risk unfit patients with more limited disease not suitable for angioplasty/stent.

Aortobifemoral graft is the most durable and efficacious treatment and is indicated in patients with total infrarenal aortic occlusion, those with severe bifurcation disease or diffuse aortoiliac disease with critical ischaemia. The bifurcated graft can be sutured to the aorta either by an end-to-side technique or by an end-to-end suture after the aorta has been completely divided and the aortic bifurcation oversewn. The procedure may also be utilised in the treatment of complex aortoiliac aneurysmal disease.

End-to-end
• Better haemodynamically/less turbulence
• Lower false aneurysm rate
• Easier to cover with natural tissue in the aortic bed.

End-to-side
• Avoids sacrifice of patent inferior mesenteric artery
• Appropriate in retention of aberrant renal artery.

Incision
Vertical midline/transverse centred on umbilicus or oblique. Bilateral longitudinal groin incisions centred on the mid-inguinal point.

Procedure
• Expose the femoral vessels first, passing slings around them for control. Next expose the aorta, making a transverse incision 2cm above the umbilicus and extending to 2cm beyond the lateral border of the rectus sheath on both sides.
• Displace the omentum and transverse colon superiorly. Incise the posterior peritoneum on the left margin of the duodenum and displace it and the small bowel wrapped in a moist pack to the right in a gut bag. Expose the aorta, crossed by the left renal vein and then expose the bifurcation and the iliac arteries.
• Mobilise the aorta and pass a tape/sling around it dividing lumbar vessels as necessary. Give the patient 5000IU heparin and cross-clamp the aorta and iliac vessels as necessary.

If there is total occlusion of the aorta, transect the aorta and oversew the bifurcation with 3/0 Prolene. Now finger compress the aorta at the level of the renal vein to remove the clot and then apply the aortic clamp, flushing the stump with heparinised saline.

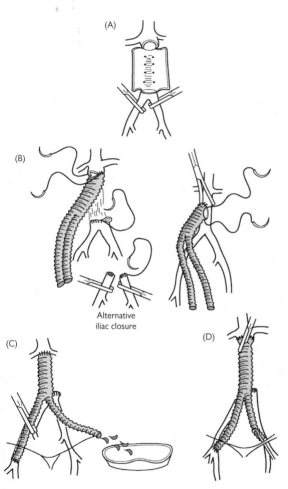

(A)

(B)

Alternative
iliac closure

(C)

(D)

Fig. 12.14 Aortobifemoral graft

- Select a Dacron bifurcation graft of an appropriate size and remove all but 2–3cm of the trunk (otherwise the legs may kink due to the sharp angle). Affect an end-to-end anastomosis between the divided aorta and graft using continuous 3/0 Prolene using the parachute technique or beginning in the middle of the posterior wall.
- Apply a vascular clamp to the graft close to the anastomotic line and test the top, releasing the aortic clamp slowly and oversewing any obvious leak to ensure the join is watertight.
- Fashion retroperitoneal tunnels to the groins by finger dissection, following the iliac artery to the common femoral in the groin and taking care not to tear the small veins just above the inguinal ligament.
- Bring the limbs of the graft to the groins ensuring maintenance of the orientation of the limbs.
- Apply vascular clamps to the common femoral, superficial femoral and deep femoral arteries. Make a longitudinal arteriotomy in the common femoral artery just above the bifurcation. Now apply gentle traction to the limb of the graft to draw out the crimping and trim the graft obliquely in order to affect and end-to-side anastomosis to the common femoral artery with continuous 5/0 Prolene. Having completed the first limb, vent the graft through the non-attached limb and flush the limb with heparinised saline before completing the 2nd limb anastomosis as for the contralateral side. Check there is adequate lower limb perfusion by visible inspection of the feet.

For an end-to-side anastomosis of prosthetic graft it may be possible to gain control of the aorta by application of a Satinsky clamp and a bulldog clamp to the inferior mesenteric artery, otherwise proceed as above. Make a longitudinal incision in the aorta, select a suitable bifurcated graft and trim the trunk as above cutting the graft obliquely to fashion a 'cobra head' and anastomose it to the aorta with a continuous 3/0 Prolene double-ended vascular stitch, starting at the heel. When the suture line is complete, clamp the prosthesis close to the suture line and slowly release the aortic clamps. Fashion the retroperitoneal tunnels and complete the femoral anastomoses as described above. Suture the peritoneum over the graft with an absorbable suture and close the abdominal wound in layers and the skin with a subcuticular suture or staples.

Extra-anatomic bypass

In these bypass procedures the prostheses pass through an anatomic pathway significantly different from that of the native vessels they bypass and include:
- Axillofemoral—unifemoral/bifemoral
- Femorofemoral
- Carotid-subclavian bypass
- Obturator bypass.

Axillobifemoral graft (5 year patency 30–85%)

Indications

This is an appropriate procedure in patients with aortoiliac disease and reasonable distal run off who are unfit for major aortic surgery. It may also be an option where direct abdominal reconstruction is prohibited by risk or a hostile abdomen, in patients with severe cardiac disease or morbid obesity. In addition it is a mechanism of revascularisation of the limbs when an infected aortic graft requires removal.

Incisions

Bilateral groin as for exposure of the femoral vessels and subclavian incision centred on mid-clavicle approximately 10cm long.

Position

The donor arm abducted and supported on a board.

Procedure (see Fig. 12.15)

The procedure may be carried out under light general anaesthesia or local anaesthesia.
- Prepare the chest and lower abdomen and both groins. Expose the axillary artery via a subclavian incision as above by splitting the fibres of pectoralis major and exposing the deltopectoral fascia. A self-retaining Travers retractor is inserted, the axillary artery identified below the deltopectoral fascia lying below the vein and brachial plexus. (Exposure of the artery may be enhanced by dividing pectoralis minor). Divide the acromioclavicular branches and mobilise a 5–6cm segment of artery controlling it with slings.

The groin dissections are as for the exposure of the common, superficial and deep femoral arteries.
- Make a small transverse incision over the 6–7th interspace in the anterior axillary line to facilitate passage of the graft from the axilla to the groins.
- Give the patient 5000IU heparin intravenously and clamp the axillary artery.
- Select a suitable Dacron graft (approximately twice the diameter of the recipient vessel—usually 8mm). Tunnel the graft subcutaneously to the groins.

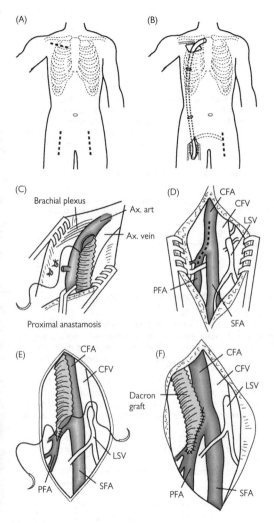

Fig. 12.15 Axillobifemoral graft

- Fashion a longitudinal arteriotomy and cut the graft obliquely and anastomosed end-to-side to the axillary artery using a continuous 5/0 Prolene suture beginning at one corner of the back wall and progressing continuously to the front. When the anastomosis is complete, clamp the graft just proximal to the suture line and release the clamps to restore blood flow to the arm.
- Next apply clamps to the common, superficial and deep femoral arteries, now apply gentle traction to the graft which is tailored and the limbs anastomosed to the common femoral artery on either side using an end-to-side technique with continuous 5/0 Prolene, the cross limb of the graft being tunnelled subcutaneously suprapubically.
- Having completed the anastomoses release the clamps ensure haemostasis and close the wounds in layers with a subcuticular suture or staples to the skin.

Femorofemoral graft (5 year patency 60–80%)

Indications
- Unilateral iliac occlusive disease not amenable to stenting.
- Patients with adequate circulation in one leg with patent iliofemoral vessels on the donor limb.

The operation can be done under local anaesthesia in unfit patients. It may be used as a limb salvage procedure in patients with a patent profunda femoris artery on the symptomatic side with rest pain but in the absence of gangrene.

Exposure
Expose the groin vessels bilaterally through vertical incisions.

Procedure (see Fig. 12.16)
- Using finger dissection or a tunnelling instrument fashion a subcutaneous tunnel suprapubically between the two groin incisions and pass an 8mm Dacron graft through the tunnel from one side to the other (Fig. 12.16A). Alternatively, the graft can be taken from the common iliac to femoral artery (Fig 12.16B).
- Give the patient 5000IU heparin and apply vascular clamps to the common femoral artery and its branches on the donor side.
- Make a longitudinal incision in the common femoral artery and carry out an end-to-side anastomosis with a continuous 5/0 Prolene suture (Fig. 12.16C and D).
- Apply a vascular clamp to the graft adjacent to the completed anastomosis and release the femoral clamps to restore circulation to the donor limb.
- On the ischaemic side make a longitudinal incision in the common femoral artery extending into the origin and first part of the profunda femoris.
- Tailor the graft obliquely applying gentle traction to reduce the crimping and fashion an end-to-side anastomosis with continuous 5/0 or 6/0 Prolene (Fig. 12.16E).
- Release the clamps and ensure haemostasis before closing the wounds in layers.

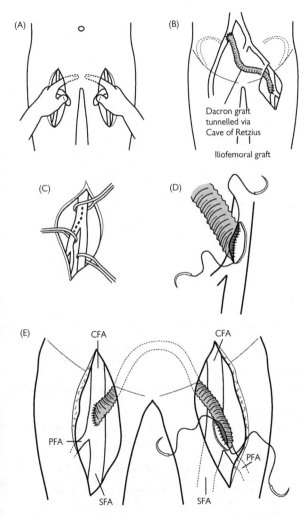

Fig. 12.16 Iliofemoral and femorofemoral graft

Iliofemoral/unilateral aortofemoral/iliopopliteal

Indications

Unilateral iliac occlusive disease, not suitable for angioplasty or stent

Incision

In flank gently curved incision from costal margin to lateral edge of rectus sheath and 2–3cm above the inguinal ligament. Distally vertical incision in the groin or lower thigh.

Procedure

- Divide the external oblique in the line of its fibres, cut the internal oblique and transversalis in the line of the incision and using finger dissection open up the retroperitoneal space, displacing the peritoneum medially.
- Identify the aortic bifurcation, common and external iliac vessels and control them with slings. Insert a self retaining retractor.
- Select an appropriate graft (8mm Dacron/PTFE). Give the patient 5000IU heparin, clamp the appropriate vessels proximally and distally and make a longitudinal arteriotomy (aorta/iliac).
- Trim the graft obliquely and fashion an end-to-side anastomosis with continuous 4/0 or 5/0 Prolene. Clamp the graft just distal to the suture line and release the vessel clamps.
- Tunnel the graft to the groin or popliteal incision, clamp the vessels proximally and distally and fashion an end-to-side anastomosis to the arteriotomy with continuous Prolene. Close the wounds in layers.

Carotid to subclavian bypass

Indications

- Subclavian steal syndrome
- Occlusive disease of the proximal subclavian
- It may be a preoperative requirement in endovascular stenting of thoracic aortic dissection or thoracic aortic aneurysm if stent placement is required to cover the orifice of the subclavian.

Position

Supine with the head turned to the opposite side and a pad under the shoulders.

Incision

6–8 cm incision parallel to and 1–2cm above the medial third of the clavicle.

Procedure (see Fig. 12.17)

- Make a supraclavicular incision 2cm above the medial end of the clavicle extending from the clavicular head of the sternomastoid. Divide the platysma and clavicular head of the sternomastoid and dissect through the fascia and the scalene fat pad (take care to avoid the thoracic duct on the left).
- Identify the phrenic nerve on the scalenus anterior and preserve it. Divide the scalenus anterior and locate the subclavian with the thyrocervical trunk and free it. The brachial plexus lies laterally in the wound.

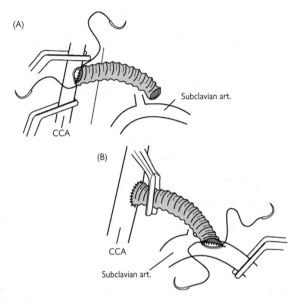

Fig. 12.17 Carotid-subclavian bypass

- Expose the carotid artery in the medial aspect of the incision by retraction of the sternal head of sternomastoid. Dissect anterior to the internal jugular vein, open the carotid sheath and mobilise the common carotid artery passing slings to control the vessel.
- Heparinise the patient with 5000IU heparin and apply clamps to the subclavian and then the carotid.
- Select a suitable Dacron graft and fashion the carotid anastomosis end-to-side first at right angles to the carotid. The graft is brought either anterior or posterior to the jugular vein and clamped adjacent to the anastomosis the carotid clamps being removed to restore cerebral circulation.
- Now tailor the graft to length and cut it obliquely to match the arteriotomy in the subclavian artery and fashion an end-to-side anastomosis to the artery.
- Secure haemostasis and close the wound in layers.

Obturator bypass

Indications

- Graft sepsis localised to the groin
- Crush injury to the groin
- Infected femoral aneurysms in IV drug abuser.

Position

Supine with the entire leg prepared to allow abduction/lateral rotation. The groin wound is covered with an adhesive drape and the skin of the thigh is prepared.

Procedure

- Expose the iliac vessels by a retroperitoneal approach. If there is no infection in the patent graft it may be used as the donor site (unlikely), otherwise use the common iliac or aorta as a donor site.
- Locate the obturator foramen just posterior to the superior pubic ramus by following the obturator nerve along the pelvic brim.
- Reflect the peritoneum from the external iliac towards the pubic ramus. Incise the obturator membrane anteriorly and medially to avoid the nerve and vessels.
- Expose the above knee popliteal artery via a vertical skin incision displace the sartorius posteriorly and mobilise the artery with slings.
- Tunnel a suitable graft to the supragenicular incision via the obturator foramen. Give the patient 5000IU heparin and clamp the iliac vessel.
- Make a longitudinal arteriotomy, cut the graft obliquely and fashion an end to side anastomosis with continuous 5/0 Prolene. When the anastomosis is complete clamp the graft adjacent to the suture line and release the iliac or aortic clamps ensuring the join is watertight. Fashion a similar anastomosis to the popliteal artery above the knee.
- Close the wounds in layers.

Infrainguinal bypass

Aims

To restore the circulation to the lower limb affected by occlusive vascular disease.

Indications

- Crippling intermittent claudication—the majority of claudicants are managed by interventional radiological procedures or conservatively
- Critical ischaemia
- Limb salvage.

These bypass procedures make use of the native long saphenous vein (reversed vein graft/in situ vein graft) or a prosthetic graft of either Dacron or PTFE or a prosthetic graft with a distal vein cuff/patch. The graft is attached proximally to the common femoral artery and distally to the above knee/below knee popliteal artery (femoropopliteal bypass) or to the infracrural vessels in the case of femorodistal bypass for limb salvage.

Preoperative preparations

Good quality arteriography to define the extent of the disease and to assess the distal run-off.

Position

Supine with the knee flexed to 45°, the hip flexed and externally rotated. Prepare the lower abdomen, groin and entire leg, placing the foot in a sterile, transparent bag. If a prosthetic graft is to be used administer a broad spectrum antibiotic at induction of anaesthetic.

Incisions

See access to major blood vessels (p392) for exposure of the groin and popliteal vessels.

Femoropopliteal bypass grafting

Procedure

- Make the initial incision vertically in the groin across the inguinal crease following the line of the long saphenous vein.
- Expose the femoral vessels in the groin and either the above knee or below knee popliteal artery.
- Mobilise the common femoral, SFA and profunda arteries as normal (ligate overlying lymphatics to avoid lymphocele). If a *reversed vein graft/in situ vein graft* is contemplated preoperative vein mapping is helpful.
- Using finger dissection expose the entire length of the necessary long saphenous vein, ligating the venous tributaries with silk or an absorbable tie (4/0) or ligaclips ensuring you do not compromise the vein by ligating too close to the main trunk.

- Leave the vein in situ until the moment of harvest. When both the donor and recipient site vessels have been exposed, mobilised, and slung with tapes, remove the vein and attach a bulldog clamp to the upper end of the reversed vein. Using a Tibbs cannula of appropriate size flush the reversed vein with heparinised saline and check for leaks before marking the vein with an ink line along its length to help avoid twisting during its passage along the subsartorial tunnel.
- Pass a tunnelling instrument subsartorially between the donor and recipient incision sites (an additional small above knee incision as for exposure of the above knee popliteal artery may help in tunnelling to a below knee site). In the case of a *synthetic graft* (usually 6/8mm Dacron/PTFE) pass the graft as above through the tunnel ensuring no kinks and straighten the leg to ensure there is a sufficient length of graft or vein to reach the target vessels without tension or excess.
- Give the patient 5000IU heparin intravenously and apply arterial clamps and fashion an arteriotomy with a 15 blade knife extending it with Potts scissors to an appropriate length.
- Spatulate the end of the vein or synthetic graft and anastomose to the distal vessel with a continuous 5/0 or 6/0 Prolene. A similar anastomosis is fashioned end-to-side to the common femoral artery using a 5/0 Prolene suture. Release the clamps and ensure good flow in the graft.
- Having ensured haemostasis, close the wounds in layers.

In situ vein graft

May be used in femoropopliteal reconstruction as above or in femorodistal grafting for limb salvage where the distal anastomosis is fashioned to the anterior tibial, posterior tibial or peroneal arteries (for exposure of these vessels see p392–5). The minimum diameter of vein acceptable as a conduit is 3mm.

Procedure (see Fig. 12.18)
- Expose the femoral vessels as above and the recipient vessels likewise. Expose the long saphenous vein throughout its length taking care not to undermine the skin flaps. Ligate the side branches and the saphenofemoral junction exposed, its branches being divided and ligated.
- Apply a paediatric Cooley clamp to the common femoral vein and the saphenofemoral junction disconnected leaving a cuff of common femoral vein exposed so that it can be oversewn with a continuous 5/0 or 6/0 Prolene suture and the Cooley clamp removed. The first valves in the long saphenous vein are divided under direct vision and clamps applied to the femoral vessels.
- Fashion a vertical arteriotomy in the common femoral artery (the site is determined by the position of the saphenofemoral junction relative to the bifurcation of the common femoral artery) and carry out an end-to-side arteriovenous anastomosis carried out with continuous 5/0 or 6/0 Prolene. After completion release the occluding clamps and blood flow is established in the vein to the next competent valve.

- Pass a Halls/LeMaitre vein valve cutter retrogradely from below through the anastomosis and withdrawn it to achieve valvulotomy evidenced by pulsatile blood flow throughout the graft (several passes rotating the cutters may be necessary). Achieve appropriate control of the distal vessels; trim the graft to length and spatulate the end. Anastomose the graft to a suitable site on the popliteal artery or one of its three branches below the knee.
- Check that the foot is perfused and for pulses either by palpation or using Doppler. Close the wounds in layers.

Adjuvant techniques in infragenicular prosthetic grafts

The patency of below knee prosthetic grafts may be improved by the use of interposition vein cuffs or patches

The Miller cuff (see Fig. 12.19)

- Harvest a segment of vein 3–4mm diameter from a suitable site (lateral tributary of long saphenous vein or short saphenous vein).
- Open the vein longitudinally along its length and place a double ended suture (5/0 or 6/0 Prolene) in the middle of the posterior wall of the arteriotomy and the middle of the vein sheet with the intimal surface innermost.
- Suture around the apex and heel of the arteriotomy until the two ends meet in the middle of the anterior wall of the arteriotomy. Trim the excess vein and sutured together the vein cuff ends. Now cut the distal end of the PTFE graft obliquely to match the length of the cuff and sutured to it with continuous 5/0 or 6/0 Prolene.

The Taylor patch (see Fig. 12.19)

- Harvest a segment of vein and open it as described above.
- Cut the PTFE graft obliquely and the heel is sutured to the proximal apex of the arteriotomy.
- Make a 2cm longitudinal incision in the toe of the graft. Trim the corners of the vein patch and suture it to the apex of the arteriotomy taking care to avoid any narrowing and continue the suturing proximally along the arteriotomy and PTFE incision.

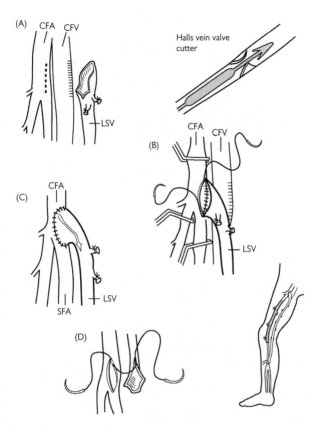

Fig. 12.18 In situ vein graft

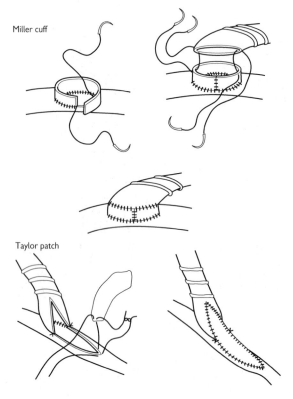

Fig. 12.19 The Miller cuff and Taylor patch

Popliteal artery entrapment syndrome

This occurs as a developmental defect, the popliteal artery passing medial to and beneath the medial head of gastrocnemius or a slip thereof leading to compression of the artery. Five anatomical variants are recognised and lead to intermittent claudication symptoms in young people. The pedal pulse classically vanishes on active plantar flexion of the foot against resistance or on passive dorsiflexion.

Preoperative findings

Angiography
- Medial deviation proximal popliteal artery
- Segmental occlusion mid popliteal artery
- Post stenotic dilatation

Any two or more of these are diagnostic of the condition. CT or MRI scan will define the anatomy precisely. The posterior approach is better for all anatomical variants and allows easy repair of the artery if necessary.

Position

Prone on the table under general or epidural anaesthesia with the leg slightly flexed.

Incision

Lazy S incision with the horizontal portion in the popliteal crease.

Procedure

- Deepen the incision and divide the deep fascia longitudinally taking care to avoid damage to the sural nerve.
- Identify and protect the tibial nerve passing a sling around it to allow gentle traction. Identify the popliteal vein, the artery is not in its usual position and is best identified high in the popliteal fossa as it exits from the adductor canal.
- Trace the artery inferiorly and divide the compressing band of muscle/ fascia, mobilising the entire length of the artery. Fix the transected head of gastrocnemius to the femur with an absorbable suture.
- If the artery is occluded or its wall thickened or fibrotic, apply bulldog clamps proximally and distally and resect the damaged segment after administration of 5000IU heparin.
- Harvest a suitable length of long saphenous vein and replace the damaged segment of artery with a reversed vein graft sutured end-to-end to the divided artery ends with continuous 5/0 Prolene.
- Ensure haemostasis and close the wound in layers without drainage.

Peripheral aneurysms

The majority affect the femoral or popliteal artery and are often associated with aortic aneurysmal disease.

Carotid aneurysm

These are rare and are either true aneurysms or post traumatic, the bifurcation being the commonest site of true aneurysm disease. The choice of treatment is dependent on the size and location, resection and reconstruction with an autogenous conduit being the preferred method, particularly if infection is suspected.

Procedure

See pp386–7, 406–7

Femoral artery aneurysm

Two principal types:
- Confined to the common femoral
- Involves origin of profunda.

Indications

Surgery is usually carried out if size greater than 2.5cm diameter or for complications (embolisation/thrombosis/rupture) or symptoms (pain/venous or neural compression).

Position

Supine with lower abdomen and entire leg prepared and draped with foot in a sterile, translucent bag.

Incisions

Rutherford Morrison incision as for control of the external iliac artery and vertical incision in groin for mobilisation of femoral vessels.

Procedure (see Fig. 12.20)
- Make an oblique incision in the iliac fossa lateral to the edge of the rectus sheath and divide the abdominal wall muscles to expose the peritoneum. Mobilise the peritoneum medially to expand the retroperitoneal space identifying the ureter.
- Mobilise the external iliac artery and pass a sling around it for control. Now make a vertical incision in the groin and mobilise the common femoral artery, profunda femoris, and the superficial femoral vessels passing slings for control.
- When proximal and distal control have been achieved give the patient 5000IU heparin, apply arterial clamps to the inflow and outflow vessels and incise the aneurysm sac, evacuating thrombus and atheroma.
- Now sew an interposition 8mm Dacron/PTFE graft end-to-end to the distal external iliac/common femoral artery with continuous 3/0 or 4/0 Prolene beginning in the middle of the posterior wall. If the aneurysmal disease does not involve the origin of the profunda make a similar end-to-end anastomosis to the common femoral artery above the bifurcation.

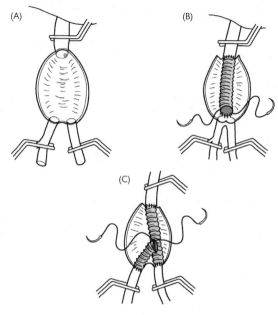

Fig. 12.20 Femoral aneurysm

- In the case of involvement of the profunda origin it may be possible to tailor the graft to cover the origins of both the profunda and superficial femoral or alternatively a separate interposition graft to the profunda may be required.
- Check the graft for haemostasis and the limb for perfusion and close the aneurysm sac over the graft with an absorbable suture before closing the wound in layers.

Popliteal aneurysm

Debate continues as to the correct timing of intervention for asymptomatic popliteal aneurysm disease. Surgery is performed for complications (embolisation or thrombosis) or rapid expansion.

Approaches
- Medial approach—most frequently used
- Posterior approach—lazy S incision but disadvantage of separate incision for vein harvest.

Position
Supine as for femoropopliteal bypass surgery.

Incisions
As for exposure of above and below knee popliteal artery over site of previously mapped long saphenous vein.

Procedure (see Fig. 12.21)
- Fashion incisions as above taking care to avoid the underlying long saphenous vein. Deepen the upper end through the deep fascia and deflect the sartorius muscle inserting a self retaining retractor.
- Expose the above knee popliteal artery and mobilise a sufficient length of the vessel as it leaves the adductor canal, passing slings around the vessel for control. The distal popliteal artery below the knee is approached via a vertical incision parallel to and just below the tibia. Continue dissection between the medial head of gastrocnemius and the tibia to reach the neurovascular bundle.
- Mobilize the popliteal artery and a sling passed. Harvest a suitable length of long saphenous vein, between the two incisions and tunnel it orthotopically in a reversed state between the above and below knee vessels. (If no suitable vein is available use 6 or 8mm PTFE as the conduit.)
- Heparinise the patient and apply arterial clamps to the popliteal artery making an appropriate sized arteriotomy.
- Fashion an end-to-side anastomosis of the conduit to the above knee distal superficial femoral artery. The distal anastomosis can be fashioned end-to-side/end-to-end to the below knee popliteal artery or tibioperoneal trunk. When both anastomoses are complete release the occluding clamps on the proximal and distal ends of the graft to restore flow in the graft and check the circulation.
- Remove the occluding clamps on the aneurysm and ligate the native artery proximal to the aneurysm and proximal to the distal graft anastomosis. Close the wounds in layers.

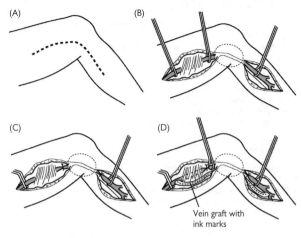

(A)   (B)   (C)   (D)

Vein graft with
ink marks

Fig. 12.21 Popliteal aneurysm

Pseudoaneurysms

These may be iatrogenic or secondary to infection, trauma or post surgery and occur when there is disruption of arterial continuity with extravasation of blood into surrounding tissues with formation of a fibrous tissue capsule.

Indications
- Active haemorrhage with increase in size
- >3cm diameter
- Impending skin necrosis
- Pain/femoral nerve compression
- Not suitable for percutaneous closure with fibrin.

Most iatrogenic are located in the femoral or brachial artery.

Iatrogenic pseudoaneurysm
Procedure
- Make a vertical incision over the pulsatile mass (in the case of a femoral pseudoaneurysm proximal control may be achieved through a separate retroperitoneal incision in the iliac fossa).
- Enter the aneurysm sharply and evacuate the layered thrombus to reveal the vessel in the base and the pinpoint arterial defect.
- Control the bleeding by finger compression of the defect. Usually only one or two 5/0 Prolene sutures are required to secure the vessel.
- Evacuate residual haematoma.
- Close the wound in layers with a suction drain.

Femoral anastomotic aneurysm
Position
Supine with the leg prepared and the foot in a sterile, translucent bag.

Incision
Repair through the previous groin incision (proximal and distal control should not be compromised and the iliac vessels may need to be exposed by an oblique retroperitoneal approach).

Procedure
- Expose the pseudoaneurysm anteriorly via the groin incision and identify and isolate the limb of the graft above the aneurysm.
- Identify the native vessels if possible and free them, passing a sling around each to gain control. If unable to free the native vessels they may be controlled with balloon catheters from within the aneurysm sac.
- Give the patient 5000IU heparin and clamp the graft. Open the aneurysm sac by a longitudinal incision and insert controlling balloon catheters if necessary.

- Oversew the orifice of the native common femoral artery with 3/0 Prolene and select a new Dacron graft of the same diameter and tailor the distal end to form a 'cobra head'. Suture the tailored distal end to the orifices of the superficial femoral and profunda vessels with 3/0 Prolene beginning at the heel and progressing around both sides to the toe. Cut the graft to length and suture it end-to-end to the previous graft limb. Now release the occluding clamps and check for haemostasis and adequate limb perfusion.
- Close the wound(s) in layers.

Fasciotomy

Indications

The treatment of compartment syndrome (a group of clinical symptoms/signs associated with pathological increase of tissue pressure within the osseofascial compartments of the extremities usually following trauma or post ischaemia and involving the skeletal muscles).

Signs

Pain, swelling (tense) and tenderness diminished sensation.

Treatment effective only if performed correctly.
- Lower limb requires 4 compartment release
- Upper limb requires 2 compartment release

Procedure

Lower limb

- Make a lateral incision in the leg one fingerbreadth anterior to the fibula and extending from the fibular head to the ankle.
- Divide the deep fascia throughout the length of the incision.
- Make a medial incision one fingerbreadth posterior to the tibial border dividing the deep fascia to the ankle.

Upper limb

- Make a curvilinear incision in the forearm extending from the anticubital fossa to the palm. The tense muscles will bulge through the divided fascia.
- Assess the colour of the muscles/bleeding and contraction.
  Non-contractile non-bleeding tissue is excised.

Wound management

Frequent changes of non-adherent sterile dressings and delayed primary closure may be feasible. Alternatively skin grafting may be required to close the skin defect.

Renovascular access surgery

Aims
Provision for dialysis access.

Preoperative assessment
Full cardiac history required and preoperative assessment of inflow vessels.
- Stenosis.
- Pulse volume.
- Consistency of the artery wall.
- If absent ulnar pulse perform Allen's Test—if positive, risk of steal?
- Check skin for MRSA colonisation.
- In the obese female with little visible veins explore wrist vessels—may need to superficialise a vein.
- Straight configurations tend to have fewer problems than those tunnelled in a curve.
- The preferred conduit is autogenous vein if available.

Anaesthesia
Options include:
- Local anaesthesia—majority performed by this method
- Brachial plexus block—adds temporary sympathectomy and vasodilatation
- General anaesthesia—increased risk, altered pharmacokinetics in CRF.

Procedure
Snuff box AV fistula
- Make a 3–4cm incision over the anatomical snuff box and isolate the distal cephalic vein. Mobilise it and transect the vein spatulating the end.
- Infiltrate further anaesthetic below the extensor retinaculum and mobilise the distal radial artery, dividing the small branches with diathermy or 4/0 Vicryl ties. Pass short segments of silk tie to act as slings and apply Yasergill/Maryfield clamps.
- Flush the divided cephalic vein with 20ml heparinised saline (papavarine 400mg/L) and make a small arteriotomy in the radial artery.
- Fashion an end-to-side AV anastomosis with continuous 6/0 or 7/0 Prolene. Check there is a palpable thrill and haemostasis is secure.
- Close the wound in layers with 4/0 PDS.

Radiocephalic (Cimino) fistula
- Infiltrate the skin of the wrist overlying the radial artery with 1% xylocaine and make a 3–4cm incision in the skin. Isolate and mobilise the cephalic vein passing a silk tie as a sling.
- Transect the vein distally to allow a sufficient length of vein to be swung to the radial artery taking care to avoid spiralling or twisting of the divided vein.
- Flush the vein with heparinised saline and apply a Maryfield clip to the vein.

- Mobilise the radial artery dividing any small branches either with diathermy or 4/0 ties and fashion a 1cm vertical arteriotomy using iris scissors and perform an end-to-side AV anastomosis with continuous 6/0 Prolene.

A radiocephalic fistula may be fashioned at almost any site in the forearm although the radial artery becomes progressively deeper in the upper arm.

Brachial AV fistula

- Infiltrate 10–15ml of local anaesthesia into the skin of the cubital fossa from just lateral to the palpable brachial pulse laterally.
- Make an oblique/transverse incision in the skin to expose the superficial veins. The venous anatomy is variable but options include:
  - End-to-side using the median cubital vein
  - Deep perforating vein if it will reach the artery
  - If median cephalic thrombosed mobilise proximal cephalic to reach.
- Infiltrate further anaesthetic and divide the deep fascia and the biceps aponeurosis to expose the brachial artery which is mobilised over a sufficient length and slings passed. (If high bifurcation use the radial/ulnar.)
- Divide the vein ligating the distal end and spatulating it proximally applying a Maryfield clip to prevent backbleeding.
- Apply bulldog clips to the brachial artery and fashion a 1cm arteriotomy with iris scissors. Join the spatulated vein to the arteriotomy with a continuous suture of 6/0 Prolene and release the occluding clips on the brachial artery. Check the haemostasis and for the presence of a thrill.
- Close the wound in layers with 4/0PDS.

Basilic transposition AV fistula

The basilic vein lies deep within the limb close to the brachial artery and is often spared from venepuncture or infusion injury.

- Expose the vein is exposed by a longitudinal incision along the medial border of the biceps muscle extending the major part of the length from the elbow to the axilla. The side branches are divided and the vein mobilised throughout its length taking care to preserve the median cutaneous nerve of forearm and the median nerve. Tunnel the mobilised vein subcutaneously to lie adjacent to the brachial artery or superficialise it.
- Apply bulldog clips to the brachial artery and divide the vein proximally and spatulate its end. Make a 1cm arteriotomy in the brachial artery and fashion an end-to-side AV anastomosis with continuous 6/0 Prolene.
- Close the subcutaneous tissues below the superficialised vein and close the wound in layers with an absorbable suture after ensuring the presence of a palpable thrill in the fistula.

Lower limb AV fistula

The long saphenous vein of >3.5mm diameter in the thigh can be used as a suitable conduit if there are no suitable veins in the arm. The preferred configuration is a straight transposition onto the anterior thigh.

- Expose the long saphenous vein in the proximal thigh through a vertical incision along the desired length.

- Transpose the mobilised vein subcutaneously to lie over the distal superficial femoral artery in the mid to distal thigh.
- Expose the SFA and apply bulldog clips to the artery and fashion a 1.5cm arteriotomy. Now join the spatulated vein end to the arteriotomy with a continuous 6/0 Prolene and release the occluding SFA clamps.
- Close the wound in layers.

Prosthetic access grafts
Indications
Synthetic arteriovenous bridge if no adequate vein exists. The usual prosthetic material is PTFE. Requirements for a synthetic graft are suitable arterial inflow and a vein to provide adequate venous outflow.

A variety of anatomical graft configurations are possible:
- Straight radiobasilic
- Brachiobasilic forearm loop
- Brachioaxillary graft
- Thigh loop (common femoral/femoral vein).

Grafts require a brief period of consolidation (7–10 days) but are prone to infection or thrombosis.

Brachioaxillary PTFE graft
Position
Supine with the arm extended on a table with the hand in a sterile, translucent bag.

Procedure
- Make a transverse incision in the axilla and mobilise the axillary vein passing slings around the vessel.
- Now expose the brachial artery at the elbow either by a vertical incision just below the edge of biceps or by an oblique cubital fossa incision.
- Mobilise the artery and pass slings around it for control. Using a tunnelling instrument fashion a subcutaneous tunnel between the two incisions and pass a length of unsupported 6mm or 8mm PTFE graft along the tunnel.
- Give the patient 5000IU heparin and clamp the axillary vein with bulldog clips.
- Make a 1.5cm venotomy, tailor the graft obliquely and suture the graft to the venotomy with continuous 6/0 Prolene. Now apply bulldog clips to the brachial artery and fashion a 1.5cm arteriotomy, anastomosing the graft to the artery in a similar fashion end to side with 6/0 Prolene. Release the arterial clamps and check for haemostasis at the suture line then release the clamps on the axillary vein.
- Close the wounds without drainage in layers.

Amputations

Despite use of embolectomy, arterial bypass surgery and catheter-directed thrombolysis the annual amputation rate has not decreased, peripheral vascular disease being responsible for 90% of amputations performed in England and Wales.

Aims
Restoration of mobility, relief of pain life saving procedure.

Indications
Chronic ischaemia
Elderly who do not walk with flexion contractures or non-reconstructable disease (rest pain) and ulceration or gangrene affecting a considerable part of the weight bearing surface.

Acute ischaemia
Limb loss following acute ischaemia is 9–30% with a mortality >18%. Amputation appropriate when ischaemia fails to respond to surgical or medical measures and to prevent septicaemia resulting from gross tissue necrosis.

Infectious gangrene (diabetics)
When gangrene is 'dry' amputation is performed when there is a clear line of demarcation established. When 'wet' gangrene is present, preoperative control of infection is needed by use of antibiotics. Infection is usually polymicrobial and adjunctive treatment with broad spectrum antibiotics necessary (cephalosporins/ aminoglycosides/metronidazole).The foot is not salvageable when infection has destroyed the plantar architecture or if debridement results in no functional weight bearing surface. MRSA is today a likely problem.

Level of amputation (see Fig. 12.22)
Aim
- Remove the infected/dead part
- Site with good potential for healing
- Successful rehabilitation
- Prosthetic device fitting.

Ultimate objective is to identify the most distal site at which healing will reliably occur. Vascular reconstruction may allow healing at a lower level and better rehabilitation potential.

Basic principles
- Careful, precise surgical technique
- Bones transected at comfortable distance above skin flap (no tension)
- Nerves divided sharply (nerve catheters for analgesia)
- Avoid mass ligatures
- Haemostasis essential (closed system suction drains).

Foot
Digital amputations
The flaps may be fish mouth, plantar based, dorsal based or circular but should be tension free to allow closure over the bone stump. Never

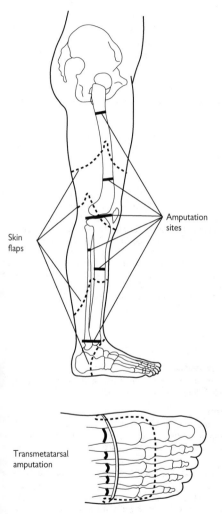

Amputation sites

Skin flaps

Transmetatarsal amputation

Fig. 12.22 Amputations in the lower limb

carry out amputation by disarticulation through a phalangeal joint, but rather transect the proximal phalanx leaving a button of bone.

Ray amputation
- Use a racquet incision with the vertical component on the dorsum of the foot to expose the metatarsal head and carry out incision distally to encircle the toe.
- Divide the distal metatarsal shaft at its neck and all the attached tendons and nerves. Secure haemostasis.
- Approximate the skin flaps are approximated accurately and without tension using non absorbable sutures.

Transmetatarsal amputation

Indications
- Gangrene of foot confined to the toes
- The plantar skin of the foot must be healthy.

Procedure
- Make a slightly curved dorsal incision from one side of the foot to the other just distal to the anticipated point of bone division in the middle portion of the metatarsal shafts. Extend the incision at the base of the toes across the plantar surface of the foot in the metatarsophalangeal crease. Deepen the dorsal incision down to the metatarsal shafts.
- Excise the plantar flap from the metatarsal shafts and divide the metatarsal bones with a Gigli or oscillating saw. The bone ends are smoothed with a rasp and the plantar flap tailored, thinned, and redundant muscle excised.
- Approximate the flap and skin edges by a tension free skin closure using interrupted sutures.

Postoperatively
- No weight-bearing for 7–10 days
- No specific prosthesis required but shoe modification.

Lisfranc forefoot amputation
Similar to above but makes use of a short dorsal and along plantar flap, the bones being divided along the base of the metatarsals.

Symes amputation
Seldom indicated for the truly ischaemic limb but may be applicable in diabetics with forefoot gangrene. Not greatly favoured by prosthetists or patients (BKA better). A healthy heel pad is a prerequisite.

Procedure
- The incision creates a long posterior flap incorporating the heel pad the dorsal incision extending across the ankle from the medial to lateral malleolus. Make the plantar incision at 90° angle to the dorsal incision and extend it in the plantar aspect of the foot distal to the heel cutting all layers to the bone (take care not to cut the posterior tibial artery on the sole).
- Enter the capsule of the tibiotalar joint. Divide the tibialis posterior and plantar flex the foot forcibly to allow division of the ligaments and

dislocate the talus. Dissect the calcaneus sharply from the heel pad and divide the Achilles tendon at its insertion. Divide the malleoli flush with the joint surface.

- Swing the posterior heel pad flap forwards and tailor its length and affect a tension free closure with interrupted Nylon sutures.

Below knee amputation

This is the best amputation for rehabilitation and mobility but is contra-indicated when there is extensive lower limb infection or gangrene close to the tibial tuberosity or involving the posterior calf skin. There should be no flexion contracture of the knee and it is contraindicated in those with no prospect of walking.

Two principle types:
- Burgess flap
- Skew flap.

Burgess flap used most often and less complicated than skew flap procedure.

Burgess flap (see Fig. 12.23)

Procedure

The level of tibial transection is 10–12cm (approx. a hand's breadth) below the tibial tuberosity.

- Make a skin incision at this level for two thirds of the circumference of the leg down to the tibia and exposing the muscles of the lat-eral/anterior compartment and extend it on either side inferiorly to the limits of healthy calf skin. Divide the muscles of the anterior compartment and isolate the anterior neurovascular bundle. Divided and separately ligated allowing the divided nerve to retract superiorly.
- Transect the fibula using a Gigli saw 1–2cm proximal to the point of tibial division. Now divide the tibia with a steep 45° bevel anteriorly.
- Expose and divide the posterior tibial and peroneal neurovascular bundles.
- Fashion the posterior myocutaneous flap leaving the gastrocnemius and soleus muscles as a base and smooth the bone ends with a rasp. Tailor the myocutaneous flap removing excess muscle and approxi-mate it over a suction drain to the anterior tibial fascia and the tibial periosteum with absorbable sutures.
- Close the skin with interrupted Nylon sutures or a subcuticular absorbable suture (4/0 PDS).

Postoperative

Postoperative analgesia can be facilitated by the insertion of a tibial nerve catheter for infusion of analgesic. Ensure the patient practises extension and flexion of the knee joint such that the joint can be straightened. A flexion contracture makes fitting of a prosthesis impossible.

Skew flap (see Fig. 12.23)

Procedure

The length of the stump measured to the point of bone division is 10–15 cm from the tibial plateau.

- Draw a circumferential line on the skin at the defined level of bone division. On this line mark a point 2cm lateral to the subcutaneous tibial crest to identify the junction point of the anteromedial and posterolateral flaps. Draw on the skin a quarter circumference arc to mark the minimal distance of the flaps. Along this circumference incise the skin, subcutaneous tissue, fat and periosteum.
- Divide and ligate the long and short saphenous veins.
- Deepen the incision through the anterior tibioperoneal muscles dividing the anterior tibial nerve and allowing it to retract. Ligate the anterior tibial vessels separately and expose the tibia and fibula on the interosseus membrane. Divide the fibula with a Gigli saw and the tibia with an anterior bevel. Having divided the bones, expose the posterior tibial and peroneal vascular bundles and ligate them separately.
- Dissect the skin flap on the distal leg distally to reveal the gastrocnemius/soleus mass which is extricated from the distal leg.
- Fashion a myoplastic flap and thin it leaving only aponeurosis over the distal few millimetres (bleeding from the soleus venous plexus and small arteries will require control or oversewing. Trim excess muscle and smooth the bone ends with a rasp. Wash the site out with saline and fold the flap upwards and suture it to the anterior tibial fascia and tibial periosteum over a suction drain using an absorbable suture.
- Approximate the skin and fat with interrupted nylon or an absorbable subcuticular suture.

Through knee amputation

Most commonly performed for trauma, provides a long stump for balance if bilateral amputee

Flaps/incisions

- Long anterior flap
- Equal length anterior and posterior flaps
- Sagittal equal length anterior/posterior flap—most common in ischaemia.

Position

Supine with a 'bump' in the operating table to elevate the thigh, and with the knee flexed.

Procedure

- Outline skin flaps with a skin marker and incise. Dissect anterior to the insertion of the patellar tendon and divide it. Continue the dissection medially to divide the four hamstring tendons. Laterally divide the biceps femoris and iliotibial band.

Skew flap

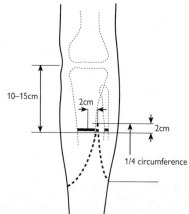

10–15cm

2cm

2cm

1/4 circumference

Burgess flap 'Rule of thirds'

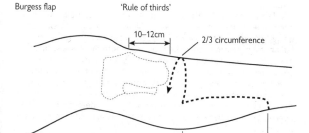

10–12cm 2/3 circumference

1/3 circumference

Fig. 12.23 Below knee amputation

- Enter the knee joint from the front and cut the cruciate ligaments. Locate the popliteal vascular bundle and ligate it and divide it. Divide the tibial and peroneal nerves and allow them to retract. Place the patellar tendon in the intercondylar notch and sew it to the cruciates with an absorbable suture and similarly the semitendinosus and biceps tendon. A drain is optional.
- Close the skin without tension using an absorbable subcuticular suture.

Above knee amputation

3 levels—supracondylar/mid thigh/high thigh.

The longer the femoral shaft the greater the mechanical advantage regarding transfer, balance etc.

Incision

Fish mouth or circumferential.

Procedure

The proximal extent of the incision is at the intended level of femoral division and the length of the flap is approximately half the anteroposterior diameter (ensure no tension—better a loose flap than an ischaemic flap).

- Incise through the skin, subcutaneous tissue, and fascia and identify the femoral vessels in the subsartorial canal, separately ligate and divide them.
- Divide and retract all anterior and posterior muscles. Isolate the sciatic nerve and divide it under tension and allow it to retract. Insert a sciatic nerve catheter and anchor it with an absorbable suture. Transect the femur at a higher level than the flap and smooth the edges with a rasp. Test closure to ensure it is tension free—if not shorten the femur.
- Secure haemostasis and suture the anterior and posterior muscles over the femoral end. (Suction drain optional, brought out through healthy skin remote from amputation site.)
- Approximate the anterior and posterior layers of deep fascia with interrupted absorbable sutures and the skin closed with interrupted or subcuticular stitches.

Varicose veins

Varicose veins occur in the long and short saphenous systems secondary to valvular incompetence possibly as a consequence of degenerative fibrosis of the vein wall and/or valve ring. They may also be secondary to perforator vein incompetence usually after deep vein thrombosis.

Indications
- Relief of symptoms—chronic ache, night cramps, itching, restless legs
- Complications—varicose eczema, ulcer, recurrent phlebitis
- Cosmetic.

Preoperative preparation

The groin and leg are shaved (especially in men). The veins are marked on the skin, with the patient standing, using a felt pen prior to surgery. Points of incompetence and sites of perforators are marked. In the case of recurrent varicose veins or where there is doubt as to the sites of major incompetence a preoperative Duplex scan assessment is mandatory and vein mapping immediately prior to surgery may be helpful.

Trendelenberg procedure

Position
Supine with the legs abducted and the knee flexed. The skin of the lower abdomen legs and groin is prepared.

Incision
Medial to the femoral pulse and approximately 5cm long below and parallel to the inguinal ligament (in the obese this may be above the skin crease).

Procedure (see Fig. 12.24)
- Insert a West's self retaining retractor to spread the skin edges apart. Identify the long saphenous vein and ligate and divide all its tributaries (the anatomy is variable, but tributaries include; superficial epigastric, superficial and deep external pudendal, and superficial circumflex iliac veins).
- Divide the long saphenous vein after clear identification of its junction with the femoral vein at the cribiform fascia (the junction is usually crossed inferiorly by a small artery branch from the adjacent femoral artery). Then transfix and ligate the proximal end with 3/0 Vicryl, the needle of the transfixion suture entering the long saphenous vein approximally one half of the long saphenous vein diameter away from the saphenofemoral junction so that the transfixion suture will lie flush with the femoral vein and any constriction of the femoral vein is avoided.

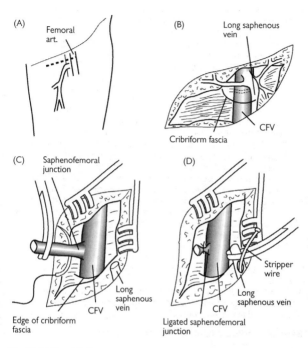

Fig. 12.24 Trendelenburg operation (saphenofemoral disconnection)

- Pass a vein stripper distally to the below knee level. Extract the stripper through a small stab incision at that site and pull distally until the small knob at its upper end is flush with the cut end of the vein. Then ligate it with a long (one metre) length of 2/0 thread, firmly anchoring the stripper wire in the vein. The long length of thread is left intact so that when the stripper wire passes through and extracts the invaginated long saphenous vein, the thread remains in the track of the long saphenous vein. Should the full length of the long saphenous vein not have been removed, traction on either end of the thread tents the skin and allows a stab incision to be made to reach the residual segment which can be grasped with its contained thread. Then pull a tape soaked in 0.5% bupivacaine and 1:200 000 adrenaline through the track of the extracted long saphenous vein and leave it in situ till the operation is complete and then removed (this reduces post operative haematoma and aids analgesia).
- Then identify any other marked varicosities and deliver them through 3mm stab incisions made in the long axis of the leg penetrating the dermis only by using fine mosquito forceps or a Mueller vein hook. Pull the vein to the surface and deliver it as a loop and divide it between forceps. Apply gentle traction until a segment of vein is delivered with each forceps, applying another forceps close to the skin as the further segment of vein emerges. Continue this process until the vein breaks off. Make a new incision further down the marked vein to pick up the vein again and repeat the process until the entire length of the marked varicosity is removed.
- Infiltrate the edges of the groin wound with 0.5% bupivacaine and approximate the subcutaneous tissues with an absorbable deep suture.
- Close the skin with an absorbable subcuticular suture. The stab wounds are either left unclosed or closed with Steristrips, occlusive dressing applied and the leg bandaged with crepe bandages from ankle to groin.

Saphenopopliteal ligation and/or stripping
(Short saphenous disease)

Preoperative preparation
The evident varicosities are marked with a skin pen as before, with the patient standing. A preoperative Duplex scan or the use of hand held Doppler will have allowed the accurate identification of the site of the saphenopopliteal junction.

Position
Prone.

Incision
Transverse skin crease incision placed 1cm distal to the site identified by Duplex scan or Doppler as the site of the saphenopopliteal junction.

Procedure
- Insert a small self-retaining retractor to separate the skin edges. Expose the deep fascia and open it transversely.
- Grasp the short saphenous vein with forceps and follow it to the junction, dividing the gastrocnemius veins and a vein coursing upwards to the posteromedial vein of the thigh. Achieve a transfixion ligation of the saphenopopliteal junction in a similar manner to that described

above for saphenofemoral ligation. Take care throughout the dissection to avoid damage to the sural nerve.

- Stripping of the short saphenous vein is achieved as for the long saphenous vein by passing a stripping wire down the calf. The stripper wire is retrieved via an incision of sufficient size to clearly define the vein from the adjacent sural nerve and thus avoid inadvertent neural damage. Remove remaining marked varicose tributaries via stab incisions as described above.

- Close the popliteal wound in layers, the deep fascia and subcutaneous fat with an absorbable suture and the skin with an absorbable subcuticular stitch after infiltration of the wound with 0.5% bupivacaine. Close the stab wounds with Steristrips and dressings and a crepe bandage applied.

Multiple stab phlebectomy

This may be applied in isolation when there is evidence of distal varicosities but no evidence of saphenofemoral or saphenopopliteal incompetence on Duplex scanning. It is conducted as described above through multiple 3mm stab incisions placed at appropriate points along the marked vein in the long axis of the leg. Perforating veins can be dealt with similarly or ligated flush with the deep fascia when exposed through larger incisions placed directly over the marked sites.

Recurrent varicose veins

When previous groin/popliteal exploration has been carried out and there is evidence of recurrence it is mandatory prior to any further re-exploration that Duplex assessment of the sites of incompetence is performed. Fibrosis around the previous surgery makes re-exploration through a standard approach difficult and hazardous.

Procedure

Vascular clamps should be available in case there is injury to the femoral vein.

- The saphenofemoral junction is best approached through either a vertical incision, as to expose the femoral arterial vessels, or through the old transverse incision but exposing the femoral artery first.

- Expose and identify the femoral artery and the adjacent common femoral vein. Follow the common femoral vein superiorly until the saphenofemoral junction is seen and expose the femoral vein for approximately 1cm above and below the site of the saphenofemoral junction. *Carefully* mobilise the junction. When you are sure you have completely mobilised the junction all round, pass Lahey forceps around the junction and apply a vascular clamp to the junction adjacent to the femoral vein. Above this clamp apply an artery forceps leaving a reasonable length of vein between to allow safe division of the junction. Oversew the junction with a 5/0 Prolene suture without compromise of the femoral vein and transfix and ligate the other end of the divided vein with an absorbable suture. If there is a persistent long saphenous vein, identify it and strip it as in a Trendelenberg procedure. Otherwise the residual varicosities are dealt with by multiple stab avulsions as above.

Perforator surgery

Indications

Chronic venous disease:
- Pre-ulcerative venous disease and Duplex evidence of perforator incompetence
- Healed yet recurrent ulcers
- Active ulcer that does not respond to compression therapy.

These may be performed in conjunction with surgery for primary varicose veins.

Options
- Cocketts procedure
- Dodds procedure
- Subfascial endoscopic perforator surgery (SEPS).

Cocketts procedure

Incision

Parallel to the subcutaneous posterior border of the tibia and 1cm behind it. The incision is vertical and extended distally as required.

Procedure
- Deepen the incision and divide the deep fascia in the same vertical plane. Reflect the edges of the wound so formed until the perforating veins are seen. Ligate and divide the perforators flush with the fascia.
- Close the wound in layers and apply a dressing and a crepe bandage.

Dodds procedure

Position of patient

Prone with the leg prepared from mid-thigh to ankle and with the foot in a glove.

Incision

Stocking seam in the mid calf extending from 2cm below the popliteal skin crease to the level of the malleoli.

Procedure
- Deepen the incision and divide the deep fascia vertically the length of the incision, taking care not to injure the sural nerve and the short saphenous vein.
- Using finger dissection, sweep the flaps laterally below the deep fascia as far as the attachment of the deep fascia to the borders of the tibia to expose the perforating veins.
- Divide and ligate the perforating veins below the fascia.
- Secure haemostasis and close the deep fascia with a series of spaced interrupted absorbable suture and close the skin with an absorbable subcuticular suture. Apply dressings and a crepe bandage.

Subfascial endoscopic perforator surgery (SEPS)

Instruments

CO_2 insufflator, rigid endoscope, 3 chip video camera, light source and monitor, balloon dissector, two 10mm laparoscopy ports, reusable clip applicator.

Position

Under general anaesthesia and in Trendelenberg position with knee slightly flexed.

Procedure

- Make a 10mm incision in the skin 4cm medial to the tibia and 10–15cm below the popliteal crease.
- Dissect the subcutaneous tissue and make a small incision in the fascia. Introduce the balloon retractor into this space and direct it towards the medial malleolus. The balloon is inflated to 200–300cc to open up the space and then deflated and CO_2 insufflated to a pressure of 15mmHg. The zero degree telescope is introduced and a separate 5mm/10mm working port inserted in the mid calf under direct vision to allow passage of the clip applicator and scissors. The working port should be placed as posteriorly as possible but not through the gastrocnemius muscle. All accessible perforators are clipped and divided if necessary.
- Close the skin incisions and apply compression bandages applied as above.

Endovenous vein closure

This technique is currently being evaluated for the treatment of long saphenous disease in situ, in place of surgical stripping, using a Closure System (VNUS Medical Technologies). The system has been applied to LSV of 12mm diameter and uses electrodes to apply locally confined temperature changes to the vein wall resulting in a small thrombus plug in a contracted vessel with de-endothelialised wall and an obliterated vein lumen.

Urology

Q. King and C. Harding

Debridement of Fournier's necrotising fasciitis

Indication

Fulminating polymicrobial fasciitis involving the Colles', Dartos and Scarpa's fascia often as a consequence of perianal or periurethral sepsis.

Position

Supine or in lithotomy or extended lithotomy position, or with legs in Lloyd Davies supports.

Preparation

- Resuscitation and supportive care
- Intravenous fluids, broad-spectrum antibiotics and analgesics
- May require intensive care, invasive monitoring.

Procedure

- Incise through the affected skin and subcutaneous tissue. Use a combination of sharp and blunt dissection to identify the plane of separation between vital and necrotic tissue. The fasciitis seldom involves deep structures of penis, spermatic cords, testes and adnexae or investing fascia of the abdominal musculature. Corpus spongiosum may be involved if the process began as a urethral condition.
- Excise tissue until a bleeding edge is encountered. Where there is extensive undermining of apparently healthy skin by necrotic fascia, undermined tissue is unlikely to survive, and it may be wise to excise some of it.
- Superiorly, necrosis may extend as high as the clavipectoral fascia and clavicles. Inferiorly, it may surround the anus, but seldom involves the thighs.
- If possible, cover the testicles by placing them in thigh pouches superficial to fascia lata—if not, bring them together inferior to the penile root. If this is not done, the testes will retract into the vicinity of the external ring, producing a most unsatisfactory cosmetic result.
- Insert urethral or suprapubic Foley's catheter.
- Defunctioning colostomy may be required.

Complications

Patients are often very ill, and may develop any of the complications of haemorrhage, acute sepsis and multiple system organ failure.

Follow-up

- Intensive medical, nursing and nutritional supportive treatment.
- In the majority of cases, one or more subsequent debridement will be required.
- Reconstruction methods will depend on the extensiveness of fascio-cutaneous defect, but in general, thick split skin grafting of the penis and meshed thin skin grafting of the testes will produce a surprisingly acceptable appearance.
- More elaborate cosmetic or urodynamic surgery may be indicated, and will be tailored to the individual case.

Exploration of the 'acute scrotum'

Indications

Acute orchalgia where torsion of the spermatic cord cannot be emphatically excluded from the differential diagnosis.

Position

- Supine, Lloyd-Davies, or lithotomy.

Preparation

- Attempt manual detorsion.
- Obtain consent for orchidectomy if necessary. Counsel appropriately.
- Pre- or intra-operative ultrasound scan may be helpful but avoid delaying exploration in order to obtain one.
- Prep the genitalia and groins with antiseptic solution and shave appropriately.

Procedure

- Examine properly under anaesthesia.
- If there is no suspicion of testicular neoplasm, make a median scrotal incision or a transverse one crossing the midline. If neoplasm is suspected, approach as described under 'Inguinal orchidectomy.'
- Incise through Dartos and the scrotal septum, and explore the affected testis first.
- Develop the avascular plane around tunica vaginalis and incise it.
- Deliver testis and adnexae (Fig. 13.1A). Intravaginal torsion of the spermatic cord is obvious unless detorsion has occurred. Ecchymosis, congestion, and oedema, together with a generous, or narrow pedicle, provide sufficient justification to fix the testis.
- Torsion of a testicular appendage should be managed by removal of the appendage, but there is no need to explore the contralateral testis.
- If spermatic cord torsion is diagnosed, reduce the torsion, and wrap the testis within a warm moist swab while the contralateral testis is explored and fixed.
- Fix the testis by everting the tunica vaginalis in the manner of Jaboulay, and place three nonabsorbable sutures between the tunica albuginea of the testis (the medial side of the upper pole is safest) or paratesticular tissue and Dartos (Fig. 13.1B).
- If the torted testis becomes pink, it is treated similarly. If it is obviously necrotic, ligate cord structures and remove it. If its viability is uncertain, we leave it in situ, and obtain a Doppler ultrasound scan after 24 to 48 hours.
- Close Dartos and skin in layers using absorbable sutures.
- Where an unsuspected testicular neoplasm is discovered, management will depend on the patient's age. In the prepubertal child, testicular conservation may be appropriate and frozen section should be obtained. This situation is fraught with medico-legal hazard, and informed consent is worthwhile taking some time over.

Complications
- Infection
- Haematoma
- Testicular atrophy, anti-sperm antibody production
- Recurrent torsion.

Follow-up
- At least one outpatient appointment is arranged for counselling and examination
- Laboratory investigations only where clinically indicated.

(A)   (B)

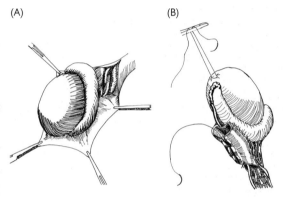

Fig. 13.1 (A) Exposure and (B) fixation of testis.

Suprapubic catheter placement

Trocar and cannula technique for Foley's catheter insertion.

Indications
Bladder drainage where the urethral route is unavailable or undesirable (e.g. stricture).

Position
Supine.

Preparation
- The bladder should be palpably full or sonographic guidance should be obtained.
- Abdominal and pelvic examinations should precede placement of the cannula unless contraindicated or impossible (e.g. compound fractured pelvis).
- Prep the lower abdomen and suprapubic area with antiseptic solution.

Procedure
- Identify and mark the site of cannula insertion at a point a short distance above the symphysis pubis or equidistant between the fundus of the bladder and the pubis.
- Remember that the bladder strips the anterior peritoneum from the abdominal wall as it fills, but that perivesical surgery, trauma or pathology may result in fixity and the interposition of bowel between bladder and abdominal wall. If in doubt use sonographic guidance.
- Infiltrate the skin and subcutaneous tissue with 1% lignocaine.
- Confirm site by aspirating via a small-gauge needle.
- Make a stab incision with an 11 blade, as deep as linea alba.
- Place trocar and cannula in the incision, and firmly, but with fine control and accuracy, insert it into the bladder—keep in mind the anatomical relations of the bladder.
- Remove the trocar and guide the Foley's catheter into the bladder, inflate the balloon and remove the guide.

Complications
- Bleeding
  - From the bladder
  - From an enlarged intrusive prostate
  - From perivesical venous plexus
  - From the iliac vessels
- Rectal or enteric injury—peritonitis or retroperitonitis
- Extravasation of urine
- Displacement or blockage of catheter
- Infection
  - UTI
  - Systemic sepsis
  - Symphysitis pubis (now fortunately rare).

Follow-up

- If the suprapubic catheter is regarded as definitive management, then simple replacement after an interval is possible without anaesthetic or special equipment.
- Silicone catheters may be left in situ for three months and latex catheters for one month.
- Special dressings are not necessary. Patients wear a cotton singlet, changed daily.
- If the placement of a suprapubic catheter was a temporising measure, then, it may be removed when the primary condition has been satisfactorily treated.

Reduction of paraphimosis

Position
Supine.

Preparation
- Analgesia, penile block, or general anaesthesia
- If the condition has been neglected and become brawny, ulcerated, or inflamed give antibiotics
- Prep the skin with antiseptic solution, and drape.

Procedure
- Gradual manual compression may be brought to bear on the oedematous foreskin as illustrated in Figs. 13.2A, B.
- When the volume of the foreskin has been reduced, simultaneous traction may effect reduction.
- If this is not possible, make a dorsal slit:
  - Identify the constriction ring in the midline dorsally and incise it through skin and Colles' fascia (Fig. 13.2C).
  - Extend the incision proximal and distal to the constriction ring until all tension is removed.
  - Obtain haemostasis and suture the longitudinal incision transversely (Fig. 13.2D).

Complications
- Failure to relieve the constriction may result in ischaemia of the glans and necrosis
- Infection bleeding and haematoma formation.

Follow-up
Most patients are offered a definitive procedure such as circumcision, electively.

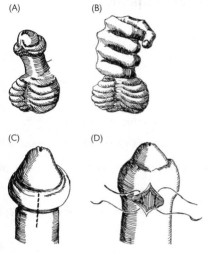

Fig. 13.2 Management of paraphimosis

Shunt procedures for priapism

Indications
Low-flow priapism that has not responded to medical interventions and less invasive procedures such as cavernosal aspiration, irrigation, or intra-cavernosal vasoconstrictor injection.

Position
Supine.

Preparation
- Prep from umbilicus to mid-thigh including groins and genitalia with antiseptic solution, and drape.
- A suprapubic or urethral catheter may be inserted for convenience and comfort postoperatively.
- Broad-spectrum antibiotics are given with induction.

Procedures
The Winter procedure T
- Use a Tru-Cut® biopsy needle to create cavernosum-spongiosum venous shunts at the glans.

The El-Ghorab shunt (Fig. 13.3A)
- Incise the dorsum of the glans transversely over the 'domes' of the cavernosal distal ends and dissect off the spongy glanular tissue over a small area.
- Grasp each 'dome' with locking tissue forceps, or place a strong stay suture for traction.
- Excise a disc of tunica albuginea penis from each side, with a 5mm diameter and close only the skin of the glans with absorbable suture (Fig. 13.3B).

Cavernosospongiosum shunt
- Expose the corpus spongiosum and one corpus cavernosum by the incision of skin, Colles' and Buck's fascia—just distal to the penoscrotal junction or more proximally.
- Separate corpus spongiosum from corpus cavernosum for a short distance, then excise an ellipse of investing tissue from each, exposing spongy tissue.
- Create a vascular anastomosis between the two corporal openings using continuous polypropylene 5/0 suture
- Close skin and fascia in layers

Cavernososaphenous shunt
- Incise as for cavernosospongiosum shunt, and a second incision over the saphenous hiatus on the same side.
- Expose the saphenous vein, mobilise it for about 15cm, and divide it inferiorly between ligatures.
- Tunnel the saphenous vein between the two incisions and excise a disc of tunica albuginea.

- Trim the vein to length and make a vascular anastomosis with 5/0 polypropylene.
- Close skin and fascia.

Complications

Immediate
- Bleeding
- Cavernositis, loss of phallus
- Persistent or recurrent tumescence

Long-term
- Erectile dysfunction from venous leak and/or fibrosis of spongy tissue.

Follow-up
- Immediately post-operatively, intermittent penile compression may improve shunt patency rates. The use of a paediatric Dynamap® machine may be helpful
- Long-term follow-up depends on outcome, potency, aetiology of the priapism and patient expectations

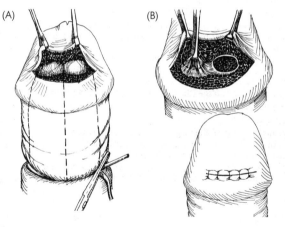

(A)   (B)

Fig. 13.3 The El-Ghorab shunt

Surgical approaches to the kidney, upper ureter, and adrenal gland

Surgical anatomy

- The kidneys lie in the retroperitoneal space on the posterior abdominal wall with average dimensions of 11cm × 6cm × 3cm.
- The right kidney is found approximately 1cm more caudal than the left.
- Each kidney is surrounded by a true fibrous capsule and a layer of perinephric fat, all enveloped by the perirenal or Gerota's fascia.
- Posteriorly both kidneys are related to the diaphragm, quadratus lumborum, psoas major and transversus abdominis muscles.
- Three nerves also lie posterior to each kidney. These are the subcostal (T12), iliohypogastric and ilioinguinal (L1) nerves.
- Anteriorly the right kidney is related to the liver, the second part of the duodenum and the ascending colon.
- Anterior to the left kidney lie the stomach, spleen, tail of pancreas, and descending colon.
- The adrenal glands cap each kidney at its upper pole.
- The blood supply to the kidneys is via the renal arteries, which are paired branches of the aorta.
- Venous drainage is via the paired renal veins into the vena cava. The left renal vein arches in front of the aorta prior to joining the inferior vena cava. The left renal vein has both the left gonadal and left adrenal vein as tributaries.
- The blood vessels are found at the level of the renal hilum, which is situated at the middle of the medial border of each kidney.
- The renal pelvis also leaves the kidney at this level, which is found at the transpyloric plane (the level of the first lumbar vertebra).

Commonly used approaches to the kidney, adrenal, and upper ureter

- When deciding on the surgical approach to be used, consideration should be given to the operation to be performed, underlying pathology and the patient's body habitus.
- The four most commonly used approaches to the kidney are flank, transabdominal, thoracoabdominal, and dorsal lumbotomy.

Flank incision

Advantages

- Minimal disturbance of other viscera (retro- or transperitoneal approach can be used)
- No contamination of the peritoneal cavity in retroperitoneal approach
- Useful in obese patients
- Can be extended for greater exposure.

Disadvantages

- Large muscles divided
- Increased risk of nerve injury
- Poor exposure of the renal hilum
- May be unsuitable for patients with respiratory disease (patient position).

Position
- Lateral position on operating table
- Upper leg extended, lower leg flexed at the knee
- 20°–40° break on operating table.

Incision and approach
- Incise 1cm below the inferior border of 12th rib or directly over it if the rib is to be excised.
- Extend the incision anteriorly towards the lateral edge of the rectus sheath—a slight caudal curvature to the lower part of the incision avoids intercostal nerve damage.
- Incise skin and subcutaneous fat.
- Incise and divide the superficial layer of muscle consisting of latissimus dorsi and external oblique.
- Divide the deeper muscle layer, consisting of serratus posterior inferior and internal oblique in the same fashion.
- Divide the musculofascial layer (consisting of lumbodorsal fascia posteriorly and transversus abdominis muscle anteriorly), and push the peritoneum medially.
- Gerota's fascia is now exposed.
- Insert a self-retaining retractor e.g. Finochietto's, to retain exposure.

Procedures
Procedures such as simple or partial nephrectomy, pyeloplasty, nephrolithotomy, and adrenalectomy can all be performed via this route.

Closure
- 'Unbreak' the table
- This incision is normally closed in layers
- Drains can be brought out through a stab incision below the wound.

Transperitoneal abdominal approach
Median and subcostal incisions are described.

Advantages
- Good exposure of renal pedicle
- Allows control of great vessels
- Rapid, and allows full abdominal exposure in trauma situation.

Disadvantages
- Longer period of postoperative ileus
- Limited access in obese patients
- Long term risk of bowel adhesions.

Position
- Patient is supine
- Padding under operating side with break in table especially if a subcostal approach is used.

Incision and approach
- Median incision
  - Incise in the midline from the xiphoid process, skirting the umbilicus inferiorly

- Divide skin and subcutaneous fat
- Incise linea alba
- Open peritoneal cavity in the direction of original incision
- Divide and ligate the ligamentum teres of the liver.
- Anterior subcostal incision
  - Make an incision from tip of 11th rib posteriorly, curving upwards to a point a third of the distance from the xiphoid to the umbilicus
  - Incise and retract skin and subcutaneous fat
  - Incise the most superficial musculofascial layer, consisting of rectus sheath medially and external oblique muscle laterally
  - Bluntly dissect through internal oblique and underlying transversus abdominis
  - Incise peritoneum in the line of the incision.

Procedures

- Most upper urinary tract operations can be performed via abdominal incisions
- The transperitoneal approach is essential in radical renal or adrenal surgery.

Closure (musculofascial)

- May be closed in layers of polydioxanone or nonabsorbable suture material
- Sometimes mass abdominal closure for midline incision.

Thoracoabdominal approach

Advantages

- Advantageous for large tumours (especially right sided)
- Good exposure of upper pole and adrenal gland
- Access to retroperitoneal lymph nodes.

Disadvantages

- Involves pleurotomy and therefore insertion of a chest drain may be necessary
- Time consuming incision and closure
- Longer hospital stay.

Position

- Semi-oblique position on operating table
- Pelvis flat whilst upper torso is rotated approximately 30°, elevating the affected kidney
- Flank directly over 20–40° break in operating table.

Incision and approach

- Make an incision over the 9th or 10th rib, or the interspace between them. This runs from the costal angle posteriorly, across the costal margin, to the mid-point of the contralateral rectus muscle in the epigastrium.
- Incise skin and subcutaneous fat.
- Divide the superficial layer of muscles (latissimus dorsi, serratus posterior inferior, external oblique and rectus abdominis) in the line of the skin incision.

- Incise intercostal muscle or strip periosteum and remove the pertinent rib. At the costal margin, divide or separate the costal cartilages.
- Anteriorly, divide the deeper layer of muscle (internal oblique, transversus abdominis and posterior rectus sheath).
- Open pleura and incise the diaphragm circumferentially near to the chest wall.
- Complete the incision by opening the peritoneal cavity and retracting the liver or spleen superiorly.

Procedures
- Radical surgery to adrenal gland or upper pole of kidney can be performed using this approach
- This exposure is useful especially if suprarenal portion of inferior vena cava needs to be accessed.

Closure
- Diaphragm is closed with interrupted nonabsorbable mattress sutures tied on its inferior surface
- Chest wall and costal cartilage are reapproximated
- A chest drain is brought out via a stab incision in posterior axillary line, and pleura closed
- Transected musculofascial layers are reapproximated in layers after placement of retroperitoneal drain (optional).

Dorsal lumbotomy

Advantages
- Ideal for open renal biopsy, removal of small kidneys, and open stone surgery
- No muscle transection and therefore less postoperative pain.

Disadvantages
- Limited exposure
- Unsuitable for radical surgery.

Position
- Lateral position on operating table
- Both knees flexed at knee
- Optional minimal break on table.

Incision and approach
- Make a vertical lumbar incision from superior border of 12th rib inferiorly towards iliac crest
- Incise and divide skin and subcutaneous tissue
- Retract paravertebral muscles medially and incise the lumbodorsal
- The kidney, within Gerota's fascia, is now exposed.

Procedures
- Nephrectomy for small non-functioning kidney, open renal biopsy, pyeloplasty or open stone surgery (including access to upper ureter).

Closure
- Lumbodorsal fascia is reapproximated
- Retracted muscles are returned to their anatomical position.

Simple nephrectomy

Indications
- Poorly- or non-functioning kidney due to chronic infection, obstruction or trauma, and associated with symptoms (pain) or complications (recurrent UTI, hypertension)
- Treatment of renovascular hypertension
- As a quick surgical alternative to more prolonged reconstructive procedures if patient's medical condition does not permit these.

Incision
Flank, abdominal or dorsal lumbotomy (see above).

Preparation
- Fractional renal function and creatinine clearance
- Treat UTI
- Prep and drape skin.

Procedure
- Expose the perinephric space
- Incise Gerota's fascia overlying the kidney laterally
- Bluntly dissect perinephric fat to expose the renal capsule
- Mobilise the kidney and identify ureter and hilar vessels
- During mobilisation, especially near the poles, always look out for aberrant blood vessels
- Divide and ligate the ureter
- Isolate hilar vessels. Clamp, double-ligate and divide them (vein first)
- Free remaining adhesions and remove the specimen
- Close wound as described above
- An optional retroperitoneal tube drain may brought out via stab incision below the wound.

Complications
- Bleeding
- Atelectasis/pneumonia
- Prolonged ileus
- Wound infection/dehiscence
- DVT/PE
- Incisional hernia.

Follow-up
- Initial wound and biochemistry check
- Further follow-up depends on original indication.

Inguinal orchidopexy

Indication
- Imperfectly descended testes
- Inguinal orchidopexy is done for ectopic, annular or canalicular testis
- The current standard of care is that it should be done before 18 months of age.

Position
Supine.

Preparation
- Imaging may be used to confirm the approach is appropriate if the testis is impalpable
- Prep and drape the lower abdomen and genitalia.

Procedure
- Make a small incision from the superolateral margin of external inguinal ring, extending laterally for 2–4cm in the skin crease
- Dissect through subcutaneous and Scarpa's fascia, taking care not to injure an ectopic testis
- Incise and reflect the external oblique aponeurosis (Figs. 13.4A, B)
- Grasp the tunica vaginalis and divide its attachments to adjacent structures, preserving cord and its coverings
- Mobilise them to their emergence at the internal inguinal ring above inferior epigastric vessels
- Divide cremaster muscle fibres and strip them from the cord (Fig. 13.4C)
- Identify the processus vaginalis, and dissect it upwards as illustrated, pushing the cord structures posteriorly away from peritoneum above the internal ring. Ensure it is empty, and ligate it flush with peritoneum (Fig. 13.4D)
- Open the tunica vaginalis and evert it
- Digitally develop a tunnel from the inguinal region into the scrotum, and incise the skin (Fig. 13.4E)
- Develop a space within the Dartos fascia (Fig. 13.4F) and insert a haemostat through it into the groin wound
- Draw the testis into the Dartos pouch which should retain it (Fig. 13.4G)—additional fixation is often helpful
- Close the groin wound in layers and skin (scrotal and groin) with fine subcuticular undyed absorbable sutures.

Complications
- Haematoma, wound infection
- Injury to vessels, resulting in testicular atrophy
- Unsatisfactory position.

Follow-up
- Ensure position is satisfactory—a second procedure may help
- High risk of neoplasia must be acknowleged—encourage vigilance.

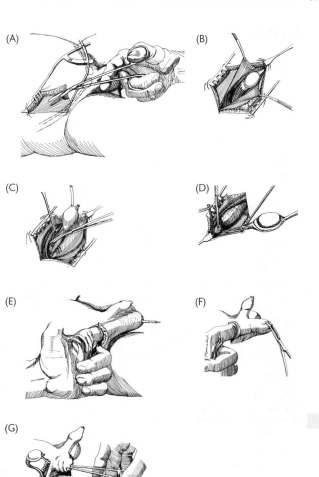

Fig. 13.4 Inguinal orchidopexy

Circumcision

Indications
- Phimosis
- Religious or cultural.

Position
Supine.

Preparation
- Genitalia are prepared with antiseptic solution and the field draped
- Keep some aqueous antiseptic for cleaning under the prepuce.

Procedure
- Dilate the phimosis and separate prepucio-glanular adhesions using a blunt probe or artery forceps, and clean away smegma (Fig. 13.5A shows planned incision)
- Compress the prepubic fat pad to show true penile length and mark out the planned external skin incision at the level of the coronal sulcus, with a V-shaped extension ventrally (Fig. 13.5B)
- Retract the foreskin and superficially incise the inner surface of the foreskin proximal to the fusion of Colles' and Buck's fascia
- Divide the frenulum, ligate or coagulate frenular vessels
- Reduce the foreskin and incise the external skin as marked (Fig. 13.5C)
- Dissect in Colles' fascia to excise the skin between the two incisions
- Secure meticulous haemostasis using ligatures and cautery (bipolar is safer)
- Use a neat row of fine fascio-cutaneous interrupted absorbable sutures, with a 'triangulation suture' in the midline ventrally (Fig. 13.5D)
- A dressing may be applied but will often fall off in the recovery room.

Complications
- Bleeding
- Infection
- Acute urinary retention
- Adhesions, meatal stenosis
- Urethrocutaneous fistula.

Follow-up
Wound and histology check.

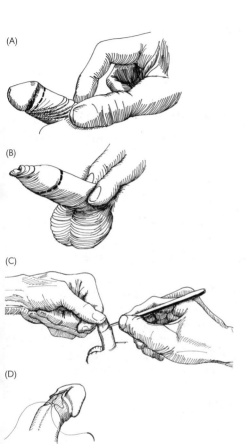

(A)

(B)

(C)

(D)

Fig. 13.5 Circumcision

Correction of hydrocele

Jaboulay correction

Position
Supine or in lithotomy.

Preparation
- Preoperative ultrasound scanning may be necessary to exclude a malignant cause
- The lower abdomen and external genitalia are prepared with antiseptic solution.

Incision
Midline sagittal or unilateral transverse scrotal incision.

Procedure
- Incise through skin and Dartos muscle
- Meticulously deal with bleeding vessels encountered
- Dissect in the avascular plane between spermatic fascia and Dartos to expose the hydrocele, and partly or completely deliver it.
- Incise tunica vaginalis and its fascia away from the epididymis and vessels
- Excise excess hydrocele sac
- Oversew the cut edge of the remaining sac with a continuous haemostatic absorbable suture
- Prevent re-apposition of the edges by suturing the sac edges behind the testis and cord (see Fig. 13.1B)
- Return the testis to the scrotum
- Drainage is optional and seldom necessary
- Close the scrotum with two layers of absorbable suture
- Non-adherent dressing and scrotal support is applied.

Complications
- Haematoma formation
- Injury to cord, testis or adnexae
- Recurrence is rare.

Follow-up
Wound check only.

Vasectomy

- Many methods of performing this procedure exist including the 'no scalpel' technique, favoured by one of the authors. A standard vasectomy is described
- Most vasectomies are performed under local anaesthetic on a day-case basis
- Careful preoperative counselling must be provided.

Indications

Permanent contraception.

Position

Supine.

Preparation

- The external genitalia are prepared with antiseptic solution
- The vas is identified by palpation and manipulated to a superficial position directly under the scrotal skin
- Local anaesthetic is introduced around the isolated vas
- It may be helpful to secure the vas with an Allis clamp.

Incision

A stab incision made directly over the vas, and may be enlarged by opening the jaws of a small arterial clamp.

Procedure

- The surrounding sheath is bluntly dissected off the vas
- A small segment of the vas deferens is excised (for histology)
- The epithelium of the cut ends is fulgurated (the suture needle can be used to do this), and ligated
- Fascial interposition techniques are often used providing a physical barrier between the two ends of the vas-spermatic fascia is closed over the caudal end, while the cephalad end is sutured to the external surface of spermatic fascia
- The Dartos and skin do not need to be sutured.

Complications

- Haematoma
- Fertility!
- Sperm granuloma
- Chronic scrotal pain.

Follow-up

- Alternative contraception must be used until semen analysis twice confirms azoospermia (usually at 16 and 18 weeks post-op)
- Histological proof that vas has been removed from both sides.

Radical nephrectomy and nephroureterectomy

Indications

- Malignant tumours of the kidney
- Nephroureterectomy is performed for urothelial tumours of the upper urinary tract

Position and approach

- Dependent on size and location of tumour and body habitus
- Commonly used approaches are transabdominal and thoracoabdominal (see above)

Procedure

- For left sided operations reflect the colon medially via incision of the line of Toldt and divide the splenocolic ligaments.
- Divide the lienorenal ligament and retract the spleen and pancreatic tail upwards.
- For surgery on the right side mobilise the colon to the hepatic flexure and Kocherise the duodenum.
- Expose the renal pedicle and double ligate the vessels.
- Ligate the arteries first and palpate veins for tumour thrombus before ligation.
- Tumour thrombus can extend as far proximally as the heart and must be removed before ligation of the vein, so cardiothoracic or vascular specialists may be needed.
- Large right renal tumours overlapping the vena cava may restrict access to the renal artery or arteries at the hilum. Retract the left renal vein upward and the vena cava towards the right to obtain access, and ligate the inter-aortocaval right renal artery in continuity. See Fig. 13.6.
- In radical nephrectomy, ligate and divide the ureter where convenient.
- In radical nephroureterectomy, dissect the ureter distally—a second incision may be required. Alternatively circumcise the ureteral orifice endoscopically using the Colling's knife, then retrieve the distal ureter by blunt dissection from above. Avoid tumour spillage. Drain the bladder and perivesical space for 10 days.
- Mobilise the kidney within Gerota's fascia, and divide the adrenal vessels.
- Remove the specimen, check the renal bed for bleeding.
- A classical radical nephrectomy involves a regional lymphadenectomy and ipsilateral en-bloc adrenalectomy but these are probably not necessary unless (in the case of adrenalectomy) the tumour involves the upper renal pole or there is suspected adrenal involvement.
- Closure depends on approach used (see above).

Complications

- Haemorrhage
- Injury of spleen, pancreas, cisterna chyli (chylous ascites) or bowel, or inadvertent ligature of superior mesenteric artery

- Thrombo-embolic complications
- Post-operative chest, wound or urinary tract infection
- Persistent urinary leak from the bladder in nephroureterectomy (rare)
- Wound complications such as hernia, neuralgia or sagging of the flank due to nerve damage
- Local recurrence.

Follow-up

- Adjuvant therapy in selected cases dependent on histology
- Initial wound and biochemistry check at 2 months
- Annual creatinine clearance and urinary protein excretion and:
- TCC—surveillance according to risk-stratified protocols for superficial urothelial malignancies may involve cystoscopies, upper tract imaging and urinary cytology
- RCC—controversial: stage-based recommendations have been made.
  - pT1   History and physical examination (H&P), liver functions (LFT) and chest X-Ray (CXR) every year
  - pT2   H&P, LFTs, and CXR every 6 months for 3 years, then yearly. Thoracoabdominal CT scan at 24 and 60 months
  - pT3   H&P, LFTs, and CXR at 3 months, then every 6 months until 3 years, then yearly. CT at 24 and 60 months

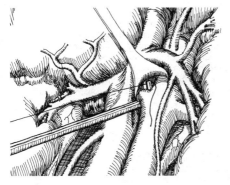

Fig. 13.6 Exposure of renal vessels

Partial nephrectomy

- Preoperative imaging for full and accurate staging and anatomical information is essential if this procedure is contemplated
- This operation can be performed extra-corporeally with auto-transplantation into the groin.

Indications

- Bilateral tumours or inherited predisposition towards multiple renal tumourigenesis (eg Von Hippel–Lindau disease)
- Small solitary renal tumours (controversial)
- Reduced renal reserve or solitary kidney
- Benign tumours.

Position and approach

Any described above, but vascular pedicle access has to be excellent.

Procedure

- The renal pedicle is dissected and the vessels prepared for soft-clamping
- Crushed ice and mannitol may be used to prevent renal ischaemic damage. Safe warm ischaemic time is 30min. *Effective* renal cooling increases this six-fold but is not easily achieved.
- The tumour or moiety is identified
- Vessels are clamped
- The capsule may be reflected, and parenchyma is incised and a polar or wedge resection taken with a 1cm margin around tumours.
- The collecting system is repaired watertight, often over a ureteral stent
- Arteries and veins are meticulously suture-ligated.
- Venous clamps are removed, the renal parenchyma is closed and the incised capsule repaired with bolsters or an omental flap, then the arterial clamp is removed. Observe for a while to confirm haemostasis is near perfect.
- Drains and a catheter are often left post operatively
- The wound is closed in layers.

Complications

- Haemorrhage, including major vessel injury
- Thrombo-embolic complications
- Loin pain secondary to clot colic or obstruction
- Postoperative chest, wound or urinary tract infection
- Leakage from collecting system causing urinoma or fistula
- Renal failure.

Follow-up

- Initial wound and biochemistry check
- Follow up for cancer and familial syndromes involves regular imaging influenced also by pathological stage and margins
- Nephrological care may also be required.

Radical cystectomy

In men this is usually a cystoprostatectomy, and in women an anterior pelvic exenteration.

Indications
- Muscle invasive but locally confined tumours of the bladder
- High grade superficial tumours or carcinoma in situ of the bladder not responsive to bladder sparing treatments
- As part of a pelvic exenteration for advanced pelvic malignant disease
- Palliative treatment of haematuria, chronic pain or recurrent infection.

Position
- Supine with stirrups or leg braces
- The operating table has a break at the level of the umbilicus producing additional lumbar lordosis and is tilted slightly head-down.

Preparation
- The risks and alternatives and the types of reconstructions are discussed.
- The abdomen, perineum and genitalia (including vagina) are prepared with antiseptic solution
- A catheter is placed in the bladder.

Incision
- A midline lower abdominal incision is made skirting around the umbilicus
- Circumcision of the female urethral meatus, or total urethrectomy in the male may precede cystectomy.

Procedure
- Incise skin, subcutaneous fat, and superficial and deep fascia.
- Continue through anterior rectus sheath, following blunt separation of the rectus muscles, transversalis fascia, and peritoneum.
- Divide the median umbilical ligament and the peritoneum along each side of the bladder. In females divide and ligate round ligament and ovarian vessels.
- Take down adhesions to the bladder, especially from the descending or sigmoid colon.
- In the male ligate and divide the vasa deferentia.
- Perform pelvic lymph node dissection. Ligate or clip lymphatics.
- Identify the ureters and divide them with their distal ends tied.
- Ligate and divide superior and inferior vesical pedicles.
- Mobilize anteriorly by teasing away perivesical and periprostatic fat, incising endopelvic fascia and dividing the pubo-urethral or -prostatic ligaments (see Figs. 13.7A, B).
- In females incise the vagina at the posterior fornix (a swab in the vagina helps—see Fig. 13.7C)). The vaginal incision is continued inferiorly on each side to join the urethral dissection. Use haemostatic clamps and oversew vaginal vessels later.

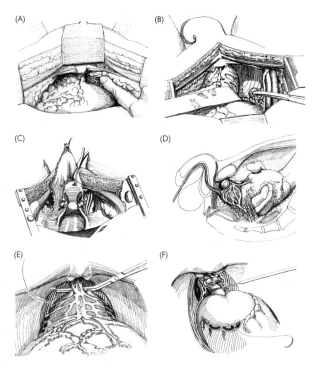

Fig. 13.7 Radical cystoprostatectomy

- In males, ligate the 'dorsal venous complex' anterior to the urethra using the manoeuvres illustrated in Figs. 13.7D, E.
- Oversew the proximal end of the dorsal vein complex, and divide the urethra as shown in Fig. 13.7F.
- In males, retract the prostate using the urethral catheter, while dividing prostatic pedicles and dissecting Denonvilliers's fascia off the rectum.
- Remove the specimen and pack the pelvis for a few minutes before securing final haemostasis and repairing vagina.
- A urinary diversion or reconstruction is now be performed see Bladder substitution.
- Closure is in layers with continuous or interrupted sutures or clips to skin.

Complications

- Vessel or bowel injury (especially rectal)
- Pulmonary, wound, or urinary infection
- Thrombo-embolic complications
- Erectile dysfunction, vaginal stenosis
- Local recurrence.

Follow-up

- Initial wound check and histology review
- Regular upper tract surveillance and biochemistry monitoring
- May include adjuvant therapy.

Radical retropubic prostatectomy

Indications

Prostate cancer in patients who are likely to benefit by virtue of
- The disease being probably significant, but surgically curable, and
- The patient having appropriate life-expectancy and performance status.

Position

Supine with stirrups or leg braces and a 20° break opening the abdominopelvic angle

Preparation

- The entire lower abdomen, perineum, and genitalia are prepared with antiseptic solution
- Autologous blood is taken for subsequent reinfusion, and volume replaced
- A catheter is placed in the bladder
- Antibiotics are given with anaesthetic induction.

Incision

- Low median, Pfannenstiel, or Turner Warwick
- The approach is extraperitoneal.

Procedure

- Deepen the incision is through skin, sub-cutaneous fat, and superficial and deep fascia.
- Continue through anterior rectus sheath and, following blunt separation of the rectus muscles, transversalis fascia.
- Apply retractors and dissect in the retropubic space.
- Carry out pelvic lymphnode sampling or dissection, removing external iliac, common iliac and obturator nodes.
- Incise the endopelvic fascia lateral to the prostate (as marked in Fig. 13.8A).
- Divide the puboprostatic ligaments.
- Separate the 'dorsal venous complex' from the urethra (Figs. 13.8B, C), ligate and divide it, and oversew both ends for security (Fig. 13.8D).
- In nerve-sparing procedures the 'neurovascular bundle' posterolateral to the urethra is preserved during this and subsequent dissection.
- Divide the urethra below the prostatic apices.
- Posterior blunt dissection separates Denonvilliers's fascia and prostate from rectum and exposes seminal vesicles and posterior bladder neck (Fig. 13.8E).
- Incise the bladder near the bladder neck, and extend the dissection to separate bladder from prostate, taking care not to injure the ureters which are close by.
- Tailor the bladder neck if necessary, and evert bladder mucosa, before making a urethrovesical anastomosis over a large Foley's catheter. Use 6–8 interrupted sutures, placed as illustrated in Fig. 13.8F.
- Drain the retropubic space and close the wound closed in layers.

Complications
- Intra-operative haemorrhage, vessel damage, rectal, or ureteral injury
- Pulmonary, wound, or urinary infection
- Thrombo-embolic complications
- Anastomotic leak or later a stricture
- Urinary incontinence
- Erectile dysfunction.

Follow-up
- Catheter is left a variable length of time
- Some surgeons perform post-op cystourethrography
- Pelvic floor exercises reduce incontinence
- Regular biochemical and possibly radiological surveillance.

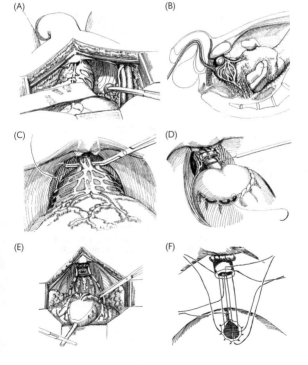

Fig. 13.8 Radical retropubic prostatectomy

Inguinal orchidectomy

Indications

Malignant tumours of the testes.

Position

Supine.

Preparation
- Ensure tumour markers have been sent off preoperatively
- Lower abdomen and external genitalia are prepared and draped.

Incision

2cm above and parallel to medial two thirds of inguinal ligament.

Procedure
- Incise through the sub-cutaneous fat, Camper's, and Scarpa's fascia
- Incise external oblique from the external inguinal ring, parallel with its fibres
- Identify and preserve the ilioinguinal nerve adjacent to the cord
- Dissect the cord is to the internal ring and clamp it
- Deliver the testicle from the scrotum, and its scrotal attachments ligated and cut
- Inspect the testis without opening the tunica vaginalis
- Ligate each component of the cord structures at the internal ring doubly and remove the specimen
- Closure is in layers with an undyed absorbable monofilament suture to skin.

Complications
- Haemorrhage
- Infection.

Follow-up
- Initial wound check
- Histology, imaging, and interval repeat tumour markers
- Subsequent management will include intensive surveillance or chemotherapy, radiotherapy, lymph node dissection or combination.

Partial penectomy

Indications
- Carcinoma of the penis involving the glans and distal shaft
- Severe penile trauma.

Position
Supine or lithotomy.

Preparation
- Penis and scrotum are prepared
- The tumour is invariably infected and is excluded from the operative field
- A tourniquet is placed at the base of the penis
- Antibiotics are given.

Incision
- The skin incision is circumferential (Fig. 13.9A)
- Allow at least 2cm margin from tumour.

Procedure
- Ligate all longitudinal blood vessels
- Incise Buck's fascia and tunica albuginea penis, and transect the corpora cavernosa but preserve corpus spongiosum at this level (Fig. 13.9B).
- Separate corpus spongiosum and urethra from the specimen, for about 1cm distally
- Suture the tunica albuginea penis and Buck's fascia as shown in Fig. 13.9C.
- Remove the tourniquet and spatulate the urethra (Fig. 13.9D).
- Fashion a urethrocutaneous anastomosis using absorbable sutures and approximate skin dorsally (Fig. 13.9E).
- Insert a Foley's urethral catheter for 24 hours and apply non-adhesive dressing.

Complications
- Haematoma formation
- Infection
- Meatal stenosis.

Follow-up
- Initial wound and anastomosis check
- May involve further surgery e.g. further radical penile surgery or lymph node dissection.

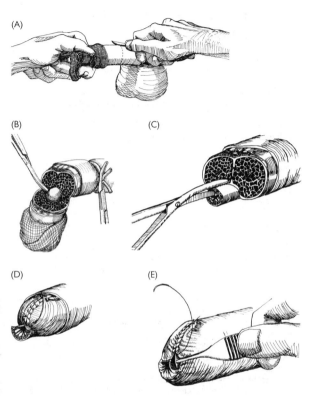

(A)

(B)

(C)

(D)

(E)

Fig. 13.9 Partial penectomy

Transurethral resection of the prostate (TURP)

Indications
- Bothersome lower urinary tract symptoms unresponsive to medical therapy
- Complications of prostatic bladder outflow obstruction:
  - Recurrent acute or acute-on-chronic urinary retention
  - Recurrent urinary tract infections
  - Upper tract decompensation (renal failure or dilatation)
  - Intractable haematuria of prostatic origin.

Position
Supine with the legs in lithotomy or Lloyd-Davies supports.

Preparation
- Urine culture. Treat with appropriate antimicrobials preoperatively if infected
- Antibiotics are given at induction of anaesthesia
- Prep the external genitalia with antiseptic solution and a TUR drape allowing access for rectal manipulation of the prostate
- Glycine (1–1.5%) or Mannitol (3%) solution are so-called non-haemolytic irrigants, and are the visual medium for resection.

Procedure
- Calibrate the urethra with Lister sounds and dilate or perform internal urethrotomy with the Otis urethrotome if necessary.
- Insert the resectoscope, either by using the obturator or under endoscopic vision.
- Perform endoscopic examination of bladder and prostatic urethra taking note of landmarks (verumontanum, bladder neck, ureteral orifices).
- Begin at the bladder neck and, using the wire loop electrode, resect the median lobe until the circular fibres of the bladder neck can be seen, then resect the lateral lobes in a stepwise manner. Finally, remove apical and anteriorly situated adenoma. Prevent damage to the external sphincter by resecting only proximal to the verumontanum. Attend to haemostasis throughout resection to maintain excellent visibility.
- Remove resected tissue 'chips' with Ellik's evacuator.
- Ensure excellent arterial haemostasis by cautery, if necessary using the rolling-ball electrode
- Insert a large-calibre (22–24Ch) triple-lumen Foley's catheter and set up *saline* irrigation. Intermittent traction on the catheter can be used to arrest venous bleeding if necessary.

Complications
- Haemorrhage (intra-or postoperative) with subsequent clot retention.
- Injury to bladder or rectum.

- TUR syndrome.
  - This is a syndrome of mental confusion, nausea and vomiting, hypertension and bradycardia, with low serum sodium concentration (typically less than 125mEq/dL) secondary to absorption of irrigant via the opened venous channels of the prostate.
  - The risk is greater during resections taking more than one hour.
- Postoperative chest or urinary tract infection.
- Thrombo-embolic complications.
- Sexual dysfunction—retrograde ejaculation (common), erectile dysfunction (rare).

Follow-up

- Outpatient symptom review, physical exam, histology review after a few weeks. Investigations as clinically indicated.

Transurethral resection of bladder tumour (TURBT)

Indications
- Curative treatment and/or staging for newly diagnosed or recurrent bladder tumours
- Palliative treatment of haematuria secondary to bladder neoplasm.

Position
As for TURP.

Preparation
- Preoperative upper tract evaluation for synchronous tumour is performed
- Antibiotics are given at induction of anaesthesia
- The external genitalia are prepared and draped as for TURP.

Procedure
- Perform bimanual examination under anaesthesia, via vagina or rectum.
- Avoid overdistension of the bladder and inadvertent resection of infolded bladder wall because of under-distension.
- Resect all exophytic tumour using a cutting current and resectoscope loop.
- Take care to resect deeply at the tumour base so that accurate, representative histology is obtained for staging.
- Where 'high risk disease' is suspected (not otherwise), take additional biopsies from bladder urothelium and prostatic urethra.
- Specimens may be separated (tumour, base of tumour, selected-site biopsies) for examination.
- Obtain haemostasis, examine for bladder perforation.
- Repeat bimanual EUA if tumour was present before resection.
- Place a large calibre triple lumen Foley's catheter, and set up bladder irrigation if necessary.
- Document position and size of all lesions.

Complications
- Haemorrhage
- Bladder perforation—small and extraperitoneal perforations may be managed by catheter drainage
- Urinary tract infection
- Thrombo-embolic complications.

Follow-up

- Immediate, postoperative intravesical Mitomycin C instillation reduces the risk of early recurrence of superficial transitional cell carcinoma.
- Guidelines have been published detailing surveillance strategies for superficial bladder cancer according to risk of disease recurrence and progression. Risk assessment is commonly based on histological stage and grade, tumour size and multiplicity, and frequency of recurrence. Surveillance will involve various combinations of endoscopy, upper tract imaging and urine cytology.
- Muscle-invasive tumours or high-risk superficial cancer may require radical surgery, radiotherapy or chemotherapy, or combinations thereof.

Transurethral litholapaxy

Indications
Bladder calculi—the stones are often associated with bladder outlet obstruction and this procedure can be combined with TURP.

Position
As for TURP

Preparation
- As for TURP
- Exclude and treat those metabolic abnormalities sometimes associated with bladder stones (hyperparathyroidism, malnutrition).

Procedure
- Keep the bladder adequately filled and continuously irrigated.
- The stone is grasped and crushed manually with stone crushing forceps or lithotrite. Avoid including bladder wall or bladder neck in the jaws of the instrument.
- Intravesical pneumatic or ultrasonic lithotripsy and lasers can also be used.
- Remove fragments with an Ellik's evacuator.
- Thoroughly examine the bladder for injury and stop any bleeding.
- Perform TURP or bladder-neck incision if indicated.

Complications
- High complication rates have been reported from this operation both in isolation and in combination with TURP
  - Haemorrhage
  - Bladder injury
  - Urinary tract infection
  - Urethral stricture
- Thrombo-embolic complications.

Follow-up
Depends on aetiology:
- If obstructive, as for TURP
- If metabolic, refer appropriately.

Bladder augmentation: ileocystoplasy

Many techniques have been developed. One method of augmentation, and one type of continent catheterisable stoma are described (see Bladder reconstruction—Mitroffanoff appendicovesicostomy). The two are often used together.

Indications

Poorly compliant, high pressure and or small volume bladder often associated with neuropathic conditions.

Position

Supine.

Preparation

- The patient should be capable of performing self-catheterisation and bladder washout
- Check renal function is adequate for metabolic consequences of urine reabsorption
- Bowel prep
- Prep and drape the abdomen
- Antibiotics with induction.

Incision

- Low median, or Pfannenstiel
- Transperitoneal approach.

Procedure

- Choose a 20–25cm segment of ileum reaching the pelvis, avoiding the terminal 20cm.
- Isolate and mobilise this on its mesenteric pedicle.
- Restore ileal continuity using any proven anastomotic technique and close the mesenteric defect above the isolated segment.
- Wash out the isolated segment and incise the antimesenteric border.
- Configure the opened segment like an inverted 'U' and suture adjacent edges using continuous all-layers absorbable suture.
- Now fold the reconfigured segment so that the superior and inferior margins are approximated, and suture part-way down each side from the fold towards the open end inferiorly to make a 'cup'.
- Bivalve the bladder using a midline sagittal incision from near the bladder neck anteriorly to just above the interureteral ridge posteriorly. The ureters should be cannulated to avoid injury during dissection.
- Suture the ileal 'cup' to the bladder, beginning at the apex of the bladder incision posteriorly, and using 3/0 continuous absorbable sutures.
- Insert large-calibre urethral and/or suprapubic Foley's catheters and perivesical peritoneal drain/s.
- Close the abdomen in layers.

Complications
Perioperative
- Thromboembolic disease
- Anastomotic leak
- Graft necrosis
- Wound, urinary tract, or chest infection.

Complications of the use of bowel in the urinary tract
- Chronic bacteriuria
- Urolithiasis
- Metabolic alterations
  - Acidosis
  - Bone demineralization
- Disturbances of gastrointestinal function
  - Diarrhoea
  - Anaemia
  - Reservoir rupture
- Malignancy.

Follow-up
- Initially 8 hourly bladder washouts are done to remove mucus. After 14–21 days the catheters are usually removed—consider cystogram to confirm integrity
- Confirm that bladder emptying is adequate or start intermittent self catheterisation
- The support of stoma therapist or specialist nurse is standard practice
- Urinary tract imaging is done at 6 weeks, 6 months and 1 year
- Renal function and urine culture are done 3 monthly for 1 year, then annually
- Annual endoscopy should be done after 5 years.

Bladder augmentation: Mitroffanoff appendicovesicostomy

Many methods have been described. One type of continent catheterisable stoma is described, often used together with the method of augmentation previously described (see Bladder augmentation—ileocystoplasty).

Indication
- An elegant means of access for intermittent catheterisation of a continent reservoir, applicable to native bladder, augmented bladder, or continent pouch
- Montie has described a similar technique using a tube of ileum—reconfigured so the plicae run longitudinally—instead of appendix

Preparation
As for Ileocystoplasty.

Position
Supine or as appropriate for primary procedure.

Incision
As dictated by primary procedure—usually Pfannenstiel, Turner-Warwick or median.

Procedure
- The appendix is mobilised on its pedicle. Additional length can be obtained by including part of the caecum (Fig. 13.10A).
- The distal end of the appendix is placed into the reservoir in such a way that it forms a catheterisable conduit with a flap valve configuration for continence (Fig. 13.10B).
- The caecal end is passed through the abdominal wall and sutured to skin using various means to make the anastomosis inconspicuous and resistant to stenosis e.g. VQZ flap, V flap. It may be concealed in the umbilicus.

Complications
- As for the primary procedure, *plus*
- Appendiceal necrosis
- Stoma leakage
- Stenosis at skin level
- Urinary fistulas
- Mucus retention, chronic UTI and urolithiasis.

Follow-up
As for augmentation cystoplasty or continent urinary diversion.

(A)

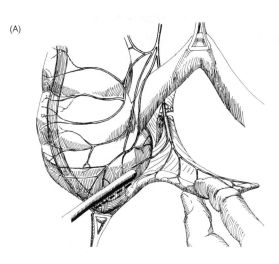

(B)

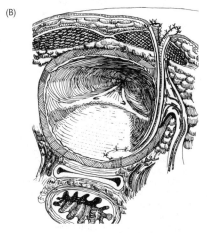

Fig. 13.10 Bladder augmentation: Mitroffanoff appendicovesicostomy

Urinary tract reconstruction after cystectomy

There are three commonly used groups of reconstructions:
- Conduit urinary diversion
- Continent urinary diversion
  - Using the anal continence mechanism
  - With continent catheterisable stoma
- Orthotopic neobladder

Conduit urinary diversion—the ileal conduit

Position

As appropriate for the primary surgery (cystectomy), or supine.

Preparation

- Appropriate counselling, marking of stoma site by stoma therapist
- Bowel prep
- Antibiotics with induction
- Prep and drape the abdomen.

Procedure

- Via a midline transperitoneal incision, incise the posterior peritoneum and mobilise ureters distally, preserving their blood supply.
- Digitally develop a tunnel through the retroperitoneum behind the sigmoid mesocolon, and pass the left ureter through it into the right iliac fossa
- Isolate a 12–15cm segment of ileum preserving its and adjacent bowel blood supply. Avoid using the distal 20cm of ileum. The pedicle should be longer towards the distal than the proximal end of the segment (Fig. 13.11).
- Restore ileal continuity using any proven anastomotic technique and close the mesenteric defect above the isolated segment.
- Spatulate each distal ureter for about 15mm and approximate adjacent edges of each spatulated portion using running full-thickness absorbable 4/0 suture.
- Pass a size 8Ch infant feeding tube or purpose-made ureteral stent up each ureter and fix to the inside of the lower ureter with absorbable suture. Pass the free ends through the conduit.
- Anastomose the proximal end of the conduit to the common ureteral opening using watertight continuous or interrupted 4/0 absorbable suture.
- Excise a disc of skin at the stoma site and make a cruciate incision through subcutaneous fascia, rectus sheath, and transversalis fascia.
- If possible, develop a space between the parietal peritoneum and the abdominal wall so that the conduit can be retroperitonealised.
- Bring the distal end of the conduit out via the stoma incision for about 4–6cm and fix it to rectus sheath with 6 interrupted absorbable seromuscular sutures.
- Evert the end of the conduit and suture to the dermis.
- Drain the abdomen and retroperitoneum.
- Close the abdomen in layers and apply stoma appliance.

Complications
Very similar to those of Ileocystoplasty (see pp536–7)

Follow-up
- Drains can usually be removed after about 5 days. If copious drainage persists, check creatinine level of drain fluid to exclude urine leak.
- The stents are removed after about 14 days.
- The support of stoma therapist or specialist nurse is standard practice.
- Imaging is done at 6 weeks, 6 months, and 1 year.
- Renal function is checked 3 monthly for 1 year, then annually.
- Follow up also according to the primary disease (e.g. bladder cancer).

Continent urinary diversion—using the anal continence mechanism—the Mainz II sigma rectum

Indications
- Continent urinary diversion in patients unsuitable for other techniques of continent reconstruction or conduit diversion
- Note:
  - High frequency of serious sequelae limits its application
  - The reconfiguration of the sigmoid reduces luminal pressure and increases capacity
  - Renal and liver failure are contraindications.

Position
As appropriate for the primary surgery/cystectomy, or *supine*.

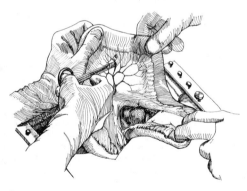

Fig. 13.11 Preparation of ileal conduit

Preparation
- Colonic assessment (colonoscopy), and assessment of anal continence mechanism (retain a 300ml soft-porridge enema for 2 hours)
- Otherwise, as for Ileal conduit.

Procedure
- Incision and ureteral mobilisation as for ileal conduit (except that the left ureter is not transposed)
- Open the sigmoid colon along a taenial line for 12cm, so that the sigmoid resembles an inverted 'U' shaped trough
- Approximate the adjacent free edges of the U with 2 layers of absorbable 3/0 suture to form the posterior wall (Fig. 13.12)
- Tunnel the distal ureters through a taenium, and then submucosally for 4–5cm, and suture the spatulated ends to colonic mucosa. Stents may be placed and brought out through the rectum with a large rectal tube
- Close the anterior wall of the reservoir, place abdominal drains and close the abdomen

Complications
See under Ileocystoplasty (p537), but also
- Stoma-related problems (kinking, stenosis, false passage), and note that
- Metabolic acidosis requiring treatment, and
- Development of malignancy (rectal carcinoma) are much commoner.

Follow-up
- As for Ileocystoplasty, *and*
- Annual colonoscopy
- Follow-up appropriate to the primary disease (e.g. urothelial cancer).

Continent urinary diversion with continent catheterizable stoma—the Mainz pouch

Preparation
- Requires a highly motivated patient fully informed about pouch maintenance, complication, and reoperation rates, and with normal manual dexterity
- Otherwise as for Ileal conduit (p540).

Procedure
- Mobilize ureters as for Ileal conduit.
- Isolate a segment of bowel consisting of caecum (15cm) and adjoining ileum (50cm) and mobilise on its vascular pedicle (Fig. 13.13A).
- Restore ileocolic continuity and close the mesenteric defect.
- Open the caecum longitudinally anterior to the ileocaecal valve and the ileum for 30cm along its antimesenteric edge.
- Make a window in the mesentery beginning where the ileal incision ends (Fig. 13.13B).

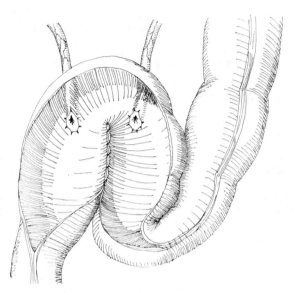

Fig. 13.12 Mainz II Sigma rectum: preparation of sigmoidcolon

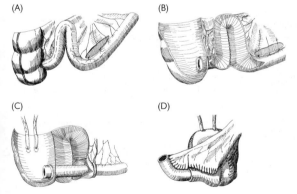

Fig. 13.13 The Mainz pouch

- Reconfigure the ileal and caecal segments as illustrated to create a hemisphere, leaving the ileocaecal valve intact.
- Intussuscept the ileal segment and draw the intussusceptum through the ileocaecal valve. The linear stapling device is usually used to fix this segment in place (Fig. 13.13C).
- The free end of the ileum is brought out as a flush stoma for self catheterisation.
- Spatulate and implant ureters into caecum, via a 4–5cm submucosal tunnel, and make a stented mucosal anastomosis.
- Leave a large bore catheter in the reservoir via the catheterisable stoma, and bring the ureteral stents through reservoir and abdominal walls.
- Close the reservoir as illustrated (Fig. 13.13D).
- Place abdominal drains and close the abdomen.

Complications
As for Ileocystoplasty.

Follow-up
- As for Ileocystoplasty, and appropriate to the primary diagnosis (e.g. urothelial cancer)

Orthotopic bladder substitution—the Studer Ileal neobladder with proximal ileal conduit

Indications
As for Mainz pouch (above) but contraindications for retention of the native urethra and its continence mechanisms must not exist, and the patient must be highly motivated and desirous of orthotopic diversion, and prepared to acknowledge and accept the risk of associated complications.

Preparation
As for Mainz pouch.

Procedure
After cystectomy with preservation of urethra and its continence mechanism
- Mobilise a 56cm segment of ileum, avoiding the terminal 15cm.
- Restore ileal continuity and close the mesenteric defect above the segment.
- Close the distal end.
- Open the isolated segment on its antimesenteric side, from a point near the (closed) distal end, for about 40cm, leaving the proximal 15cm tubular as the isoperistaltic 'afferent limb' to prevent ureteral reflux.

- Configure the opened segment like a 'U', and suture adjacent walls.
- Anastomose ureters onto the afferent limb. A technique like that described above under Ileal conduit is acceptable.
- Bring the stents out through the wall of the 'afferent limb' and the abdominal wall, and drain into a urostomy appliance.
- Anastomose the urethra to the edges of an incision made in the dependent portion of the detubularised ileal segment, using six to eight 3/0 monofilament absorbable sutures, and place a large calibre Foley's urethral catheter across the anastomosis and insert a large suprapubic catheter through abdominal wall and the anterior wall of the neobladder.
- Close the anterior wall of the neobladder to form a spherical reservoir.
- Drain the pelvis and close the abdomen.

Complications
- As for Mainz pouch, *plus*
- Urinary incontinence (stress and overflow type and nocturnal incontinence)
- Urethroileal anastomotic stricture.

Follow-up
- Perioperative care as for Ileocystoplasty and Mainz pouch
- Begin pelvic floor exercises immediately postoperatively
- Remove drains when drainage diminishes, stents after 1–2 weeks
- Remove urethral catheter and clamp suprapubic catheter after 1–3 weeks
- Thereafter as for Mainz pouch.

Surgery for vesicovaginal fistula

Vaginal approach

Indication
Benign vesicovaginal fistula.

Position
Extended lithotomy.

Preparation
* Prep the vagina and vulva with antiseptic solution. Shave if necessary
* Place appropriate retractors e.g. Scott ring retractor and Auvard weighted retractor.

Procedure
* Perform cystoscopy, and cannulate ureteral orifices if necessary.
* Make an inverted U incision in the anterior vaginal wall, including the fistula, and raise a flap of vaginal skin.
* Mobilise the fistulous tract through the perivesical fascia and excise it.
* Separate bladder, perivesical fascia, and vagina for a small distance.
* Close the bladder defect in the midline using interrupted absorbable sutures.
* Close the perivesical fascia transversely.
* Excise the free end of the vaginal skin flap, and advance it to cover the repair. Suture with interrupted absorbable suture material.
* Additional security can be obtained by the interposition of pedicled tissue flaps.
* In each case, the flap is tunnelled deep to vaginal skin and sutured in place to separate vaginal and vesical repairs.
* The labial incision is then closed.
* A vaginal pack is left in place for 24–48 hours.

Complications
* Fistula recurrence
* Urinary tract infection
* Ureteral injury
* Haemorrhage, infection, thromboembolic disease.

Follow-up
* Indwelling urethral or suprapubic catheter for 14–21 days. A cystogram may be obtained before removal of catheter.

Abdominal approach

Position
Lithotomy

Preparation
* The abdomen, vulva and vagina prepped with antiseptic solution and draped
* Cystoscopy is performed, the ureters maybe cannulated.

Incision
Pfannenstiel or median (better for omentoplasty)

Procedure

- Mobilise the bladder anteriorly in the perivesical space and bivalve it sagittally.
- Dissect between bladder and vagina until the fistula tract can be excised leaving healthy bladder, perivesical fascia and vagina separated for a distance around the fistula.
- Repair bladder and perivesical fascia, taking care not to incorporate ureters into the repair and repair vagina if possible.
- Mobilise the right hemicolon.
- Separate the greater omentum from the transverse colon and mobilise it as a pedicled flap based on the right gastroepiploic vessels.
- Place the omental flap behind the mobilised right hemicolon and fix it in place between vagina and bladder using absorbable sutures.
- Place a suprapubic or urethral catheter and abdominal drains.
- Close the abdomen in layers and insert a vaginal pack for 24–48 hours.

Complications

As for vaginal approach plus abdominal wound complications.

Follow-up

As for vaginal approach.

Ureteroneocystostomy

Indications
- Refluxing megaureter associated with perceived risk of reflux nephropathy
- Trauma or disease involving the lower third of the ureter.

Position
Supine, with 25° of additional lordosis at the lumbosacral level.

Incision
- Pfannenstiehl, Turner Warwick, median, paramedian or Gibson
- Transperitoneal or retroperitoneal approach.

Procedure
Many variations exist, whose specific application depends on the clinical setting and surgeon's preference—the Politano–Leadbetter procedure will be described as an example:
- Make a vesicotomy.
- Insert a traction suture into the ureter at the ureteral orifice and circumcise the mucosa around it.
- Incise the trigonal smooth muscle and attachments to Waldeyer's sheath, and then bluntly mobilize a length of ureter in the perivesical space.
- Pass a right angled or curved clamp through the ureteral hiatus, into the perivesical space, cephalad for a distance equal to 5 times the ureteral diameter.
- Incise the bladder urothelium over the tip of the instrument and spread the jaws to create a new hiatus.
- Draw a strong suture from the new through the original hiatus and attach it to the end of the ureter, then draw the ureter up and into the bladder via the new hiatus.
- Close the original detrusor hiatus with absorbable suture, leaving the urothelial defect open.
- Make a suburothelial tunnel from the original hiatus to the new, and draw the ureter through it.
- Anchor ureteral to trigonal smooth muscle and make a mucosa-to-mucosa ureterovesical anastomosis.
- Close urothelium over the new muscular hiatus.
- This ureteroneocystostomy is usually stented for a few days or weeks.
- Close the vesicotomy with continuous absorbable suture.
- Drain the perivesical space or (if opened) peritoneal cavity, and leave a urethral or suprapubic catheter for 7–10 days.

Complications
- Bleeding, injury to adjacent organs
- Ureteral kinking, stricture or necrosis
- Wound, urinary or chest infections
- Thromboembolic disease
- Persistent or recurrent vesicoureteral reflux.

Follow-up

- For vesicoureteral reflux, continue prophylactic antibiotics until the stent has been removed and cystography has confirmed reflux has ceased.
- Upper tract imaging at 6 weeks to exclude obstruction.
- Children with established reflux nephropathy potentially need life-long nephrological follow-up.

Pyeloplasty

Indications

Urodynamically significant, complicated, or symptomatic pelviureteric junction (PUJ) obstruction.

Preparation

- Radioisotope studies of renal function to confirm the diagnosis and that the kidney is salvageable—a period of ureteral stenting may be appropriate.
- Otherwise as for nephrectomy.

Incision

- Flank, dorsal lumbotomy or subcostal depending on patient habitus and surgeon's preference.
- Approach can be transperitoneal or retroperitoneal.

Procedure

Anderson–Hynes pyeloplasty is described here

- Expose the upper ureter, pelviureteric junction and renal pelvis taking care not to interfere with the ureteral blood supply (Fig. 13.14A—note here the kidney is retracted forwards to expose its posterior aspect).
- Identify a roughly diamond-shaped area of renal pelvis incorporating the PUJ, and place stay sutures at these points.
- Transect the ureter at the appropriate level and spatulate it by incising laterally for a distance appropriate for the planned anastomosis.
- Excise the redundant renal pelvis tissue as marked.
- Make a pelviureteric anastomosis as illustrated, starting by suturing the apex of the inferior pelvic flap into the V of the ureteral spatulation. Continue with a running fine absorbable suture along one side of the ureteral spatulation and then the other. (Fig. 13.14B). Complete the repair by closing the renal pelvis above the ureteropelvic anastomosis including a 3-point suture incorporating ureter (Fig. 13.14C).
- The repair may be stented. Drain the perirenal space.

Complications

- Haemorrhage
- Injury to adjacent structures—spleen, pancreas, duodenum, colon, great vessels, pleura, cisterna chyli
- Urinoma or urinary fistula
- Urinary, chest or wound infection
- Thromboembolic disease
- Recurrent PUJ obstruction.

Follow-up

- Remove urethral catheter after 48 hours and drains when drainage is minimal
- Ureteral stents are removed after about 2–6 weeks
- No universal follow up protocol exists. Urogram or renogram at about 6–12 weeks seems sensible with repeat imaging at 1 year and 5 years or as clinically indicated.

(A)

(B)

(C)

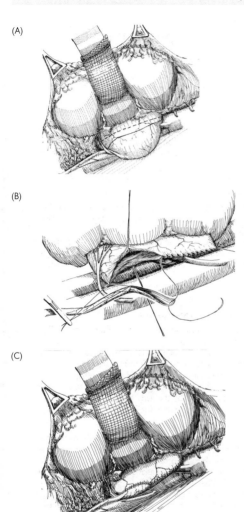

Fig. 13.14 Anderson–Hynes pyeloplasty

Procedures for hypospadias and chordee

This is a large topic and many techniques are used. Essential principles are described here. Techniques include:

MAGPI

Meatal advance and glanuloplasty (Duckett 2002).

- Here the urethral meatus is advanced and the glans reconfigured to give an approximation of the normal appearance
- It can only be applied where there is subcoronal hypospadias and no chordee
- It is a one-stage procedure and no stent or catheter is required.

Onlay island flap

- Can be used when the meatus is rather proximal on the penile shaft, but there is little or no chordee and a good quality urethral plate is present distally
- An island of dorsal preputial skin on a proximally based pedicle of Colles' fascia can be raised and transposed anteriorly where it is sutured to the urethral plate and forms the anterior wall of the 'neo-urethra'
- Glans wings are raised and approximated over the flap, and penile skin is transposed from dorsally and sutured ventrally.

Parameatal based flap (Mathieu)

- For distal hypospadias with minimal chordee and healthy, well-perfused anterior skin and fascia
- A distally-based fascio-cutaneous flap is raised, based around the urethral meatus and sutured to the urethral plate
- Glans 'wings' are raised and approximated over the flap
- Redundant dorsal penile and preputial skin is transposed anteriorly to make up the deficit created by the flap
- A catheter or dribble tube is left in for 2 days.

Tubularized flap techniques

- May be used for one-stage repair in cases of proximal hypospadias where release of chordee results in proximal displacement of the urethral meatus and disruption of the urethral plate. Pedicled flaps of preputial and penile skin can be tubularised over a stent or catheter and anastomosed to healthy urethra
- The distal end may be tunnelled through a glans channel or glans 'wings' can be raised and approximated over the tubularised flap.

Incised plate hypospadias repair

- This technique has been advocated for:
  - Cases of distal hypospadias without chordee and where a good quality urethral plate exists, *and*
  - Cases of more proximal hypospadias where severe ventral curvature is not present after penile degloving, and where a good quality urethral plate is present
- The urethral plate is deeply incised ventrally to near the corpora cavernosa and tubularised over a 6Ch stent
- A pedicled dartos flap is used to cover the repair, and glans flaps are raised and approximated over the urethra
- Dorsally based penile skin flaps are transposed ventrally to cover the shaft.

Hypospadias free grafts

- Where genital skin is unavailable or insufficient (such as after failed surgery), tubularised free grafts or onlay grafts of extragenital tissue can be used.
- These include bladder mucosal grafts, and buccal mucosal grafts (the latter appears superior in durability and in having less tendency to shrink.
- A well-vascularised recipient bed is essential which may necessitate mobilising pedicled flaps such as tunica vaginalis.

Urethral surgery for stricture: urethroplasty

Many procedures have been developed and are in common use. The essentials of some commonly used techniques are:

Position

Lithotomy or extended lithotomy.

Preparation

- A full urethral assessment may include proximal and distal urethroscopy and urethrography
- Urinary infection must be treated preoperatively if possible
- Suprapubic access is an advantage
- Shave perineum and scrotum, prep with antiseptic and drape, carefully excluding the anus
- Use a Scott retractor or sutures for retraction in the perineum.

Incision

Depends on the site and extent of stricture and the technique to be used—usually either circumcision incision or perineo-scrotal inverted Y incision or both.

Procedure

- Incise the skin and subcutaneous tissue.
- Perineo scrotal incisions
  - Separate the bulbospongiosus muscles
  - Mobilise the urethra (Fig. 13.15)
  - Using sounds or flexible cystoscope, identify the site and extent of the stricture.
- Penile incisions
  - Circumcise and deglove the penis by dissecting deep to Colles' fascia
  - Identify the site and extent of stricture, incise Buck's fascia and mobilise the urethra as necessary.

Techniques used include:

One stage procedures

- Stricture excision and primary reanastomosis.
  - Usually for relatively short strictures proximal to the penile suspensory ligament.
  - The urethral ends are spatulated for a centimetre (proximal end dorsally, distal end ventrally) and re-anastomosed over a catheter or stent using one or two layers of absorbable suture material.
  - Proximally, additional functional length can be obtained by means such as separating the crura of the corpora cavernosa, resecting part of the inferior aspect of the symphysis pubis, or transposing urethra behind one of the corpora cavernosa.

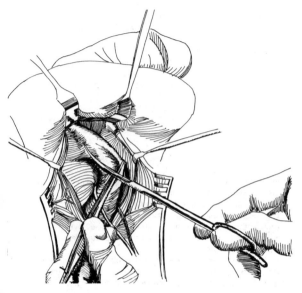

Fig. 13.15 Mobilising the urethra for urethroplasty

- Dorsal or ventral onlay pedicled flaps or free grafts.
  - Penile or preputial skin is mobilised, usually on a proximally based pedicle of Colles' fascia and transposed to bridge a defect where urethra has been incised.
  - Normal urethral calibre is restored. The repair remains stented for a period depending on the technique and surgeon's preference.
  - Free grafts of split skin, bladder mucosa or buccal mucosa are used in the same setting, quilted to Buck's fascia covering the tunica albuginea of the penis.
- Tubularized pedicled flaps or free grafts.
  - In general these are associated with higher complication and attrition rates than onlay grafts or flaps.

Two stage procedures

- In principle, transposed tissue is given time to 'bed in' and acquire local blood supply before being tubularised to restore continuity.
  - In the penile urethra, the availability of hairless skin makes it possible to incise skin and urethra in the midline, and suture urethral mucosa and corpus spongiosum to adjacent Colles' fascia and skin edge. After a minimum of 6 months eccentric flaps of medially (periurethrally) based skin are raised, tubularised over a catheter, and covered with Colles fascia and skin. Eccentric flaps are used so suture lines are not superimposed.
  - In the bulbar urethra, hairless split skin, bladder, or buccal mucosa is used to augment the opened urethra, and subsequently tubularised under bulbospongiosus muscle, fascia and scrotum.

Complications

- Wound or urinary tract infection
- Recurrent stricture—all techniques have a 'rate of attrition'
- Urinary extravasation, urethrocutaneous fistula.

Follow-up

After catheter removal, interval uroflowmetry, and endoscopy are prudent measures as symptoms may be misleading.

Procedures for stress urinary incontinence

Burch colposuspension

Indications
Genuine stress urinary incontinence with urethral and bladder neck hypermobility.

Position
Lithotomy with legs abducted.

Preparation
- Counsel regarding the possibility of urinary retention and need for self catheterisation
- Treat UTI preoperatively
- Prep and drape lower abdomen, vulva and vagina and drape excluding anus.

Incision
- Low median, Turner-Warwick, or Pfannenstiel
- Extraperitoneal approach.

Procedure
- Perform cystoscopy and place a large Foley catheter in the bladder with the balloon inflated—use this to help locate the bladder neck. Also place a suprapubic catheter.
- Place appropriate retractors and develop the retropubic perivesical space.
- Tease away perivesical and perivaginal fat, until the endopelvic, perivesical and perivaginal fascia and pectineal ligaments are demonstrated (Fig. 13.16A).
- Insert two fingers or a sponge-stick into the vagina to elevate it, and place a suture into vagina laterally at the level of mid urethra, on each side, excluding 'mucosa'. Pass each suture through the pectineal ligament also, but do not pull up yet—apply clamps (Fig. 13.16B).
- Do the same with at least one more suture on each side, at the level of the urethrovesical junction, but lateral to it. There may be considerable venous bleeding during this manoeuvre.
- Ensure that bladder and urethra have not been included in any suture, and then approximate the vagina and pectineal ligament by tightening the sutures while elevating vagina from within.
- The correct position has been achieved when the urethra and bladder neck are suspended behind the symphysis pubis, but are not compressed. The vagina need not be in contact with pectineal ligament (Fig. 13.16C).
- Place perivesical drains and close the abdomen. Remove the urethral catheter.

Complications
- Haemorrhage and haematoma
- Bladder or urethral injury

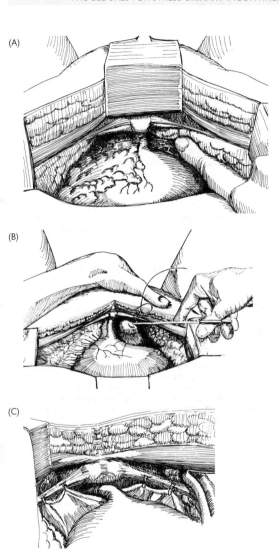

Fig. 13.16 Burch procedure for stress urinary incontinence

- Vesicovaginal fistula
- Delayed voiding or urinary retention requiring long-term intermittent catheterisation
- Venous thrombosis or embolism
- Wound or urinary tract infection.

Follow-up
- Drains are removed after a day or two when the drainage diminishes
- Clamp the suprapubic catheter and monitor post-void residual bladder volumes as soon as the patient is comfortable and mobile
- In the event of delayed voiding, she will commence self-catheterisation until the residual volumes decrease
- This can be followed up by a specialist nurse or stoma therapist, and at outpatient clinics.

Sling procedures
Indications
Genuine stress urinary incontinence as a consequence of urethral and bladder neck hypermobility as well as intrinsic sphincter dysfunction.

Position and preparation
- As for the Burch colposuspension
- Some synthetic slings may be placed under local anaesthesia.

Procedure
- Variations exist:
  - Using autologous tissue, processed cadaveric tissue, processed xenografts, semi-synthetic or synthetic materials, *and*
  - Placing the sling at the level of the bladder neck or mid urethra *and*
  - Via retropubic or vaginal approaches, or by means of a combination of vaginal, endoscopic and percutaneous techniques.
- In principle, the sling is placed (via a vaginal incision) deep to the vaginal skin and fascia, and passes through the pubocervical fascia on each side, literally slinging the urethra or urethrovesical junction.
- Tension is counterproductive—the sling is designed to restore the urethrovesical junction or bladder to the correct anatomical position, not to compress it.
- The sling is held in position by friction and subsequent fibrosis, or by fixation to the abdominal wall or pelvis.
- Cystoscopy may be used to ensure that bladder and urethra have not been injured.
- A urethral or suprapubic catheter may be left *in situ* for a period postoperatively.

Complications
- Inadvertent injury to adjacent structures (bowel, iliac vessels)
- Bleeding, haematoma
- Urinary retention or delayed voiding
- Urethral erosion, vesicovaginal or urethrovaginal fistula.

Follow-up
As for Burch colposuspension

Procedures for Peyronie's disease

Techniques used depend on the patient's erectile function and phallus size, and on the expertise and experience of the operator. They include plication of tunica albuginea penis, excision of the plaque and substitution with dermis, or insertion of a penile prosthesis. Penile plication is described.

Indication
Used for severe angulation of the penis, where length and erectile function are acceptable.

Position
Supine or in lithotomy with legs abducted.

Preparation
- Antibiotics with induction of anaesthesia if prosthesis is to be used
- Thromboembolism prophylaxis
- Prep and drape penis and scrotum.

Incision
Circumcision with degloving proximally, deep to Colles' fascia.

Procedure
- Produce artificial erection by application of tourniquet and intracavernosal sterile saline injection
- Estimate the number and size of the ellipses that must be excised opposite the plaque in order to produce straightening of the penis.
- Mark these on the penis and then check the effect by grasping the tunica albuginea penis with Allis clamps so as to produce reversible plication. Urethral mobilisation may be required
- When the correct effect is produced, incise Buck's fascia, excise ellipses of tunica albuginea as marked and close the defects with strong nonabsorbable or polydioxanone suture material
- Obtain haemostasis then replace Colles' fascia and skin and suture as for circumcision.

Complications
- Haematoma
- Urethral injury
- Cavernositis
- Over- or under-correction
- Shortening of the penis (a given complication)
- Waisting with loss of erectile turgour distally or abnormal flexibility at the waist
- Loss of penile sensation.

Follow-up
Review at specialised andrology or male sexual dysfunction clinic.

Percutaneous surgery of the upper urinary tract

Indications
- Drainage of collections outside the urinary tract
  - Perinephric abscess, urinoma
- Percutaneous nephrostomy
  - Urgent proximal drainage of the upper urinary tract in the presence of renal failure or sepsis, usually anticipating definitive treatment
  - Antegrade placement of ureteral stents (eg when the ureteral orifice cannot be cannulated retrograde)
- Percutaneous nephrolithotomy (PCNL)
  - Management of upper tract stones not appropriate for *ESWL* (see below) because of
    — Large size or complexity (staghorn calculi)
    — Hardness (cystine, calcium oxalate monohydrate)
    — Calculi in calyceal diverticula
- Percutaneous treatment of infundibular, PUJ, or ureteral stenosis (see Ureterorenoscopic procedures)
- Percutaneous management of upper tract transitional cell carcinoma (controversial).

Position
- Generally prone or semi-prone
- Retrograde placement of ureteral guidewires or catheters may require the lithotomy position initially.

Preparation
- Inform the patient of pertinent risks and alternatives
- Attempt to optimise their fitness for the procedure by means such as stopping anticoagulants, treating hypertension or UTI etc. However, the urgency of the situation (pyonephrosis for example) may make this impractical and delay unwise
- Give broad-spectrum intravenous antibiotics regardless of whether local or general anaesthesia is to be used
- Prepare the area for percutaneous access and position fluoroscopic tube and monitors
- For PCNL:
  - General anaesthesia is given
  - A ureteral balloon catheter is advanced via a cystoscope over a guidewire and inflated at the PUJ to occlude it, *and*
  - A Foley's urethral catheter is inserted to drain the bladder
  - The patient is repositioned, prepped, and draped as above.

Procedure

Access

- Fluoroscopy and ultrasonography are used to guide the placement of the appropriate guidewires, cannulas and catheters.
- For drainage of pyonephrosis, generally a lower pole posterior calyx is punctured for convenience and safety.
- For other indications, the placement of a retrograde ureteral catheter allows opacification and dilatation of the pelvicalyceal system, and the most appropriate calyx or calyces are punctured. Note that more than one tract may be used.
- A guidewire is advanced into the collecting system, and an attempt made to manoeuvre it down the ureter.
- The nephrostomy tract is dilated by a variety of techniques:
  - For placement of nephrostomy catheters or antegrade placement of ureteral stents, graduated fascial dilators are advanced over the guidewire until the correct calibre is obtained.
  - For percutaneous surgery involving nephroscopy further dilatation is achieved with telescopic dilators, coaxial dilators or (most safely) with a balloon dilator, over which a 30 Ch sheath is advanced to maintain the tract. The balloon—but not the guidewire—is removed.

Nephrostomy tube drainage

- Usually, a pigtail nephrostomy catheter is advanced over the guidewire to the appropriate position under fluoroscopy, and the guidewire is removed. The tube is secured within the collecting system by its 'pigtail' curl (which may have a strong 'memory' or a locking mechanism to prevent unravelling) and at skin level.
- A similar technique is used for perinephric abscess or urinoma.

PCNL

- A large sheath is placed to maintain the tract.
- The rigid nephroscope is passed though the sheath alongside the guidewire. Saline is the usual irrigant.
- Stones or fragments less than 10mm in diameter can be grasped and removed.
- Larger stones are fragmented using ultrasonic, electrohydraulic, laser or pneumatic lithotripsy and removed piecemeal. The balloon catheter at the PUJ prevents fragment migration during this procedure.
- All stone is removed—sometimes via several tracts. Flexible nephroscopy and fluoroscopy confirm stone clearance and exclude major collecting system injury.
- The ureteral balloon catheter is removed.
- A purpose-made double pigtail ureteral stent with attached coaxial large-bore nephrostomy catheter (Councill) is placed antegrade.
- Haemorrhage from the nephrostomy tract may be tamponaded with a Kaye balloon catheter.

Complications
- Haemorrhage, loss of renal parenchyma or kidney
- Perforation of the collecting system
- Loss of access to the collecting system
- Injury to adjacent structures—bowel, pancreas, liver, spleen, major vessels
- Urosepsis
- Persistent obstruction and urinary fistula.

Follow-up
- Intensive monitoring in the immediate postoperative period
- Urography after 24–48 hours to confirm stone-free status and urinary tract integrity
- Further procedures may be required including further nephroscopy or ESWL
- The nephrostomy tube and ureteral stent can be removed if imaging result is favourable and bleeding insignificant
- After a few hours observation, discharge for outpatient follow up in a fortnight.

Extracorporeal shockwave lithotripsy (ESWL)

Indications

- Small urinary tract calculi (<2cm in the kidney, <1cm in the ureter), in the absence of obstruction or acute urinary tract infection.

Note—Hard stones may be difficult to fragment and the management of small lower pole calyx calculi remains controversial.

Position

- Depends on the stone position within the urinary tract and the type of lithotripter (not all can accommodate a prone patient)
- Supine for renal and upper ureteral stones
- Prone for lower and midureteral stones and bladder stones
- Ensure excellent contact between the patient's skin and the shockwave transmitting device.

Preparation

- Confirm appropriateness of procedure and exclude (relative or absolute) contraindications
  - Pregnancy
  - Abdominal aortic aneurysm
  - Bleeding diathesis or anticoagulation
  - Urinary tract infection or obstruction
- Antibiotics may be given orally preoperatively
- For non-opaque calculi, urinary tract opacification may be achieved by intravenous or retrograde pyelography
- Stone localisation may be achieved using biplanar fluoroscopy and/or ultrasonography
- The need for sedation and analgesia or anaesthesia depends on the patient and the type of lithotripter to be used.

Procedure

- Position the patient so that the calculus is at the focal point of the shock wave
- Commence treatment at low power if the patient is awake
- Repeat imaging at intervals to confirm that the stone is still within the focal point, and to monitor fragmentation.

Complications

- Failure to fragment calculus, or clear fragments
- Uro sepsis
- Steinstrasse—a logjam of fragments, usually near the vesicoureteral junction or PUJ
- Haematoma, haematuria
- Significant injury to adjacent structures (growth-plates in children, lung, bowel, panceas, liver, spleen, uterus, ovaries)—fortunately very rare.

Ureterorenoscopic procedures

Indications
Diagnostic
- Ureterorenoscopy (using rigid or flexible instrument)
- Urothelial biopsy

Therapeutic
- Removal or fragmentation of upper tract urinary calculi
- Resection or destruction of upper urinary tract urothelial neoplasms
- Treatment of obstructive lesions (congenital or acquired) of
  - Calyceal infundibulum
  - Ureteropelvic junction
  - Ureter.

Position
Dorsal lithotomy.

Preparation
- If endopyelotomy is contemplated imaging of the related vascular anatomy is prudent
- Appropriate counselling and consent
- Arrange intraoperative fluoroscopy
- Treat UTI
- Antibiotics with anaesthetic induction
- Prepare perineum and genitalia with antiseptic solution, perform EUA, and drape.

Procedure
- Perform rigid cystoscopy, and, if appropriate, retrograde pyelography.
- Pass a guidewire into the ureter.
- Dilatation of the ureteral orifice and intramural ureter—if necessary— may be done most safely using a balloon dilator.
- A ureteral access sheath may be helpful, especially for flexible ureteroscopic procedures, and is placed, using the Seldinger technique over a tapered dilator and guidewire. The dilator is then removed.
- Pass the ureteroscope either over the guidewire, or alongside it, under direct endoscopic vision with fluoroscopic control.
- Choose the device most appropriate for the job and pass it along the working channel of the ureteroscope.
- Visibility is achieved by irrigating through the ureteroscope. Irrigant flow is improved by intermittent pressure provided by a blood pump or manually using a syringe or other device.
- Small calculi can be retrieved using a variety of graspers or wire baskets.
- Larger calculi (>5mm) are fragmented using one of the following:
  - Electrohydraulic, laser (pulsed-dye or holmium YAG), ultrasonic or ballistic (Swiss lithoclast) lithotripsy.
  - The first two can be used with flexible or rigid instruments, the last two with rigid instruments only.

- Biopsies can be taken using cold forceps.
- Tumour can be vaporised using the holmium YAG laser or resected using a ureteroscopic resectoscope.
- Strictures can be dilated using balloon dilators, or incised either under endoscopic vision using cold knife, electrosurgical knife, laser, or the Accucise device.
- It is not necessary to place ureteral stents after endoureteral procedures without ureteral trauma or dilatation, but they should be used when there has been traumatic manipulation or extravasation. For endopyelotomy, special endopyelotomy stents are used.

Complications
- Ureteral avulsion
- Urinary extravasation, urinoma
- Haemorrhage, 'clot colic'
- Injury to adjacent structures (iliac vessels, duodenum)
- Infection
- Stricture.

Follow-up
- Urolithiasis
  - Remove stents after a few days
- Endoureterotomy, endopyelotomy
  - Remove stents after 6 weeks
  - Thereafter as for pyeloplasty
- Urothelial neoplasms
  - Confirm disease-free status or plan definitive treatment
  - Strict surveillance protocols are used, similar to those for bladder cancer, and involving imaging, urine cytology, and endoscopy.

Laparoscopic urology: introduction

- Laparoscopic surgery is one of the most rapidly progressive areas of urology.
- There is increasing evidence that surgical outcome is at least as good when certain major procedures are performed laparoscopically rather than using conventional scalpel surgery.
- Evidence supports the following procedures being performed laparoscopically:
  - Orchidectomy for intra-abdominal testes
  - Ureterolithotomy
  - Pyeloplasty
  - Simple nephrectomy
  - Radical nephrectomy
  - Nephroureterectomy
  - Adrenalectomy
  - Renal cyst decortication.
- Currently, laparoscopic radical prostatectomy and live donor nephrectomy are also becoming established but long term results are awaited.
- Recent reports of major reconstructive procedures such as enterocystoplasty and ileal conduit urinary diversion have been described in the literature.
- Benefits of laparoscopic surgery include:
  - Shorter hospital stay
  - Less analgesia required
  - Fewer complications
  - Quicker return to functional normality.

Performing laparoscopic operations

- Careful patient selection is essential such as the consideration of existing respiratory disease, obesity, organomegaly, coagulation problems or previous surgery that may make laparoscopic procedures unnecessarily difficult.
- Pneumoperitoneum can be achieved either by open (Hassan) or closed (Veress) techniques.
- CO_2 is the most commonly used insufflant due to its inertness and solubility in blood.
- The intra-abdominal CO_2 pressure is generally kept at around 15mmHg.
- Trocar placement depends on the procedure being performed.
- Transperitoneal or retroperitoneal approaches are commonly used.
- Trocars vary from 3–20mm in diameter and can be disposable or non-disposable.
- Trocar sheaths can accommodate many instruments including:
  - Laparoscope
  - Graspers
  - Dissectors
  - Scissors
  - Scalpel
  - Electrocautery

- • Retractors
- • Suction
- • Needle holders
- • Suturing devices.
- Instruments also exist for specimen extraction, and often removal is achieved manually using a Pfannenstiel incision.
- Port-site closure is usually in layers with a subcuticular suture to skin.

Laparoscopic radical nephrectomy

Indications
- Malignant tumours of the kidney
- Renal vein or IVC involvement necessitates open surgery
- Large, polar tumours may be better served with conventional open surgery.

Position
Modified flank position with table break at the umbilicus.

Incision
Ports are umbilical, lateral (edge of the rectus sheath) and upper midline.

Procedure (principles)
- The colon is reflected and on the right the duodenum is Kocherised
- The ureter is identified and dissected
- The renal lower pole is mobilised
- Hilar dissection and vessel ligation is performed
- The upper pole is mobilised
- The specimen is extracted (it may be morcellated first).

Laparoscopic pyeloplasty

Indications
- Pelviureteric junction obstruction.
- Long-segment obstruction or associated calculi may contra-indicate laparoscopic surgery.

Position
- Initially, cystoscopy and retrograde pyelography are performed, and a ureteral stent is inserted with the patient in dorsal lithotomy position.
- Modified flank position is used for laparoscopic procedure.

Incision
- For a retroperitoneal approach, a subcostal port is primarily sited beneath the tip of the 12th rib with secondary ports anterior (above the iliac crest in the anterior axillary line) and posterior (at the lateral border of paravertebral muscles).
- Ports for transperitoneal approach have been described above.

Procedure (principles)
- The procedure is usually performed retroperitoneally.
- Ureteral identification and proximal dissection is fundamental whichever approach is used.
- The renal pelvis and upper ureter are fully mobilised.
- Dismembered procedures such as the Anderson–Hynes procedure (pp550–1) are most commonly performed but other procedures such as the Foley V-Y plasty have been reported.
- The renal pelvis is transected circumferentially and excess pelvis removed.
- The proximal ureter is spatulated and anastomosed to the cut edge of the renal pelvis.
- Renal pelvis above the anastomosis is closed with a running suture.
- A drain is often placed as the repair is seldom watertight.

Laparoscopic retropubic radical prostatectomy

Indications

- Clinically localised prostate cancer.
- Prior open prostate surgery is an absolute contra-indication and previous TURP may make laparoscopic radical prostatectomy impossible.

Position

Supine with lower limbs in lithotomy.

Incision

Five ports are placed in an upward-pointing chevron with the apex at the umbilicus.

Procedure (principles)

- The retropubic space is explored and the vasa deferentia are identified and divided
- The seminal vesicles are mobilised and the prostate dissected off the rectum.
- Anterior perivesical dissection, with division of the urachus, allows incision of the endopelvic fascia.
- The dorsal venous complex is suture-ligated.
- The bladder neck is opened starting anteriorly and the seminal vesicles are seen when bladder neck and prostate are separated posteriorly.
- Prostatic vascular pedicles are divided.
- Attempts are made to preserve the postero-lateral neurovascular bundles.
- Finally the urethra is divided at the junction with the prostate
- The urethrovesical anastomosis is performed and the specimen removed.

Laparoscopy for cryptorchidism

- Diagnostic laparoscopy is often necessary for location of an undescended testis.
- Prior to laparoscopy confirmatory re-examination under anaesthesia should be performed.
- An umbilical and two lateral ports are used to allow all of the abdomen to be examined.
- Atrophic testes can be removed, but normal-looking testes are identified can be placed in the scrotum by a variety of procedures.

Complications of laparoscopic urology

Failure to obtain pneumoperitoneum
- Equipment failure
- Pre-peritoneal placement of trocar
- Leakage of insufflant around trocar (especially with open placement)
- Bowel insufflation
- Air embolism from blood vessel insufflation.

Bowel injury
- During primary port placement
- Subsequently, including entrapment of intestine on exiting the abdomen.

Vessel injury
- Abdominal wall vessel injury—usually inferior epigastric vessels
- Major vessels such as aorta or iliac arteries are infrequently injured

Diathermy injuries
Can be occult so vigilance is necessary.

Urinary tract injury
Bladder and ureteral injuries.

Bleeding
Can be from the sheath site or direct vessel injury.

Acute hydrocele
Due to accumulation of irrigant in the context of a patent processus vaginalis.

Cardiac arrhythmias

Hypothermia
The insufflant used is generally not warmed so prolonged procedures may result in decreased core temperature.

Postoperative complications
- Subcutaneous emphysema
- Thrombo-embolic complications
- Postoperative chest, wound or urinary tract infection
- Wound complications such as incisional hernia at port sites.

Paediatric surgery

P. Raine and G. Walker

Surgery on the newborn

Newborns may need surgery for an antenatally or perinatally diagnosed congenital anomaly (e.g. duodenal atresia, multicystic kidney) or an acquired problem (e.g. necrotising enterocolitis, testicular torsion). Whatever the underlying diagnosis, common principles apply to pre-, peri- and postoperative assessment and management. A series of investigations and monitoring/supportive procedures may be indicated.

Admission procedure
- Full history
  - Maternal—age, previous/intercurrent illness, drugs
  - Obstetric—parity, previous pregnancies
  - Pregnancy/delivery—complications, mode of delivery, gestation
- Examination
  - Full clinical examination (head to toe)
  - Weight, length, head circumference—plotted on growth chart
- Consent
  - Informed consent from both parents for principle operation and secondary procedures (e.g. central venous long line)

Investigations
Necessary to establish baseline normality and for ongoing management:
- Blood tests performed on venous or capillary (heel-prick) specimens
  - Full blood count
  - Serum urea and electrolytes, liver function tests, glucose, C-reactive protein
  - Blood gas analysis (arterial or capillary): pO_2, pCO_2, pH, base deficit clotting screen
  - Blood culture—if any suggestion of infection.
- Radiology: chest and abdomen (both on one 'babygram' film).

Vascular access
Choice depends on likely duration/volume of infusion and on type of intravenous fluid.
- Peripheral venous access via cannula in dorsum of hand, antecubital fossa, dorsum of foot or scalp vein.
- Central venous access via peripherally inserted central line (epicath)—forearm/lower leg.
- Formal jugular vein (external or internal) cutdown and tunneled catheter from anterior chest wall.
- Arterial line (radial) if intravascular blood pressure monitoring and arterial blood gases needed.

Fluid and electrolyte requirements
Fluid requirements for the newborn take account of:
- High glomerular filtration rate and physiological diuresis
- Large surface area/body weight ratio and high insensitive losses
- High total body water (up to 75%)
- Blood volume 80 to 100ml/kg depending on maturity or prematurity.

Water requirements range from:
- 100mls/kg on day 1 to 175ml/kg on day 7 for a very premature baby (birth weight <1250gm);
- 60mls/kg on day 1 to 150ml/kg on day 7 for a mature baby (>3000gm).

Electrolyte requirements are approximately 2–4mmol/kg/day of sodium and chloride, 2mmol/kg of potassium, 1–2mmol/kg/day of calcium and phosphate, and 0.5mmol/kg of magnesium.

The most suitable fluid for normal maintenance is usually 0.225% sodium chloride with 10% dextrose.

Acid/base balance

Acid/base balance (normal pH and bicarbonate) is essential for normal metabolic and respiratory function. The commonest and most significant derangement (metabolic acidosis) should be corrected before submitting a neonate to anaesthesia and surgery using the formula:

8.4% $NaHCO_3$ solution (ml) = weight (kg) × base deficit × 0.3

Initially use half amount then repeat after rechecking gases.

Nutritional requirements

A newborn cannot withstand any period of calorie starvation without detriment to healing and growth. Gut feeding is usually started with continuous low volume administration via a nasogastric tube. Unless enteral feeding can be started within 24 hours of surgery, intravenous nutrition will be needed.

Positive nitrogen balance is achieved with >75kcal/kg/day and 100kcal/kg/day is the normal requirement. A balanced intake of carbohydrate, lipid, protein (amino acids), vitamins and trace elements is needed in addition to water and electrolytes.

Blood and blood products

It is often advisable to group and save a baby's blood at initial venesection so that a cross-match can be done rapidly if needed.
- Blood products—fresh frozen plasma, cryoprecipitate and platelets— may be needed to counteract problems of coagulation disorder and disseminated intravascular coagulation caused by sepsis.
- Red blood cell replacement is normally made using packed red blood cells on the basis of a circulating blood volume of between 80–100mls/kg.
- Excess circulating volume and cardiac overload is managed by frusemide infusion (1mg/kg) and hypoglycaemia may need to be corrected by a break in blood transfusion for dextrose administration.

Antibiotic prophylaxis

The argument for prophylactic antibiotic use in clean, non-contaminated surgery is stronger for neonates because of decreased immunity. Whenever possible, the policy should be guided by bacteriological cultures but 'best guess' antibiotics are:
- Cefotaxime/metronidazole for enteric organisms (gentamicin/ amoxycillin/metronidazole if more complex)
- Flucloxacillin for staphylococci (vancomycin for multiple resistance MRSA and coagulase-negative staphylococci).
- Antifungals should be considered after prolonged antibiotic use and in additionally compromised patients (cardiac defects, urinary obstruction).

Anatomy of the child

The surgeon should recognise the essential differences between the anatomy of the child and that of the adult and be aware of the importance of allowance for body weight and surface area.

Weight

Most calculations in paediatrics are dependent on knowing the weight of the child. In the emergency situation where the weight is not known, an estimated weight can be derived from the following equation (in children between 1 and 10 years):

$$\text{Weight (kg)} = (\text{age} + 4) \times 2$$

In children and infants weight should be plotted on a centile chart. In older children this can be correlated to height, and in infants to length and head circumference.

Surface area

The proportions of the head, body, and limbs vary throughout childhood. Head and body are proportionately greater in relation to limbs than in adults. To establish body surface area, a specialised chart should be used which will take into account the age of the child (Lund and Bowder).

Abdomen

The abdomen in the child is as broad as it is long, and is more square than rectangular as in adults. This partly explains the preference for transverse incisions for abdominal access.

Small bowel

In neonates the total length of small bowel is approximately 6× crown-rump length. This equates to around 150cm in a term neonate.

Large bowel

The caecal pole is often higher in children so appendicectomy incisions should not be placed too low. The rectum should be the most distensible part of the large bowel, and if this is not the case on contrast enema, it raises the question of Hirschsprung's Disease.

Anus

In most infants, the anus should be of sufficient calibre to allow the passage of the examiner's little finger. The position of the anus in girls should be between one half and one third of the distance from the posterior fourchette to the coccyx. If it is closer to the vagina, consider an anteriorly placed ectopic anus.

Fluid and electrolyte management

Normal fluid requirements

The aim of appropriate fluid management is to maintain or achieve normal hydration in a child. The best indicator of normal hydration is an adequate urine output (neonates 2ml/kg/hr, children 1ml/kg/hr). All regimens depend on knowing the weight of the child, which ideally should be measured or can be derived from the following calculation (in children between 1 and 10 years):

Weight (kg) = (age + 4) × 2

The following table gives a guide to normal fluid requirements in children. This takes into account expected insensible losses, but increased losses (measured or occult) need to be added.

Weight	Fluid requirement for 24 hours		Sodium mmol/kg/day	Potassium mmol/kg/day
<10kg		100ml/kg	3	2
10–20kg	1000ml	+ 50ml/kg	+2	+1
>20kg	1500ml	+ 20ml/kg	+1	+0.5

For example a 22kg child needs:
100ml/kg/day for the first 10kg = 1000ml
50ml/kg/day for the next 10kg = 500ml
20ml/kg/day for the next 2kg = 40ml
Total = 1540ml in 24 hours

Electrolyte requirements

Maintenance sodium and potassium requirements are in the above table. A typical intravenous fluid to achieve this would be 0.225% NaCl with 5% dextrose with 10mmol of potassium added to each 500ml bag.

Assessment of dehydration

Levels of dehydration are conveniently separated into mild (loss of 5% body weight in fluid), moderate (5–10%), and severe (>10%). In mild dehydration children may exhibit increased thirst with dry mucous membranes and a decreased urine output. As more fluid is lost, the child will become increasingly oliguric leading to an altered conscious level, tachycardia, tachypnoea, and signs of reduced perfusion (increased capillary refill time).

Correction of dehydration

Estimated fluid deficit (% loss of body weight × weight × 10) needs to be added to normal daily maintenance and replaced over 24 hours. As, in most cases, there will have been loss of salt and water, the ideal fluid to replace the deficit is 0.9% NaCl. However, rather than administering two separate fluids, 0.45% NaCl with 5% dextrose is appropriate. Measurement of serum electrolytes is important to determine how quickly to rehydrate (over 48 hours if sodium low or high), and whether to add potassium to the solution.

Administration of fluids

If the gastrointestinal tract is functional this should be the preferred route of fluid administration. If a child will not drink, a feeding NG tube can be used. However, in cases where fasting is indicated, the intra venous route is used (see section on Venous access).

Vascular access

Peripheral lines

Commonly used sites for peripheral access include the dorsum of the hand, antecubital fossa, long saphenous vein at the medial malleolus, dorsum of foot, and the scalp in infants. Central venous access is required for certain drugs and concentrated IV nutrition fluids. Peripherally sited central lines (epicutaneous lines) can provide more prolonged period of access. Current recommendations are to ensure the tip of these lines is not advanced into the right atrium.

Intraosseous access

Placement of a specifically designed needle into the intramedullary space of the tibia can offer rapid access for resuscitation, fluids, and drugs. Demonstration of insertion should be in conjunction with formal resuscitation training (APLS, PALS).

Central access

Common veins used for central access include internal and external jugular, subclavian and femoral veins. All can be accessed percutaneously, but the following is a description of the technique for open jugular vein access.

Preoperative

Ensure no bleeding tendency. Determine if any previous central lines—consider Doppler studies or venography if numerous previous lines. Consent should include risk of bleeding, infection and inadvertent dislodgement.

Position

Supine. Head down with neck extension and facing to contralateral side.

Incision

Transverse neck incision about 2cm above clavicle.

Procedure

- If external jugular vein obvious then blunt dissection to expose it. Control of vein achieved by passage of two 3/0 Vicryl ties around it. After tunnelling the line, carry out a venotomy and insert the line. Advancement of line augmented by lateral traction of the vein by cranially sited tie.
- Gain internal jugular vein access by blunt dissection through two heads of sternocleidomastoid. Open the sheath overlying the vein. Clear the vein medially and laterally then grasp it with non-toothed forceps. Pass a right-angled dissector around the deep aspect of vein and then a silicone loop. Avoid rotation of vein by holding with forceps when loop is passed round. Repeat this action achieving cranial and caudal control.

- Make a stab incision in the anterior chest wall. Tunnel the line in the subcutaneous tissue to emerge at the neck incision—aim to place the cuff >1cm from exit site. Cut the line to appropriate length (above inter-nipple line). Flush line with heparinised saline. Deliver the vein into wound with silicone loops—aim to tent vein open with a small amount of intraluminal blood. Grasp superficial aspect of the vein with non-toothed forceps and carry out venotomy with scalpel or scissors. Advance line through venotomy and determine the position of tip with X-ray (RA/SVC junction). Ensure line aspirates and flushes easily. If required, close the venotomy with a purse-string or interrupted 6/0 non-absorbable suture.
- Closure the skin with subcuticular 4/0 or 5/0 absorbable sutures and secure the line.

Complications
- Haemorrhage
- Infection (5–10%)
- Dislodgement
- Pneumothorax in percutaneous subclavian insertion.

Oesophageal atresia

Incidence and presentation

Incidence 1 in 3000 live births. Infants often coughing and 'mucousy' at birth. May have a colour change with first feed. Unsuccessful passage of NG tube into blind ending upper oesophageal pouch (at about 12cm), radiography confirms arrest in mid-thorax (T2–3). The history may reveal maternal polyhydramnios.

Anatomy

85% have a lower pouch fistula to trachea at carina (TOF) (Fig. 14.1A). 10% will be pure oesophageal atresia (OA)—no air in stomach on X-ray.

Preoperative

Carry out continuous suction of upper pouch by Replogle tube to avoid aspiration. Investigate the child for associated VACTERL abnormalities. Renal ultrasound and echocardiography are important. If right sided aortic arch it may need to consider left thoracotomy.

Position

Right side up with right arm abducted over head.

Incision

Right posterolateral thoracotomy under angle of scapula.

Procedure

- Open 4th intercostal space. Push parietal pleura away by inserting a damp swab through space. Insert self-retainer to spread ribs.
- Continue dissection posteriorly with damp pledgets, pushing the pleura anteriorly (extrapleural approach). Identify the azygos vein and ligate it in continuity—then divide. Continue pledget dissection medially until the fistula is identified—it may be seen to inflate with ventilation. Clear the fistula with right-angled dissector and control it with a silicone loop.
- Follow the fistula cranially until its attachment to the trachea is identified. Excise the fistula at tracheal junction and close the trachea with interrupted 5/0 absorbable sutures. Check for air-tight closure under water.
- Identify upper pouch—this is helped by advancement of Replogle tube. Carry out limited mobilisation of upper pouch—but exclude an upper pouch fistula (3%). Open the upper pouch transversely ensuring mucosa is opened—the tube will advance into the field.
- Place four or five 'posterior wall' sutures with 5/0 absorbable material. Pass a 6F NG tube across the anastomosis into the stomach. Complete an interrupted single layer anterior anastomosis. (Fig. 14.1B).
- Allow the lung to reinflate and close the intercostal space. Insert an extrapleural chest drain. Close the muscle layers with 4/0 absorbable sutures. Subcuticular 5/0 absorbable sutures to skin.

Postoperative

Commence nasogastric feeds early. Carry out a contrast study at one week and encourage oral feeds if the anastomosis is satisfactory.

Complications

- Anastomostic leak (~8%)—most can be managed conservatively
- Anastomotic stricture (30–50%)—Balloon dilatation or bouginage
- Tracheomalacia—if severe may require intervention (aortopexy or tracheostomy)
- Gastro-oesophageal reflux (30%)—may require fundoplication.

The mortality rate is low if the body weight is >2.5kg and no major cardiac defect.

Management of pure OA

Preoperative work-up as above.

Management

- Managed initially by gastrostomy.
- Give good volume four-hourly feeds to encourage reflux up the distal pouch.
- Radiological assistance required to determine gap between proximal and distal pouches.
- Carry out definitive surgery as above.

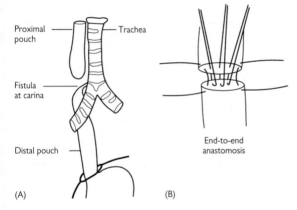

Fig. 14.1 Oesophageal atresia

Intestinal atresia

Duodenal atresia

Associated with Down's syndrome (less than one third of cases). It presents with bile vomiting and distended stomach, may have been identified on antenatal scans (polyhydramnios). There is a double-bubble on plain radiograph. The second part of the duodenum is distended and atretic. 15% are above level of bile duct—no bile is seen on aspirating the NG tube.

Procedure

- Carry out an upper abdominal transverse laparotomy.
- Identify the large baggy proximal duodenum and the small distal duodenum. Mobilise the ends with care to avoid bile duct.
- Make a transverse incision to open the proximal duodenum and open the distal duodenum longitudinally. Carry out a diamond end-to-end anastomosis with interrupted 5/0 absorbable sutures.
- Pass a transanastomotic feeding tube (transgastric or nasal). If the distal duodenum cannot be mobilized and anastomosis cannot be performed safely, use the first loop of jejunum to proximal duodenum.

Jejunoileal atresia

In this there is abdominal distension with a visible/palpable mass and vomiting (bile). The radiograph shows small bowel obstruction and ultrasound reveals a cystic dilated loop. Dilated pre-atretic bowel can be compromised by segmental volvulus.

- Type I Intraluminal membrane (serosal surface looks intact)
- Type II Obvious gap between ends but no defect in mesentery
- Type III Gap in mesentery
- Type IV 'Apple peel' distal intestine or multiple atresias (depending on classification)

Procedure

- Make a transverse mid-abdominal incision.
- Untwist any bowel volvulus. Carry out careful inspection of and irrigation through all bowel distal to atresia to establish patency of the lumen (contrast enema may have shown patent colon).
- Resect or taper any excessively dilated proximal segment.
- Carry out a primary anastomosis if possible with single-layer of interrupted, 4/0 or 5/0 absorbable sutures (end-to-end or end-to-back).

High stomas lead to fluid and electrolyte disturbances and skin problems—avoid them if possible.

Colonic atresia

This presents with bile vomiting and abdominal distension. Contrast enema will demonstrate a microcolon to level of atresia. This may be therapeutic in meconium plug syndrome where there is an intraluminal cause for the obstruction. There is an association with Hirschsprung's disease.

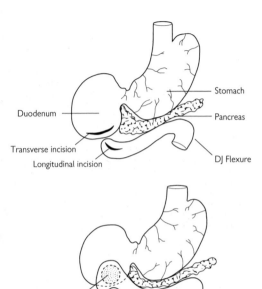

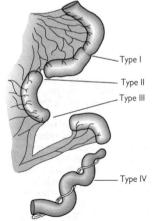

Fig. 14.2 Duodenal atresia with corrective anostomosis

Fig. 14.3 Jejunoileal atresia

Procedure
- Make a transverse mid-abdominal incision. Determine site of atresia and the condition of proximal intestine. Resect any extremely dilated areas or any areas involved in perforation.
- Treat proximal atresias by a primary single layer anastomosis with interrupted 5/0 absorbable sutures (unless more than 3:1 discrepancy in the size). Treat distal atresias (beyond splenic flexure) by forming a double barrelled colostomy and delay the anastomosis until 3–6 months later.

Anorectal atresia

This presents with recognition of a blind perineum on routine examination or with absent stool passage and distension. It is usually anorectal and often associated with a fistula to urethra (male) or vulvovagina (female), urinary tract anomalies and sacral deficiency. A radiograph (pronogram) at 24 hours shows a dilated terminal rectum and gasless (atretic) zone between the rectum and perineum—absent sacral vertebral segments suggest a poorer prognosis. Ultrasound (before gas reaches distal bowel) shows a dilated terminal bulb of atretic bowel.

Immediate management options
- Perineal operation to create neo-anus only appropriate for very 'low' atresias.
- Sigmoid or right transverse defunctioning colostomy with later reconstruction by abdomino-perineal pull-through or posterior sagittal anorectoplasty (PSARP).

Definitive procedure (PSARP)
Catheterise bladder.

Position
Prone with support beneath hips to raise the sacral area—legs abducted to give access to perineum.

Procedure
- Carry out careful assessment of external sphincter fibres with muscle stimulator and marking of skin anal site.
- Make a sagittal incision from coccyx to proposed anterior anal verge. Deepen the incision keeping strictly to the midline separating external sphincter fibres. The internal sphincter and levator muscle fibres should be seen and divided in midline.
- Enter the retrorectal space and identity posterior wall of terminal bulb of the rectum, mobilise it in the extra-serosal plane. Separation from posterior urethra and prostate difficult as anatomical plane fused.
- Identify any urethral fistula—this may be aided by opening the rectum in midline posteriorly to approach fistula directly from lumen. Divide the fistula flush with urethra and closed to avoid a diverticulum.
- Mobilise the rectum proximally/presacrally by further separation from urethra/prostate to allow advance to perineum without tension. Amputate the rectal bulb tip and anastomose with 5/0 absorbable sutures to putative anal skin site, which can be inverted. Taper the rectal lumen tapered by posterior strip resection if markedly distended.

- Carry out meticulous apposition of internal sphincter and levator fibres in midline posterior to rectum with 3/0 absorbable sutures. Appose the subcutaneous fat tissue with 3/0 absorbable sutures.
- Close the wound with 3/0 absorbable sutures with interrupted to skin.

Complications

- Anal recession and stenosis—due to tension and ischaemia—may need dilatation
- Skin excoriation—unaccustomed to frequent loose stools
- Constipation—inadequate defaecation reflex and evacuation
- Incontinence and soiling—deficient muscle and muscle control.

Gastroschisis

Incidence, anatomy, and presentation

This is a congenital abdominal wall defect to the right of the umbilicus with extruded, unprotected small and large bowel. Increasing incidence about 1 in 3000 live births. Associated with young maternal age. May be discovered on antenatal scanning. Parents should be counselled about likely clinical course. A vaginal delivery not contraindicated.

Preoperative

At birth, herniated bowel should be wrapped in impervious cover to prevent evaporative losses. Venous access should be obtained and fluid resuscitation commenced. The infant should be nursed in a position where mesentery is not on traction. Pass an NG tube.

Position

Supine.

Procedure

- Cleanse herniated bowel with aqueous antiseptic solution. Determine size of defect. Pass finger through defect and gently stretch abdominal cavity. Attempt reduction of thickened, 'matted' bowel, which may be aided by small extension of defect laterally. If the bowel reduced under minimal tension close abdominal wall.
- Undermine skin edges with diathermy dissection to reveal abdominal wall muscle which may be deficient. Clear the muscle layer to allow closure.
- If the defect is small it can be closed with pursestring 2/0 absorbable. Close larger defects linearly with interrupted 2/0 absorbable sutures. Use 4/0 or 5/0 absorbable sutures to close the skin. Some surgeons advocate reducing the bowel without general anaesthetic.

If there is doubt about intra-abdominal tension during reduction, a staged approach is advisable.

- Attach Silastic sheeting around defect and tubularise it to create a 'silo'—a ventral hernia within a prosthesis. Then suspend the 'silo' vertically and the oedematous bowel gradually reduces over the next 5–7 days.
- Once the bowel is reduced, close the defect in the above manner. Newer devices allow application of the silo without suturing—a self-expanding ring holds the sac within the defect. This can be applied in a sterile fashion without the need for general anaesthetic.

Consider placement of central (or epicutaneous) IV line at the time of surgery for parenteral nutrition.

Postoperative

NG tube on free drainage until reduction in bilious aspirates. The gut function is slow so feeds increased gradually—average time to full feeds 21–28 days.

Complications

- Outlook generally good.
- Extra-intestinal congenital anomalies rare—associated atresia occurs in ~10%.
- About 50% can be treated with primary closure.
- Short gut syndrome—'functional' or due to loss of bowel.
- Recognised incidence of necrotising enterocolitis.

Exomphalos (omphalocele)

Incidence, anatomy and presentation

Incidence decreasing. May present antenatally—amniocentesis advisable to determine karyotype. There are associations with chromosomal and cardiac anomalies. Caesarean section recommended to avoid rupture of sac.

Anatomy and management

Represents failure of regression of extracoelomic midgut and physiological umbilical 'hernia' results in a membrane covered mid-abdominal herniation of small bowel, large bowel, and liver. If minor (<5cm defect), surgical closure is possible but underdeveloped peritoneal cavity prevents reduction for most >5cm hernias. Conservative approach allows sac to thicken and cicatrise and results eventually in skin covering, but requires later repair of residual ventral hernia.

Meconium ileus

Presentation
Abdominal distension, visible/palpable mass and vomiting (bile). A radiograph shows small bowel obstruction and ground glass appearance of meconium/gas mixture. The obstruction is caused by viscid, meconium pellets inspissated in distal ileum. The proximal ileum/jejunum obstructed and dilated: colon empty and unused (microcolon). It can be complicated by perforation (antenatal and postnatal), segmental volvulus and atresia. Associated with cystic fibrosis (about 80%). Analyse karyotype and, if doubt remains, perform a sweat test later.

Investigation
Following plain radiography, perform water-soluble contrast enema for diagnostic and possible therapeutic reasons. The microcolon will be outlined, and if contrast enters dilated loops of bowel the diagnosis is not in doubt. The lubricating effects of the contrast material may promote passage of normal meconium and a laparotomy may be avoided in around 50% of cases.

Incision
Mid-abdominal transverse.

Procedure
- Deliver all intestine into the wound. Peritoneal calcification indicates antenatal perforation.
- Open the dilated intestine and aspirate/flush viscid meconium. Resect any severely dilated ileum or sites of perforation.
- Attempt to flush distal bowel. If flushing successful, and no severe discrepancy between ends, primary anastomosis can be carried out. However, formation of double-barrelled enterostomy is usually advised either through wound or adjacent to it.
- Other options include Bishop-Koop enterostomy (distal segment as stoma with proximal bowel anastomosed end-to-side) and Santulli enterostomy (proximal segment as stoma with distal bowel anastomosed end-to-side).

Postoperatively management
If cystic fibrosis confirmed, ensure involvement of the appropriate team. Offer parents genetic counselling for future pregnancies. Once established on enteral feeds, start pancreatic enzyme replacement to aid digestion. Use prophylactic antibiotics.

Morbidity and mortality
The outlook for children with cystic fibrosis continues to improve with current life expectancy in the 40s. The previously held opinion that infants presenting with meconium ileus represented the severe end of the spectrum is no longer appropriate.

Hirschsprung's disease

There is absence of ganglion cells (aganglionosis) of distal bowel for variable distance proximally from anus—commonly only involves rectum with transition to normal at rectosigmoid junction. About 20% extend into the sigmoid with occasional total colonic and, very rarely, whole bowel involved. If presents with delayed meconium passage and progressive distension, there is often explosive release of gas and meconium on digital examination. Radiography shows dilated colon to level of 'transition zone', coning down to normal calibre distal bowel. Confirmation by contrast enema/rectal biopsy. The condition may be syndromic with life-threatening respiratory insufficiency.

Immediate management options
- Defunctioning colostomy (right transverse) and delayed definitive procedure
- Saline bowel washouts and decompression with early progression to pull through procedure.

Definitive procedure
Options are endorectal (preserving rectal muscle coat—Soave), rectum-removing (Swenson) or retrorectal (retaining distal rectal pouch—Duhamel). The Soave procedure is described (Fig. 14.4).

Preoperative
Carry out a bowel washout to ensure complete evacuation. Give intravenous antibiotics. Insert a urethral bladder catheter.

Position
Supine on small frame to hold baby in lithotomy position and permit access to abdomen and perineum.

Approach
Procedure commonly done transanally assisted by laparoscopic biopsies and bowel mobilisation. Carry out biopsy confirmation of transition zone and level of normal ganglion cells. If laparotomy needed, perform a Pfannenstiel lower abdominal transverse incision with either retraction or cutting of rectus muscles.

Procedure
- Insert perianal retracting sutures tied over colostomy bag ring to evert and expose lower anal canal. Infiltrate the anal mucosa with adrenaline (1:100 000) solution to minimise bleeding—incised circumferentially just above dentate line.

- Develop dissection in the submucosal plane gradually everting mucosal tube. Carry out laparoscopic vessel cautery and mobilize the sigmoid colon as required. Identify the point of full thickness bowel wall eversion, at the pelvic peritoneal reflection and carry out dissection through the muscle and serosal planes into the peritoneal cavity. Draw the bowel transanally until normal biopsy site identified. Amputate the colon at this point and anastomose to anal mucosal cuff with multiple 5/0 absorbable sutures working in quadrants—avoid tension.
- If laparotomy performed, close the wound with 3/0 continuous absorbable to muscle and fascia and 4/0 subcuticular sutures to skin.

Complications

- Pelvic infection/peritonitis from perforation/contamination
- Anal stenosis/stricture from ischaemia or tension
- Constipation—suggests residual aganglionosis
- Urinary dysfunction—pelvic splanchnic nerve damage
- Enterocolitis—a risk for all Hirschsprung's cases and not removed by successful surgery.

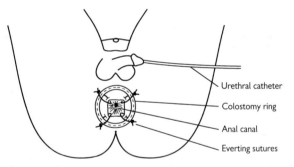

Urethral catheter

Colostomy ring

Anal canal

Everting sutures

Fig. 14.4 Soave approach for Hirschsprung's disease

Necrotising enterocolitis

This is a transmural inflammatory process occurring throughout the GI tract—probably related to ischaemia, invading bacteria and substrates in feed. Onset acute often in newborn complicated by prematurity, infection, intestinal obstruction or other cause of stress. It presents with systemic evidence of lethargy, pallor, distress with bile vomiting, abdominal distension, bleeding per rectum and signs of abdominal wall redness, oedema and tenderness, mass, crepitus on palpation. Abdominal radiograph may show intramural gas (ring and tramline signs) and free intraperitoneal gas signifying perforation. There is rapid progression to necrosis and perforation mandates surgery.

Options
- For very sick, premature, low birth weight babies peritoneal drainage alone may be safest
- Laparotomy with resection, exclusion and stoma decompression is more definitive.

Preoperative management
Correction of acidosis, hypothermia, anaemia, and coagulation disorders and give adequate fluid and antibiotic resuscitation improve the chances of successful outcome.

Position
Supine.

Incision
Transverse muscle cutting supraumbilical.

Procedure
- Aspirate faeculent and bile-stained fluid and culture for bacteria. Carefully separate and explore the inflamed, adherent and friable bowel loops. Evacuate intraloop and loculated abscesses and fluid collections.
- Make assessment of bowel viability and need for resection. Carry out multiple resections and stomas or 'clip and drop' (isolating viable, closed segments in peritoneal cavity to await later restoration of continuity). Stoma formation is invariably needed as primary anastomosis in this situation is highly risky— secondary restoration of continuity is safer. If there is very extensive ischaemic damage this may preclude resection because of 'short bowel' risks. Carry out closure and take a second look at 48 hours—close the abdomen using a prosthetic patch both relieves tension (promoting reperfusion) and facilitates second laparotomy. Bring out stomas through wound or through a separate incision.

- Persisting inflammation and wound infection is a high risk—close wound with 2/0 or 3/0 continuous absorbable sutures to peritoneum, muscle and fascia with subcuticular 4/0 continuous absorbable or monofilament sutures to skin.

Complications

- Persisting systemic problems of acidosis, sepsis, coagulation disorder
- Intraperitoneal sepsis/abscess formation
- Reactionary/secondary intraperitoneal bleeding
- Inadequate absorption and diarrhoea due to mucosal change
- Short gut syndrome following resection and need for parenteral nutrition
- Later stricture and obstruction due to partial ischaemia
- High mortality related to multi-system failure.

Sacrococcygeal teratoma

This tumour develops in utero and involves all three germ layers. It is occasionally malignant. It may be detected antenatally by raised maternal alphafetoprotein levels and abnormal ultrasound scan—occasionally there are severe complications of fetal hydrops, which require premature delivery. It often presents as a large mass in perineum/pelvis between rectum and sacrum/coccyx causing gross pelvic distortion and limb displacement. It is cystic or solid with variable vascularity (can present with high output cardiac failure and excessive bleeding). Doppler ultrasound and MRI imaging are useful to define blood supply and direct exploration to the abdomen or perineum.

Preoperative

- It is essential to have good intravenous access and blood cross-matched in case of excessive bleeding from pelvic vessels, insert a urinary bladder catheter.
- The approach to the tumour is perineal/pelvic but occasional an initial laparotomy is required to control major blood vessels.

Position

Prone with sacro-perineal area elevated with support beneath the pelvis. An iodine soaked gauze packed into rectum will help to define anatomy.

Incision

Make a chevron shaped incision with V based over lower sacrum and limbs of chevron extending either side of tumour.

Procedure

- Elevate skin flaps to expose the tumour and dissect it from posterior rectum anteriorly.
- Amputate coccyx to allow dissection of tumour in anterior sacral space. Use electrocautery sparingly to avoid pelvic autonomic nerve damage. The tumour often has pseudocapsule which aids its definition and separation from pelvic floor and viscera.
- If there is extensive intrapelvic extension, it may be necessary to turn the patient supine and explore the tumour from an abdominal approach. Carry out careful ligation of blood supply from hypogastric, presacral and internal iliac vessels before removal. Haemostasis secured by ligature and cautious electrocautery.
- Approximate the pelvic muscle layers with 3/0 absorbable sutures. Close the chevron incision as an inverted Y with 4/0 absorbable and a suction drain if large residual presacral space. Remove the gauze packing from rectum.

Complications

- Wound infection—related to major tissue disturbance at tumour removal
- Wound haematoma—large potential dead space
- Difficulty with bowel control related to major pelvic muscular dysplasia
- Problems of incontinence related to pelvic nerve distortion/damage
- Lower limb dysfunction related to initial major hip/pelvic distortion.

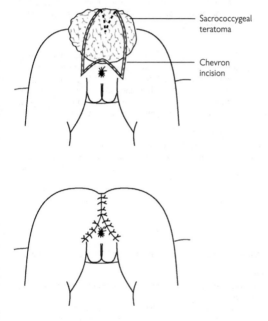

Sacrococcygeal teratoma

Chevron incision

Fig. 14.5 Excision of saciococcygeal teratoma

Congenital diaphragmatic hernia (CDH)

Incidence and presentation

About 1 in 3000 live births (includes in utero losses). Antenatal diagnosis is made in 50% if detailed scans routinely available (<20% otherwise). Postnatal presentation is with immediate respiratory compromise of newborn, which deteriorates with bag and mask ventilation (inflation of intrathoracic stomach). Intubate and ventilate the baby and pass a large (10F) NG tube. Confirm diagnosis by radiography. Small percentage diagnosed late (minor symptoms).

Anatomy

The Bochdalek defect is most common (posterolateral). The Morgagni defect (anteriomedial) is most often a late presentation. Hernia of intra-abdominal viscera into chest—commonly small and large intestine, also stomach, liver, spleen and occasionally kidney also occurs, 80–90% left sided. Pulmonary hypertension is secondary to pulmonary hypoplasia. Echocardiography aids diagnosis and can monitor treatment.

Timing of surgery and adjuncts

Delayed surgery now standard practice. It is not advisable to proceed to repair until ventilatory parameters have improved. Newer treatments include inhaled nitric oxide, surfactant, extracorporeal membrane oxygenation and sildenafil. Gentle ventilation with permissive hypercarbia is recommended. This includes high frequency oscillation.

Position

Supine.

Incision

Ipsilateral transverse upper quadrant or subcostal (1cm below margin).

Procedure

- Open peritoneum and retract upper edge of wound to reveal anterior rim of diaphragm.
- Gently deliver herniated contents from chest into wound. Carry out soft retraction of liver and gut to expose size of defect. Look into hemithorax to determine if sac present. If sac is present, excise it. Identify the posterior rim and mobilize it.
- Insert interrupted horizontal mattress sutures with 2/0 or 3/0 non-absorbable. Place each suture individually and tie after all in place. If no posterior rim and defect large, a patch (PTFE, Silicone) may be used. Cut patch to appropriate size and suture in place with 2/0 or 3/0 non-absorbable sutures. Sutures may be inserted around ribs posteriorly. Chest drains are used uncommonly.
- Close the wound in layers with 3/0 absorbable and subcuticular 4/0 or 5/0 absorbable to skin.

Mortality
Mortality of live born infants around 40%, is usually due to intractable pulmonary hypertension. Some centres report improved survival with multidisciplinary directed approach.

Complications
- Recurrence of hernia
- Chronic lung disease
- Intestinal obstruction—due to adhesions or volvulus (universal mesentery)
- Gastro-oesophageal reflux.

Diaphragmatic eventeration
The diaphragm is present but muscle atrophied. Presentation is similar to CDH although it is often less severe. Radiograph shows pronounced smooth dome of elevated diaphragm and ultrasound scanning shows paradoxical movement of diaphragm (upwards on inspiration). Treatment is by plication of diaphragm through abdominal incision or thoracotomy.

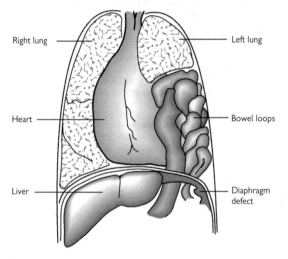

Fig. 14.6 Diaphragmatic hernia

Spina bifida

There is defective neural tube formation with exposed neural tissue at the area of failed posterior vertebral arch development often in the lumbosacral spine. It is often prenatally detected by raised maternal alphafetoprotein levels and anomalous ultrasound scan. Associated conditions are hydrocephalus (cognitive dysfunction), neurogenic bladder and bowel (incontinence) and lower limb paresis/paralysis and sensory losses. The back lesion may be 'closed' (meningocele) or 'open', leaking CSF (myelomeningocele). Open lesions expose the newborn to risks of further neurological damage and ascending CNS infection and warrant early operation to mobilize and close the meningeal membranes, fascia and skin over the exposed central nerve cord.

Preoperative

Antibiotic prophylaxis.

Position

Prone with support to upper chest and pelvis to avoid ventilatory problems related to abdominal pressure.

Procedure

- Outline the exposed neural plaque and meninges by a skin incision.
- Tabularise the nerve cord, if possible, with very fine (5/0, 6/0) absorbable continuous sutures to minimise CSF leak. Close the dura similarly with 5/0 or 6/0 absorbable. Close the fascial layer in a vertical line achieved by longitudinal incision in the erector spinae fascia which is reflected medially to the midline over the bifid spines.
- Close the skin with 3/0 absorbable in either vertical or transverse line with wide undermining to release tension—occasionally rotation or lateral release flaps are needed for a wide defect. Insert a suction drain, useful if extensive undermining of skin.

Complications

- Wound infection
- Skin necrosis/dehiscence due to excessive tension
- Ascending CNS infection and meningitis
- More rapid progression of hydrocephalus related to cessation of CSF leak.

Release of tongue tie

A tight frenulum of the tongue can restrict movement to extent of interference with feeding or speech—rarely the case if tip protrudes beyond
lower teeth. Anxiety about possible effects is a common reason for
referral. Reassurance alone is often sufficient.

Procedure

Usually under general anaesthesia but local possible as procedure takes
seconds.

- Tongue tip grasped with forceps and drawn upwards and forwards to
  expose tight border of frenulum—divided with scissors to release
  tongue. Two leaves of frenulum divided further posteriorly for greater
  advance and the frenular artery in midline avoided.
- This procedure is usually bloodless but significant bleeding requires
  suture (4/0 absorbable) to artery at base of frenulum.

Complications

- Reactionary bleeding—may demand re-exploration and suture of
  artery
- Inadequate release and residual restriction.

Ranula

Anatomy and presentation

This is a smooth, bluish, cystic swelling arising in floor of mouth beneath tongue from sublingual gland. It may cause problem with feeding, interference with speech development and cosmetic concern but there are rarely symptoms of pain/discomfort or infection.

Preoperative

Nasal endotracheal intubation improves the surgeon's access to oral cavity. Jaw opened with dental gag and hypopharynx/posterior airway packed to avoid potential aspiration.

Procedure

- Holding suture in tongue tip may help control and access.
- Excise small, discrete, well-defined cysts completely with repair of mucosa with interrupted absorbable 4/0.
- Make no attempt to excise larger cysts as risk of damage to lingual nerve and submandibular duct.
- Excise a segment of anterior cyst wall with scissor dissection or electrocautery to open and drain cyst. Outer (mucosal) and inner (duct epithelial) linings of cyst then sutured together (with continuous absorbable 4/0) to control bleeding, prevent re-adherence and produce a stoma in cyst wall (marsupialisation). Cyst then rapidly shrinks down and sublingual saliva drains via stoma.

Complications

- Infection if oral hygiene poor and foreign material lodges in cyst
- Bleeding from resected cyst wall
- Recurrence if marsupialisation inadequate.

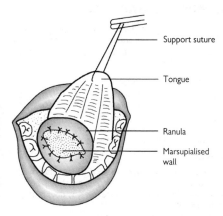

Support suture

Tongue

Ranula

Marsupialised
wall

Fig. 14.7 Marsupialisation of ranula

Preauricular skin tag and sinus

Skin tag/appendages and sinuses arise in the pre-auricular position anterior to the tragus or on the helix as remnants of the first branchial arch and cleft. Skin tags are a cosmetic issue. Sinuses may discharge or become inflamed and chronically infected.

Procedure: excision of skin appendage

- Make an elliptical skin incision in a vertical orientation around the base of the tag judging the dimensions required to produce a flat skin surface without 'dog-ears' on closure. If present, dissect a central cartilage rudiment down to its origin and core it out.
- Close skin with interrupted 5/0 absorbable or Nylon sutures.

Procedure: excision of sinus

- Remove a non-infected sinus by an elliptical incision around its orifice and dissection around the sinus to its base. The sinus tract may be defined using a fine lacrimal duct probe. It may extend as deeply as the temporo-mandibular joint.
- Close the wound with 5/0 absorbable or Nylon sutures.

An infected sinus may ramify in subcutaneous tissues and produce a complex abscess with overlying erythematous skin.

- Carry out wider exploration and excision by raising skin flaps using a Y incision with upper limbs anterior and posterior to the lower pole of the ear and the lower limb just behind the jaw line. Expose the parotid gland—take care to preserve facial nerve and branches.

Complications

- Residual/recurrent infection following incomplete sinus excision
- Facial nerve branch damage
- Temporo-mandibular joint discomfort and stiffness.

Branchial cyst/sinus

This arises from a remnant of the second branchial arch/cleft. The cyst presents as a smooth swelling around midpoint of the line of anterior border of sternocleidomastoid muscle; the sinus may extend from tonsillar fossa of pharynx to skin surface. Differentiation from other cervical masses may need US or CT scanning. Usually asymptomatic but viscid mucus may discharge from a small skin punctum. Infection leads to tenderness/abscess formation and incision and drainage followed by delayed formal excision.

Other arch remnants are very rare. First arch occasionally results in cyst/fistula at angle of jaw and around the external auditory meatus. Third and fourth arch remnants are at the level of thyroid.

Position

Supine with neck extended using a shoulder roll—head rotated to contralateral side. Slight head up tilt decreases venous engorgement (too much tilt risks air embolus).

Preoperative management

IV antibiotics at induction if evidence of infection. Sinus/fistula is best defined by inserting a fine lacrimal probe and anchoring with skin suture for traction. Dye may be instilled (methylene blue) but any spillage/leakage stains normal tissues and obscures dissection.

Incision

Neck skin crease incision over swelling or skin ellipse around sinus orifice.

Procedure

- Divide the platysma and superficial cervical fascia in the line of incision. Carry out dissection between branches of carotid artery avoiding vagus, hypoglossal and glossopharyngeal nerves. If there is close proximity to parotid, carry out careful separation.
- The tract/sinus may extend to pharyngeal wall and some times a second (higher) parallel incision is needed to follow dissection superiorly. It is important to excise deep components completely to avoid recurrence.
- Close the fascia with interrupted absorbable 3/0 sutures and subcuticular absorbable 4/0 to skin. Insert a suction drain if dead space remains.

Complications
- Local oedema/infection
- Recurrence due to incomplete excision
- Nerve or vascular damage

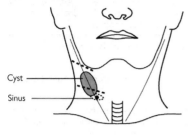

Fig. 14.8 Excision of branchial cyst/sinus

Thyroglossal cyst and fistula

Definition and anatomy

The cyst is a firm, rounded, midline, anterior neck swelling in line of descent of thyroid gland—usually above hyoid bone. It can occur lower in neck, on left of midline, or within the tongue. If in doubt about diagnosis, carry out thyroid scan (ultrasound or isotope).

It moves up and down with tongue protrusion/retraction. Infection in cyst may lead to skin fistula and discharge of 'glairy' mucus.

Position

Supine with head midline and neck extended by roll beneath shoulders.

Preparation

Check with anaesthetist that digital access to the airway is possible. A laryngeal mask is not appropriate (distorts surgical anatomy). Give IV antibiotics at induction if infection suspected.

Incision

Transversely (collar) over hyoid incorporating skin ellipse if adherent to cyst.

Procedure (Sistrunk's procedure)

- Dissect down and round central hyoid partly dividing strap muscle insertion (sternohyoid). Excise central hyoid (bone-cutter) with attached cyst. Remove central segment of hyoglossus muscle including thyroglossal tract to base of tongue (foramen caecum). Assistant's finger in floor of mouth pushes forward base of tongue to improve definition and access.
- Closure is helped by neutralising neck extension. Obliterate dead space with interrupted absorbable 3/0. If there is residual dead space or infection suspected, leave thin rubber/Silastic tissue or suction drain. Close skin with subcuticular continuous 4/0 monofilament sutures and tie-over dressing or subcuticular continuous absorbable 4/0 sutures.

Postoperative

Overnight stay to monitor airway.

Complications

- Swelling and potential upper airway obstruction if bleeding/haematoma
- Wound infection/abscess if excision incomplete or cyst/tract infected
- Incomplete excision with recurrence (5–20 % depending on whether tract or cyst alone excised)

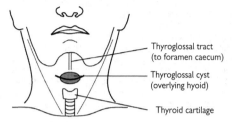

Fig. 14.9 Approach for thyroglossal cyst and fistula

Lymphangioma/cystic hygroma of neck

Cystic hygroma may develop on either side of neck (posterior triangle) in relation to defective thoracic and right lymphatic duct drainage into the venous system. It can reach a large size detectable on antenatal scans. Lymphangiomas ramify extensively between and through normal neck structures as multiloculated, cystic, diffuse masses. They may lead to respiratory distress and feeding problems and can extend into floor of mouth and base of skull. Occasionally a rapid size increase due to infection or bleeding. US or MRI scan delineates the relation to anatomical structures. They can be managed conservatively or by sclerosant injection but cosmetic problems or compression/obstruction may demand surgery.

Position
Neck extended over roll and rotated away from side of lesion.

Procedure
- Make a transverse (collar) incision in skin crease. Divide the superficial fascia and platysma and expose the multiloculated cystic lesion.
- Carry out exploration with regard to displaced position of facial and hypoglossal nerves and with care to avoid vascular damage (thyroid vessels). Meticulous time-consuming exploration may allow safe removal of entire swelling but excision often limited or partial and restricted to debulking large hygromas. Insert a tissue vacuum drain to prevent lymph accumulation.
- Close the wound with 3/0 absorbable to platysma and fascia and 4/0 subcuticular absorbable or monofilament Nylon.

Complications
- Haematoma and infection related to extensive dead space
- Cervical branch of facial nerve damage leading to droop of angle of mouth
- Hypoglossal nerve damage leading to asymmetric tongue movement and speech impairment
- Residual cosmetic problem due to irregular, puckered scar.

Dermoid cysts

Dermoid cysts are subcutaneous inclusions of dermal tissue, usually at fusion lines, which lead to development of small, firm cysts containing sebaceous secretions. Unlike epidermoid (sebaceous) cysts, there is no communication with the surface (punctum) and neither discharge nor infection occurs. Cysts are mobile with respect to both the skin and the deeper tissues. Typical sites are the outer end of eyebrow (external angular dermoid), midline of nose, suprasternal notch. Occasionally deeper (dumb-bell) extension occurs into cranial fossa or an encephalocele is associated (ethmoid).

Diagnosis
If there is any doubt about deep extension, CT scan is needed.

Incision
Make the incision in skin tension (Langer's) lines and, for an external angular dermoid, in plane of hair shafts in eyebrow.

Procedure
- Deepen the incision to reveal cyst capsule. Carry out sharp dissection in plane around capsule to allow complete mobilisation of cyst. Take care to avoid capsule breach which a) loses definition of cyst, b) risks leaving capsule tissue from which cyst may regenerate, and c) releases potentially irritant sebaceous material. Fine blood vessels may need cautery but this is often a 'bloodless' procedure.
- Close the dead space closed with 3/0 or 4/0 absorbable suture and close skin with subcutaneous continuous 4/0 or 5/0 absorbable or with Nylon/Prolene continuous 4/0 tie-over suture. Apply pressure dressing.

Complications
- Haematoma/bleeding if dead space is left
- Infection
- Recurrence if any residual cyst capsule
- Risk of serious intracranial sequelae (abscess) if deep extension left
- Unsatisfactory eyebrow scar unless incision carefully sited in hair-bearing area.

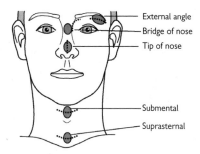

External angle
Bridge of nose
Tip of nose
Submental
Suprasternal

Fig. 14.10 Sites of dermoid cysts

Pyloric stenosis

Presentation and diagnosis

Classically presents in males (4:1) at about six weeks age with projectile, non-bilious vomiting, visible gastric peristalsis, weight loss, and hypochloraemic alkalosis. Family history may be of value. Differential diagnoses include gastro-oesophageal reflux and overfeeding although neither of these should cause alkalosis.

Confirmation: a) palpation of 'tumour', b) visualisation on ultrasound or barium meal.

Preparation

Preoperative correction of dehydration and metabolic derangement (low serum sodium, potassium, chloride, and hydrogen ion) with 0.45% sodium chloride/5% dextrose (and potassium). Correction may take 24–48 hours. Monitor resuscitation with U&Es and capillary gases. NG tube passed and stomach aspirated—saline lavage if evidence of stasis or bleeding.

Position of patient

Supine with support under upper lumbar spine.

Incision/approach

- Right upper-quadrant, transverse incision (traditional) at level of liver margin. Anterior and posterior rectus sheaths divided transversely—muscle either divided or retracted laterally.
- Umbilical approach through a curved skin incision in the upper umbilical crease and vertical midline linea alba split; leaves less conspicuous scar but access is slightly more restricted.
- Laparoscopy.

Procedure

- Deliver the pylorus through the wound by traction on the greater curve of the stomach. Stabilise the 'tumour' between thumb and forefinger of the operator.
- Make a longitudinal incision of serosa in avascular area of mid-anterior wall from the pyloroduodenal boundary (vein of Mayo) on to antral wall proximally.
- Split all thickened circular muscle fibres transversely with blunt forceps to reveal bulging external surface of mucosa.
- Test the mucosal integrity by squeezing gastric secretions or air through pylorus. Manage any suspicion of mucosal breach (perforation) by stitching tag of omentum to pyloromyotomy site, maintaining gastric tube drainage and delaying feeds for at least 24 hours.
- Use continuous absorbable 3/0 to rectus sheath and subcuticular absorbable 4/0 sutures to skin.
- Leave a NG tube in situ to decompress hypertrophied stomach. Feeds reintroduced over the next 24 hours.

Complications

Morbidity:
- Mucosal perforation (about 1%)
- Wound infection (10%)—related to poor immunity and nutritional state
- Wound dehiscence
- Persisting gastro-oesophageal reflux (not unusual). Treat with thickened feeds.

Mortality rare (<0.5%)—can follow undiagnosed perforation or milk aspiration.

Follow-up

Review at two months to assess weight gain and any persisting gastro-oesophageal reflux.

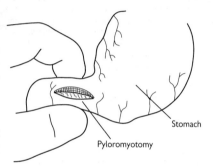

Fig. 14.11 Ramstedt's pyloromyotomy

Intussusception

Description, incidence, presentation

Intussusception is an invagination or telescoping of the terminal ileum/leo-caecal valve into caecum/ascending colon probably induced by enlargement of Peyer's patches. Commoner in males (2:1), it peaks at 3–10 months, and presents with sudden onset of severe, colicky abdominal pain and passage of redcurrant mucousy stool. Between spasms of pain, when abdominal wall relaxes, a sausage-shaped mass may be felt in the right hypochondrium. Confirmation is made by plain X-ray, ultrasound or contrast enema with air or barium.

In about 75% cases, air (pneumatic) or contrast (hydrostatic) pressure reduces the intussusception, sometimes at a second attempt after some hours. Signs of peritonitis, perforation or marked and established obstruction suggest irreducibility and surgery is then the first option. Close liaison between surgeon and radiologist is important in agreeing on indications for enema reduction, for a prolonged attempt at reduction and for a repeated attempt. Intussusception in older children, recurrent intussusception and ileoileal intussusception raise the possibility of a lead point (e.g. polyp, Meckel's) and demands surgical reduction.

Preoperative preparation

Good IV line and correction of fluid/electrolyte imbalance is essential.

Position

Supine.

Procedure

- Make a right, transverse, subumbilical, muscle-cutting incision. Note any free intraperitoneal fluid (serous, blood-stained, faecal-contaminated). Reduce intussusception partly intraperitoneally but the mass usually brought out through the wound. Note the degree of ischaemia and integrity of serosal surface noted. Attempt reduction by a combination of distal squeezing pressure and gentle proximal taxis. Serosal splitting suggests imminent rupture, and may require resection. Similarly, an obvious mass suggesting a lead-point requires resection and anastomosis. Otherwise, continue reduction and, once completed, bowel oedema and discoloration usually rapidly improves. If serious doubt remains about bowel viability, resection and anastomosis is safest option. If caecal area is entirely unaffected by oedema and inflammation carry out appendicectomy. This is sometimes to avoid any future confusion about presence of appendix.
- Close the wound with absorbable continuous 2/0 or 3/0 to anterior and posterior rectus sheaths, use absorbable interrupted 3/0 to subcutaneous tissue and absorbable continuous 4/0 subcuticular.

The laparoscopic approach has been used; most useful when completeness of hydrostatic/pneumatic reduction is in doubt and in complex cases (e.g. Henoch–Schonlein purpura). *Recurrence* is about 4%; less after surgical reduction.

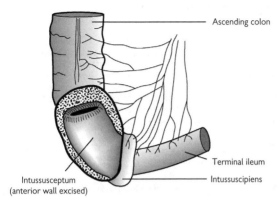

Fig. 14.12 Intussusception of terminal ileum

Meckel's diverticulum

Incidence and anatomy

This represents failure of involution of the omphalomesenteric duct. Situated on the antimesenteric border of ileum, within 100cm of ileo-caecal junction. Length between 1–8cm. Characteristically supplied by distal section of right vitelline artery (end-artery branch of the SMA). Incidence is reported from 0.3 to 4%. In asymptomatic patients, male:female ratio is 1.3:1 but complications commoner in males (3.3:1). Approximately 25% lined by heterotopic gastric, pancreatic or duodenal mucosa, which increases risk of complications.

Presentation

- Gastrointestinal bleeding
- Intestinal obstruction (intussusception/bands/volvulus)
- Perforation or inflammation.

It can also be found incidentally during laparotomy/laparoscopy.

Diagnosis

99m technetium-pertechnetate scan detects heterotopic gastric mucosa (not other diverticula). Glucagon, pentagastrin, and H2-blockers are given to augment sensitivity. Renally excreted isotope in bladder can hide uptake in a Meckel's (particularly in small children).

Preparation

Ensure normovolaemia if presentation is bleeding.

Position of patient

Supine.

Incision/approach

Right, transverse, muscle-cutting, sub-umbilical for open operation. Laparoscopic-assisted or laparoscopy approach also used.

Procedure

- Identify and ligate vitelline artery and divide it. Excise Meckel's with resection of ileal wedge/segment (2–5cm on either side). Bleeding may be from an ulcer of adjacent ileal mucosa. Close the ileum by end-to-end single-layer interrupted, inverting anastomosis using non-traumatic needle with 4/0 or 5/0 absorbable.
- Resect any incidental diverticulum (i.e. no other significant pathology—bowel not compromised)—lifetime risk of complications about 5%. If incidental diverticulum not excised, record clearly in the case-notes and inform parents and G.P.

Morbidity

Adhesive obstruction following surgery 5–10%. Long-term complications higher in previously symptomatic patients. Mortality close to zero.

Acute appendicitis

Classical symptoms: central abdominal pain, vomiting, anorexia, malaise, mild/moderate pyrexia and migration of pain to right iliac fossa.

Classical signs: right iliac fossa tenderness, guarding, rebound tenderness and rigidity.

Confusing presentations: dysuria, diarrhoea—due to unusual position of appendix, young age of child and complicating/intercurrent illness.

White cell count, ESR/CRP, urinalysis, plain abdominal x-ray, ultrasound scan and CT scan may aid diagnosis.

The discipline of 'active observation' limits both unnecessary removal of normal appendix and delayed operation with perforation and peritonitis.

Preoperative

Fluid resuscitation essential—patient may need 0.9% sodium chloride bolus followed by 0.45% NaCl, 5% dextrose and added potassium chloride (10 mmol/500ml). Immediate preoperative intravenous cefotaxime and metronidazole is required.

Position

Supine.

Incision

Transverse incision in skin crease (Langer's lines) centred on McBurney's point (1/3 of distance along line from anterior superior iliac spine to umbilicus). Incision can be extended either laterally into loin or medially if necessary to deal with difficult appendicitis or other pathology.

Procedure

- Divide superficial fascia in the line of wound. Split external oblique muscle in line of fibres extending medially to anterior rectus sheath—small nick in lateral sheath gives extra access. Split internal oblique and transversus abdominis in line of fibres to allow gridiron access.
- Insert retractors inserted and pick up peritoneum with forceps and open it—take bacteriology swab and any pus aspirated.
- Identify lower pole of caecum and base of appendix by following taenia coli. Free appendix from surrounding tissue with finger dissection. Deliver the appendix and caecum into wound.
- Remove appendix either by retrograde (starting at base) or antegradely depending on its accessibility and degree of freedom. Clamp mesoappendix, divided and ligated with absorbable 3/0 suture. Insert purse-string suture (3/0 absorbable) into caecum around base of appendix which is cross-clamped, crushed, ligated and amputated allowing stump to be buried by tying purse-string suture.

If problems arise at any stage in defining or mobilizing appendix, in controlling bleeding or potential bleeding points or in identifying or excluding other pathology, improve access by extending incision as above. If appendix has perforated, search for and remove any intraperitoneal faecolith. Peritoneal lavage with antibiotic containing, warm, saline solution is helpful in removing intraperitoneal pus and fibrin. Drain peritoneal cavity or wound (rarely needed unless significant abscess, continued oozing or retained faecolith).

Postoperative

No oral intake, NG tube aspiration and continued intravenous maintenance fluid for 24 hours or until gastrointestinal function recovers. Three doses of antibiotic over 24 hours—extended to three or five days if perforation/peritonitis especially in young children (<5 years.)

Complications

- 10% normal appendicectomy rate: minimised by careful 'active observation' policy.
- Wound infection (abscess) 5–7% overall incidence: higher with perforated appendix and free pus.
- Wound dehiscence: usually heals by secondary intention.
- Intraperitoneal collection/abscess 1–3% incidence: right iliac fossa, intraloop, pelvic, subphrenic. Usually presents at 1–3 weeks post-op.
- Secondary adhesion obstruction: requiring gut rest/nasogastric tube aspiration/IV fluids or laparotomy.
- Respiratory complications of basal atalectasis/pneumonia.

Laparoscopic approach

- Insert an infraumbilical port, left and right iliac fossae ports.
- Change camera to LIF port following initial inspection. Grasp appendix and mesoappendix divided with coagulation diathermy.
- Ligate appendix with 2 loops proximally and one loop more distally.
- Divide appendix between distal and proximal loops and removed through umbilical port.
- Close umbilical wound with 2/0 absorbable to linea alba.
  3/0 absorbable to fascia and subcuticular 4/0 absorbable.
- Close peritoneum (continuous), internal oblique (interrupted)
  2/0 absorbable: external oblique (continuous), superficial fascia (interrupted) 3/0 absorbable; 4/0 subcuticular absorbable.

Appendix abscess/mass

If, at presentation, a defined and localised right iliac fossa appendix abscess/mass without generalised peritonitis or obstruction is found, attempted laparotomy and appendicectomy not advisable. Initial management options are:

- Conservative—IV fluids and antibiotics
- Ultrasound assisted aspiration of abscess and insertion of tube drain
- Incision and drainage of abscess.

If these measures are successful, interval appendicectomy can be performed at 3–6 months.

Malrotation and volvulus

Embryology and incidence
The developing fetal intestine herniates into a physiological exomphalos during which time it lengthens. By the 12th gestational week the bowel returns to the abdominal cavity and rotates 270° anti-clockwise around the axis of the vitello-intestinal artery. Duodenum, ascending and descending colon become fixed. Failure of this rotation and fixation is termed 'malrotation'. The implications of this are a midgut, suspended on a narrow-based universal mesentery that is at risk of volvulus—almost invariably clockwise (. Quoted incidence is as high as 1 in 500 live births but this includes infants with abdominal wall defects and congenital diaphragmatic hernia.

Presentation
Bile vomiting in the neonatal period indicates intestinal obstruction and, of all possible causes, volvulus requires urgent intervention as the bowel is at risk of becoming ischaemic. In peritonitis, frank haematemesis, or PR bleeding, laparotomy should not be delayed by other investigations. Plain X-ray can be abnormal, ultrasound may show abnormal relative position of superior mesenteric vessels but upper GI contrast study is diagnostic (DJ junction on right, corkscrewing of small bowel).

Preoperative
Warn parents of possibility of catastrophic bowel ischaemia if you suspect. Cross-match blood and correct any coagulopathy.

Incision
Supra-umbilical transverse.

Procedure
- Deliver intestine completely and determine if volvulus present. If present, it is usually clockwise. If intestine is compromised, untwist and cover with warm saline packs to encourage reperfusion.
- Determine nature of malrotation. Ladd's bands may run across duodenum to attach to mobile, high lying caecum. Divide these bands following diathermy coagulation. Mobilise duodenum so that it lies relatively straight on the right side of the spine. Attempt to broaden mesentery by opening one leaf of the mesentery.
- Return intestine to the peritoneum in the non-rotated position—large bowel on the left and small bowel right. The appendix does not need to be excised but, if left in situ, the fact and position should be accurately documented and parents informed.
- If intestine found to be ischaemic with little recovery with warm packs, consider closing and performing a 'second-look' laparotomy after 48 hours.
- Layered closure with continuous 2/0 or 3/0 absorbable. Subcutaneous 4/0 absorbable. Subcuticular 4/0 or 5/0 absorbable.

Postoperative management

NG tube on free drainage until signs of ileus resolve. Consider parenteral nutrition may be required if this is prolonged.

Complications

Short gut syndrome if a large amount of small bowel resected. Early diagnosis and intervention essential to avoid this.

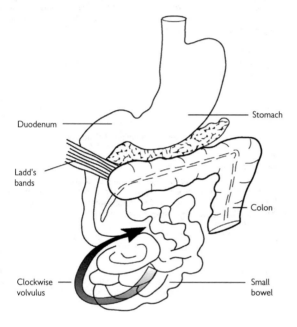

Fig. 14.13 Volvulus of small bowel

Epigastric hernia

This is herniation of extraperitoneal fat through a small defect in linea alba of upper midline abdominal wall. Commonly midway between xiphisternum and umbilicus but can be at any point. It presents either as a visible lump or due to discomfort caused by traction of tethered hernia on underlying peritoneum. Confusion at referral with the much larger, diffuse, midline swelling due to divarication of the rectus abdominis muscles, which is not a true hernia and improves and eventually disappears with spontaneous approximation of the muscles.

Preoperative

Mark hernia site carefully as it may be impossible to palpate in the anaesthetised relaxed patient.

Position

Supine.

Incision

Short transverse centred on hernia in midline of abdomen.

Procedure

- Divide subcutaneous fat and fascia transversely to reveal slightly different texture of extra peritoneal fat protruding through linea alba fascia.
- The defect often very small (2–3mm)—enlarged by lateral incisions to permit reduction of fatty hernia. If the fat amputated, supplying vessels must be ligated/cauterised. Defect closed with 3/0 interrupted non-absorbable sutures.
- Use interrupted 3/0 absorbable to fascia subcutaneous fat: continuous 4/0 absorbable subcuticular to skin.

Complications

- Bruising or bleeding if haemostasis not secured at operation
- Residual discomfort if peritoneum tethered to closure of defect.

Umbilical hernia

This is due to a residual small defect in fascial closure at the umbilical ring following cord separation in newborn. It is noted as bulge into umbilicus when infant cries or strains. It is very rarely symptomatic and often remains small. There is potential for spontaneous closure up to about 4 years of age especially if defect <1cm at 1 year of age. It is diagnosed by tip of examining finger palpating defect in umbilical ring.

Preoperative
Standard preparation for day case surgery.

Position
Supine. Local anaesthetic peri-umbilical infiltration or rectus sheath block improves post-op recovery—rectus sheath block preserves operative field for the surgeon.

Incision
Subumbilical curved (semilunar) incision in skin fold. Symmetry best achieved by small central stab incision and lateral split by opening forceps.

Procedure
- Carry out subcutaneous dissection cephalad on each side around umbilical ring and hernia to isolate.
- Divide the ring completely to open defect with tissue forceps and retract each lateral extremity of sac. Inspect it to ensure no vitello-intestinal, intraperitoneal connection at umbilicus.
- Close the defect with closely-spaced, interrupted 2/0 absorbable suture. Tack down the umbilicus to site of hernia repair with one 4/0 absorbable suture.

Closure
Use subcutaneous interrupted 4/0 absorbable to obliterate dead space and subcuticular continuous/interrupted 4/0 absorbable or adhesive strip skin closure. Pressure dressing for 24–48 hours reduces risk of haematoma.

Complications
- Bruising or haematoma related to residual wound dead space
- Infection (umbilicus harbours bacteria)
- Postoperative abdominal pain due to intraperitoneal air/blood irritation.

Inguinal herniotomy

Incidence, anatomy, and presentation

Commoner in boys (8:1) and on right side (3:1). Almost invariably indirect (through both rings of inguinal canal), through a patent processus vaginalis. Emerges above and lateral to pubic tubercle (cf. femoral hernia). Fundus varies from external ring to lower scrotum. Distinguish from hydrocoele by inability to get above swelling and no transillumination, but in neonates latter is less useful. Often presents as an intermittent swelling with a cough impulse at inguinal canal. Spermatic cord feels thickened.

Indications

In first months of life, chance of irreducibility leading to bowel strangulation and ischaemia is highest—surgery should not be delayed. After 6 months of age, herniotomy is elective unless irreducibility occurs. Parents should be warned to present urgently if hernia is red, tender or hard.

Incision

Skin crease incision (about 2cm) over inguinal canal.

Procedure

- Divide subcutaneous tissue and Scarpa's fascia in line of incision (superficial epigastric vessels retracted or divided). Expose external oblique fascia and rolled edge of inguinal ligament. Perform herniotomy either at external ring or by opening inguinal canal by splitting external oblique fibres (avoiding the ilioinguinal nerve beneath).
- Expose hernial sac by dividing external spermatic fascia (if outside inguinal canal), cremaster fibres and internal fascia in line of cord. Lift sac with the cord into the wound and posterior aspect freed after reducing contents. Separate vas (posteromedial) and vessels (posterolateral) from hernial sac—great care needed to avoid damage to these fine structures. Separate fragile, friable sac from vas and vessels with mixture of sharp and blunt dissection.
- Clear sac to the internal ring and transfixion-ligate with 3/0 absorbable (herniotomy) sutures. No muscle repair or narrowing of hernial orifices (herniorraphy) required. If testis has retracted, replace it in the scrotum. If it lies within hernial sac, it should be separated carefully and mobilised with lengthening of vessels to allow a scrotal orchidopexy.

In girls, identification of sac external to superficial ring. Divide the sac and round ligament and open to reveal contents. Inspect the ovary, if easily identified (remember rare possibility of androgen insensitivity syndrome with testis in sac). Transfix sac and close external oblique to the pubic tubercle.

Closure

Use absorbable 3/0 to close external oblique and Scarpa's fascia and subcuticular 4/0 or 5/0 sutures to skin.

Complications/consent issues

- Recurrence rare but may follow difficult herniotomy with oedematous sac
- Damage to the vas
- Testicular atrophy following irreducible/strangulated hernia
- About 10% chance of inguinal hernia on contralateral side
- In girls, abnormal 'ovary' should be biopsied to exclude testicular feminisation (androgen insensitivity syndrome).

Hydrocele

Presentation

Usually congenital due to persistence of a patent processus vaginalis. Very occasionally secondary to infection, inflammation, trauma, or tumour of testis/epididymis. Clinically distinguished from hernia by soft fluid consistency, bluish colour, position of testis within swelling, non-reducibility and ability to palpate normal cord above it. Equal incidence left and right. If communicating, it may vary in size diurnally (larger at end of day) and may resolve completely (usually before age 4 years.). Encysted hydrocoele presents as firm, discrete swelling in remnant of processus above testis— also in girls as swelling in canal of Nuck (round ligament).

Preoperative

Mark appropriate side clearly by 'X' with indelible pen.

Incision

Short (about 2cm) groin crease incision over external inguinal ring/ inguinal canal.

Procedure

- Divide subcutaneous tissue and superficial fascia in line of wound. Expose external oblique aponeurosis and divide in line of fibres to open inguinal canal or continue dissection at the external ring. Identify and preserve ilioinguinal nerve.
- Divide layers of spermatic cord (cremaster fibres and spermatic fascia) in the line of cord. Separate processus from vas and testicular vessels which lie posterior to it (medially and laterally respectively). Clamp processus and divide and clear proximally to deep inguinal ring then transfixion ligate with 3/0 absorbable. Express fluid from hydrocele/distal processus. It is not necessary to excise hydrocele sac. Return testis to fundus of scrotum by traction on scrotal skin.

Closure

Use 3/0 absorbable to external oblique fibres if divided and to superficial fascia—4/0 subcuticular absorbable sutures to skin.

Complications

- Scrotal haematoma—bleeding from cremasteric vessels
- Recurrent hydrocoele—may be transient
- Testicular atrophy—damage to testicular vessels
- Inguinal pain or dysaesthesia due to ilioinguinal nerve damage.

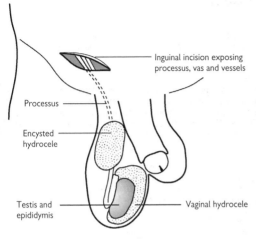

Fig. 14.14 Approach for hydrocele

Orchidopexy

Incidence

Undescended testis found in 2–4% of infant boys: percentage higher if premature. By six months of age this falls to around 1.5%. Incidence slightly higher on right side.

Examination

With the patient in supine position and relaxed. Palpate for cord structures at the superficial ring, then for the testis along line of descent. If testis palpated, attempt to manipulate into scrotum. A retractile testis can be brought to the base of the scrotum without any tension, and does not require surgical intervention.

Rationale and timing

Lower temperature conditions of the scrotum enhance spermatogenesis. A 5–10 fold increase in neoplasia may not be reduced by orchidopexy, but a scrotal testis is essential for self-examination later in life. Orchidopexy should not be planned until after the first birthday.

Preoperative

If testis impalpable, warn parents that rudimentary testis may be discovered and excised. Laparoscopic approach may be of benefit in impalpable testis, and can be combined with the Fowler-Stevens technique (initial in situ ligation/division of testicular vessels and delayed orchidopexy relying on hypertrophied blood supply via vas.

Position

Supine.

Procedure

- Make a skin crease groin incision. Open Scarpa's fascia in line of incision. The testis will be found in superficial inguinal pouch or, occasionally, ectopic in a penile, perineal or crural site.
- Grasp testis with toothed forceps and deliver into wound. With blunt dissection peel away superficial coverings and expose deep surface of cord. Once around the cord, thin out gubernacular connections with forceps watching for 'looping vas' distal to testis. Divide gubernaculum. Separate external spermatic fascia and cremaster from underlying cord structures and clear to superficial ring.
- Open inguinal canal by dividing external oblique in line of fibres. Separate vas and vessels from (patent) processus vaginalis, divide this and clear it to deep ring. Divide any lateral bands associated with vessels to give extra length. Occasionally retroperitoneal dissection is required to mobilise testis further. Identify testis by opening the tunica vaginalis over it and remove any testicular or epididymal appendages.

- Develop the route to scrotum by finger or mosquito forceps, and create extra Dartos pouch created through transverse scrotal incision with blunt dissection. Pass mosquito forceps cranially from scrotum to groin and grasp the testis and draw into scrotum. If cord under mild tension, suture from testis to midline raphe may limit retraction.

Closure

Use interrupted 5/0 absorbable to scrotum. External oblique and Scarpa's fascia closed with 3/0 or 4/0 absorbable. Subcuticular 4/0 absorbable to skin.

Morbidity

- Retraction and recurrence of undescent
- Testicular atrophy due to trauma to the vessels.

Circumcision

Natural history of the foreskin

At birth, the prepuce is adherent to the glans. Over the first few years of life the potential space develops and small retained pearls of smegma may be noted. The foreskin becomes retractable at a variable stage over the first five years of life as the adhesions lyse. Allowing this process to occur naturally, without advising regular retractions, prevents parental and patient anxiety. Balanitis and posthitis may cause scarring of the foreskin which may, in turn, stenose (phimosis). A non-retractile foreskin may respond to short term topical application of steroid ointment.

Indications

- True phimosis: note a history of ballooning on micturition and previous balanoposthitis. Balanitis xerotica obliterans (BXO) can also be associated with scarring of the glans.
- Paraphimosis: strangulation of the distal penis and glans due to retraction of a very tight foreskin over the glans. Consider dorsal slit and delayed circumcision if oedema marked.
- Recurrent UTI (controversial).
- Religious circumcision for boys of Jewish or Muslim faiths—both parents should give informed consent.

Contraindications

- Hypospadias: the foreskin may be needed for repair.
- Buried penis: circumcision may lead to inflammation of unprotected glans.

Procedure

- Local penile or caudal block is used as an adjunct to general anaesthesia.
- Retract foreskin completely and separate all adhesions. Foreskin is held in artery forceps (usually in dorsal/ventral midline) so that it can be symmetrically drawn distally—good assistance essential for this. Carefully judge amount of skin to be excised—excision either by amputation with foreskin cross-clamped distal to glans tip or by scissor dissection around glans. Trim mucosa to leave a 2–3mm cuff around corona of glans. Identify all vessels (dorsal, lateral and ventral) by retracting skin to expose denuded penile shaft and control them by bipolar diathermy or fine (5/0 absorbable) ties. Carry out accurate skin to mucosa repair around corona using 5/0 or 6/0 absorbable interrupted. Insert an '8' suture at the frenulum to secure the frenular artery.

Postoperative

Child best left without dressing to avoid trauma of removal. Apply ligno-caine gel (1%). Give regular baths after 24 hours which aids micturition and healing.

Complications

- Bleeding—reactionary and secondary can be profuse and require transfusion/exploration
- Infection around suture line—apply local antibiotic ointment
- Urethral meatal stenosis—especially if BXO present (1% hydrocorti-sone ointment) or baby still in nappies (ammoniacal dermatitis)
- Pain related to excessive skin removal
- Disturbance of sensitivity of glans.

Retraction of foreskin (adhesionolysis)

Absence of true phimosis demonstrated by lifting foreskin away from glans to demonstrate laxity of skin. Occasionally a foreskin may by partially retractable but some adhesions may limit full retraction (usually dorsally).

Procedure

General and local or topical (EMLA cream) anaesthesia.
   Develop subpreputial space by:
- Sweeping blunt probe around glans beneath foreskin.
- Separating foreskin from glans using dry swabs for traction on tissues until foreskin gradually fully retracted.
- Clean residual smegma with saline or chlorhexidine soaked swab to expose corona fully. Any persisting difficulty in retraction due to tightness of foreskin raises possibility of need for prepuceplasty. Apply Vaseline, 1% hydrocortisone ointment or lignocaine gel (1%).

Postoperative

Frequent bathing and gentle retraction of foreskin to maintain retractibility.

Complications

- Recurrent fusion (adhesion) of foreskin to glans
- Secondary phimosis due to scarring of stretched and traumatised foreskin
- Paraphimosis.

Prepuceplasty

Commonly performed in place of circumcision. Allows widening and consequent retractabilty of previously tight, phimotic foreskin. Not advisable if significant banalitis or BXO present.

Procedure

- Carry out dorsal penile or caudal block. Procedure performed under general anaesthesia.
- Retract foreskin if possible with separation of all adhesions. Identify the site of tight constricting ring around penile shaft.

Option 1 Perform a dorsal slit longitudinally through area of constricting band (about 1cm). Achieve haemostasis with bipolar diathermy. Close transversely with 5/0 or 6/0 absorbable.

Option 2 Draw foreskin distally over glans and two forceps applied to either side of dorsal midline of foreskin. Apply straight forceps forcibly to crush dorsal midline foreskin longitudinally to desired distance (about 1cm). Perform dorsal longitudinal incision of both layers of foreskin. If bleeding from dorsal vein, use bipolar diathermy or 5/0 ligature. Close incision transversely (circumferentially) with 5/0 or 6/0 absorbable.

- Ensure foreskin retracts easily over glans at end of procedure.

Postoperative

As for circumcision.

Complications

- Bleeding—reactionary and secondary
- Recurrent preputial stenosis (phimosis) due to inadequate dorsal incision
- Unsatisfactory appearance of foreskin with small lateral dog-ears of excess skin.

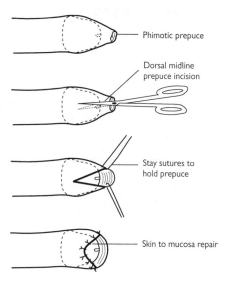

Phimotic prepuce

Dorsal midline prepuce incision

Stay sutures to hold prepuce

Skin to mucosa repair

Fig. 14.15 Prepuceplasty

Torsion of testis or appendix

Presentation and anatomy

Torsion of testis or testicular appendage (hydatid of Morgagni) are equally common—occasionally the epididymis (or its appendage) torts. Peak ages for testis torsion are perinatally or in later childhood. Extra vaginal torsion (perinatal) involves the cord whereas intravaginal torsion (later childhood) involves the testis on long mesorchium (bell and clapper anatomy). Onset characterised by abrupt and severe pain with testis in high position and excruciatingly tender. Torsion of hydatid may produce precisely localised tenderness and hard pea-sized swelling at upper pole of testis—blue tinge sometimes seen through skin. Prompt exploration is needed unless torsion can be excluded by positive evidence of epididymo-orchitis—pyuria or obvious primary infection (e.g. mumps). Torted hydatid may be treated non-operatively as infarction rapidly resolves although relief of pain may be quicker following excision.

Preoperative

Informed consent includes possibility of orchidectomy and fixation of contralateral side.

Incision

Approach tunica vaginalis either by oblique incision in hemiscrotal skin crease or through midline scrotal raphe.

Procedure

- Open tunica vaginalis to release haemorrhagic fluid and expose testis. The anatomy of torsion defined by inspection of testis, hydatid and spermatic cord.
- Detort by twisting testis in appropriate direction—usually towards midline septum. If perfusion recovers, colour of testis will improve. If testis remains dark purple/black, incise tunica albuginea to further release constriction and tension. If there is significant recovery, fix testis at 3 or 4 points to tunica vaginalis using 3/0 absorbable.
- If no recovery of colour, incise testis to assess perfusion—if no useful perfusion, excise testis with ligation of cord.
- Fixation of contralateral testis is mandatory if viability of index testis is in doubt or if anatomy is bell and clapper variety—most surgeons routinely fix contralateral testis at same operation if torsion encountered. There is no indication for contralateral exploration in a torted hydatid.

Closure

Use 3/0 interrupted absorbable to scrotal skin.

Complications

- Scrotal haematoma/abscess
- Atrophy of testis if established ischaemia
- Relative infertility
- Cosmetic issue about scrotal asymmetry—Silastic prosthesis can be placed subsequently.

Head and neck surgery

A. J. Dickenson and B. S. Avery

Tracheostomy

A tracheostomy is usually performed as an elective procedure under a general anaesthetic with an endotracheal tube in place. In patients with advanced cancers of the mouth, pharynx, or larynx, or severe infection such as Ludwig's angina, it may be necessary to do the operation under local anaesthetic. These are potentially very dangerous operations and should be performed by an experienced surgeon. In a life and death situation where the airway has been lost, no attempt should be made to perform a tracheostomy, but instead a cricothyroidotomy should be performed. This account deals with the procedure of elective tracheostomy.

Indications

There are many reasons for performing an elective tracheostomy.

- Prior to major head and neck surgery, e.g. cancers of the mouth, pharynx or larynx, maxillofacial trauma.
- The management of acute respiratory problems, e.g. acute respiratory distress syndrome (ARDS).
- Patients with severe neurological problems, e.g. head or spinal injuries/bulbar palsy etc.
- Congenital disease in children, e.g. cardiac, lung or facial deformity problems.

Equipment required

Like any operation a tracheostomy can vary from being very easy to extremely difficult and dangerous.

- Number 11 and 15 surgical blades.
- Bone cutters, monopolar and bipolar diathermy.
- Portex and/or Shiley disposable PVC tracheostomy tubes should be used. They should be cuffed and for a normal adult size 8–9mm are appropriate. The cuff should be inflated and tested together with all the anaesthetic tube connections.

Position

Supine with a sandbag under the shoulders and the head extended as far as possible. Mark the sternal notch and cricoid cartilage and use disposable sticky edged drapes to create a square around the operative area.

Incision

Make a 4cm transverse incision just below the level of the cricoid cartilage (Fig. 15.1). A longer incision may be advisable in a bull-necked individual and a vertical incision starting just below the cricoid cartilage may be useful to avoid entanglement with other procedures, such as a radical neck dissection. The area should be infiltrated with local anaesthetic and adrenaline, if safe to use, for the purpose of haemostasis. The incision will vary according to the circumstances.

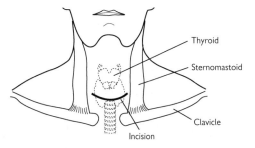

Fig. 15.1 Tracheostomy incision

Procedure
- Incise the skin and subcutaneous fat with a number 15 blade. Whilst palpating the trachea, dissect vertically in the midline down to the thyroid isthmus.
- Retract the anterior jugular veins, which lie either side of the midline, sometimes they have to be divided.
- On reaching the thyroid isthmus diathermy it in the midline with uni-polar diathermy and divide with a knife. Clean the trachea and keep the wound open with suitable Langenbeck retractors.
- Use a cricoid hook to pull the trachea upwards if there is not much space. Open it at the level of the 2nd and 3rd tracheal rings using a number 11 blade. In the elderly the tracheal rings may be calcified and bone cutters are some times required.
- Either a hole can be cut in the trachea or make a flap attached inferiorly (Fig. 15.2). Ask the anaesthetist to withdraw the endotracheal tube just beyond the top of the hole in the trachea, and insert the tracheostomy tube. Inflate the cuff and attach the anaesthetic tubes.
- Initially suture the tracheostomy tube flanges to the skin, and attach the tapes if appropriate.

Postoperative care of the tracheostomy
- Apply suction under sterile conditions. This varies according to the amount of secretions produced.
- Ensure that inspired gases are humidified.
- When room air is inspired, attach a humidifier to the tracheostomy tube.
- Change the tracheostomy tube if it becomes crusted and obstructed. Normally by 4–5 days the tracheostome is well-established and it is then easy to remove and replace the tube.

Removal of the tracheostomy tube
Deflation of the cuff may allow the patient to breathe past the tube. Alternatively the tracheostomy tube can be plugged and a fenestrated Shiley tube can be used. At the time of tube removal the secretions should be sucked out first and the tube removed. The neck wound should be covered with a hand held pack to make sure that the patient is breathing comfortably in the normal way. An adhesive dressing is used to cover the tracheostome and the wound will close spontaneously over the next 1–2 weeks.

Complications
Intraoperative
- Intratracheal fire caused by ignition of oxygen with diathermy. This is rare but well documented. The anaesthetist should be asked to insert the endotracheal tube a long way into the trachea so that the cuff is below the larynx. Inflate the cuff with saline and not air. This will avoid puncture at the time of opening the trachea, and the cuff may protect the lungs from fire. A bowl of saline should be available to douse the flames. Ask the anaesthetist to reduce the oxygen concentration when opening the trachea and avoid using diathermy at this stage if possible.

Postoperative

- *Tube displacement or blockage.* If this occurs the tube should be replaced. Normally after 4–5 days replacement is straightforward. Before this time replacement may be more difficult and good lighting is needed.
- *Bleeding* from the soft tissues may occur postoperatively. Usually it stops but it may require a return to the operating theatre for haemostasis.
- *Chest infection.* Where tracheostomy has been performed electively for surgery the risk of postoperative chest infection is increased.
- *Infection around the tracheostomy tube.* This sometimes occurs and is more likely when there has been extensive neck surgery, e.g. radical neck dissection. Appropriate treatment of the infection whilst keeping the cuff inflated will resolve the problem.

Late complications

Sometimes the tracheostome does not fully heal and air and secretions may bubble onto the neck through a small fistula. Under a general anaesthetic a fistula can be repaired by excising it down to the trachea and closing the soft tissues in layers.

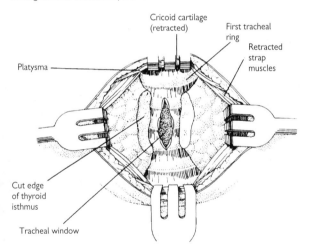

Fig. 15.2 Window created into the trachea for a tracheostomy tube

Thyroglossal cyst excision

Anatomy

Embryologically, the thyroid gland arises at the foramen caecum at the base of the tongue and descends through the anterior neck into a normal pretracheal position. Remnants of the embryological duct can persist at any point along this path of descent, forming a smooth, round swelling. It is unusual for this to be functioning endocrine tissue. On the whole, the majority (>95%) are midline, 70% below the hyoid bone. Characteristically the lesion moves on swallowing or protruding the tongue.

Indications

- Infection (5% of cases; the majority are symptomless)
- Fistula formation
- Suspected malignant change.

Equipment required

- Number 10 and number 15 surgical blades
- Monopolar and bipolar diathermy
- Bone nibblers.

Position

Supine with a sandbag between the shoulders and head supported by a head ring.

Procedure (Sistrunk's operation)

- Make a 35–45mm transverse skin crease incision over the cyst. The platysma is divided and deep cervical fascia incised vertically in the midline to exposing the cyst.
- Mobilise the sac and using gentle traction identify the pedicle passing up to the hyoid bone. During its embryological migration the thyroid tissue passes behind the posterior aspect of the hyoid bone. Resect the central portion of the hyoid to gain adequate access to the remaining tract. This can be achieved with bone nibblers.
- If there is any remaining tract dissect it bluntly up to the base of the tongue. This can be assisted by a finger placed in the mouth to displace the tongue base inferiorly and anteriorly into the neck.

Closure

Close the wound in layers over a suction drain.

Postoperative care

The drain is retained until there is no further drainage.

Complications

Intraoperative

- Haemorrhage.

Postoperative

- Haematoma
- Seroma
- Scar.

Thyroidectomy

Indications

Absolute

- Suspicion of malignant change
- Compression of the trachea by a benign lesion

Relative

- Treatment of thyrotoxicosis
- Unsightly goitre

Choice of operation

- *Thyroid nodule*: thyroid lobectomy
- *Thyroid cancer*: total thyroidectomy
- *Nodular colloid goitre* (with hyperthyroidism): subtotal thyroidectomy

Preoperative preparation

Investigations may include indirect laryngoscopy, thyroid function tests, serum calcium, ECG, thyroid antibodies, fine-needle aspiration, and ultrasound to exclude malignancy. Patients with thyrotoxicosis need preoperative preparation with carbimazole, iodine, or possibly beta blockade. Informed consent must be obtained beforehand, and in particular it should include advice on possible change in voice and possible hyperthyroidism or damage to the recurrent nerve.

Position of patient

Supine with neck extended at 20°–25° and the table foot down. Place the head on a padded ring with a pillow or pad beneath the shoulders. Place packs on either side of the neck. Use a double towel as a head set. Stand on the side opposite the lobe to be removed.

Incision (Fig. 15.3A)

Look for skin creases. Mark the incision beforehand with ink or a 2/0 thread pressed on the skin. Make a transverse incision near to midway between the thyroid cartilage and manubrial notch, in a crease if possible. The incision should reach the sternomastoid on each side.

Procedure

- Use a no. 15 blade. Deepen the incision through fat, platysma, and cervical fascia to expose the strap muscles. Reflect skin flaps proximally and distally. Begin with the knife and then use gauze dissection. Stop bleeding. Insert a Joll retractor.
- Divide the strap muscles in the midline (Fig. 15.3B).

Apply gentle traction to rotate the inferior pole to the opposite side. Wipe away the fascia on its undersurface to identify the superior parathyroid.

Now pay attention to the recurrent laryngeal nerve and the inferior thyroid artery. Move the assistant's retractor to exert a pull laterally. Apply a small swab to the gland and exert a medial pull with the left hand to expose the fascia overlying the inferior thyroid artery, the recurrent

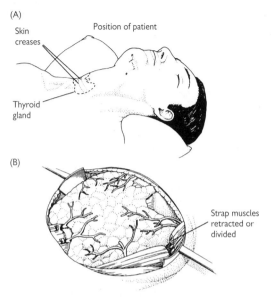

(A)

Skin creases

Position of patient

Thyroid gland

(B)

Strap muscles retracted or divided

Fig. 15.3 Incision for thyroidectomy and division of strap muscles

laryngeal nerve, and the inferior parathyroid (Fig. 15.4). Gently divide the fascia longitudinally to identify the nerve close to the ligament of Berry. Do not disturb the inferior parathyroid. Simply locate it. Ligate the artery in continuity and then the inferior thyroid veins. The lobe is now free and can be removed by dividing the isthmus, dissecting the gland off the trachea, and oversewing the isthmus with Vicryl.

In a subtotal lobectomy the gland is not dissected off the trachea. Instead, several small haemostats are applied along the lateral aspect of the gland anterior to the recurrent nerve and the tissue anterior to the forceps is excised. The remnant is oversewn with Vicryl if possible.

Total thyroidectomy

Total lobectomies are performed on each side with or without radical neck dissection. Further operative details are given in the chapter on endocrine surgery (Chapter 5)

Closure

Close in layers. Bring suction drains (one on each side) through separate stab wounds. Close the platysma with Vicryl and the skin with clips.

Postoperative care

1. Check the vocal cords postoperatively. The anaesthetist usually does this (but the appearance of the cords may be misleading).
2. Ensure an adequate airway. If haematoma develops open all the layers of the wound.
3. Remove drains on day 2. Check serum calcium daily.
4. Home on day 3–5. Surgical out-patients department and thyroid function tests after 6 weeks.

Complications

These can be early, intermediate, or late.

Early

- Thyrotoxic storm is rare after thyroidectomy for thyrotoxicosis but needs treatment with antithyroid drugs and beta blockade.
- Bleeding may be reactionary within hours of the operation and requires urgent decompression.
- Tracheal collapse is usually recognised by the anaesthetist and requires re-intubation.
- Paralysis of the recurrent nerves or superior laryngeal nerve damage usually presents as a voice change if not recognized early.

Intermediate

- Wound infection and hypocalcaemic tetany which usually occurs within a week of surgery. Always check the serum calcium preoperatively before the patient goes home. Tetany is treated by intravenous infusion of calcium and then oral administration of vitamin D.

Late

- Hypothyroidism—confirmed by measuring thyroxine levels.
- Hypertrophy of the scar.
- Keloid is rare except in the dark-skinned races.

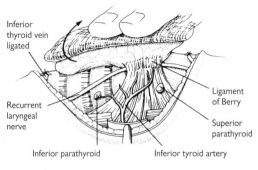

Inferior
thyroid vein
ligated

Recurrent
laryngeal
nerve

Ligament
of Berry

Superior
parathyroid

Inferior parathyroid   Inferior tyroid artery

Fig. 15.4 Exposure of recurrent laryngeal nerve

Parathyroidectomy

Indications
Parathyroid adenomas, carcinoma, secondary- or tertiary-hyperparathyroidism (all four glands).

Preoperative preparations
Frozen section facilities should be available. The laboratory should be informed.

Position of patient
Supine with the head on a neck ring, the neck extended, and a 20°–25° downward tilt.

Incision and access
The same approach as for subtotal thyroidectomy is used (p646).

Procedure
- Mobilise the thyroid gland and retract its upper and lower lobes forward. Also assess its areolar bed. The normal parathyroid glands are difficult to identify but lie posterior to each of the four poles of the thyroid. Each gland is yellowish and is flattened with a small vascular pedicle.
- If there is an adenoma carefully remove it. If the patient has secondary- or tertiary-hyperparathyroidism, remove all four glands.
- Apply tissue or dissecting forceps to the gland and dissect it free by a combination of sharp and blunt dissection. Diathermise bleeding vessels. If you are in doubt about the nature of the tissue send biopsies for frozen section. Sometimes an adenoma can be found in the mediastinal region or in relation to the superior or inferior thyroid arteries.

Closure
Layers. Clips to skin. Suction drainage.

Postoperative care
- Observe for signs of hypocalcaemia and haematoma.
- Remove the drain at 2–3 days.
- Repeat serum calcium daily to observe the trend.
- Most patients can have their sutures removed on day 4 or 5 and go home.
- Arrange surgical out-patients department appointment in 6–8 weeks.

Complications
- Haemorrhage
- Nerve injury
  - Unilateral recurrent laryngeal nerve injury: hoarseness
  - Bilateral recurrent laryngeal nerve injury: stridor
  - Superior laryngeal nerve: change in 'timbre' of voice
  - Cervical sympathetic chain: Horner's syndrome

Submandibular gland excision

Anatomy

The deep part of the submandibular gland lies under cover of the medial border of the mandible, below the oral mucosa and above the mylohyoid muscle. The superficial part is covered by deep fascia, platysma, and skin. The larger superficial and smaller deep lobe are joined around the posterior edge of the mylohyoid muscle. The submandibular duct originates from the deep surface of the deep lobe and passes forwards into the floor of the mouth where it opens as a papilla lateral to the lingual fraenum behind the lower incisor teeth. The facial artery and vein lie initially deep to the posterior pole and then run over the upper surface of the gland.

The lingual nerve lies above the gland but anteriorly loops around the infero-lateral aspect of the duct (Fig. 15.5) and can therefore be damaged during surgery causing tongue anaesthesia. The mandibular (or marginal) division of the facial (VII) nerve can be damaged during surgery causing ipsilateral weakness of the lower lip. Patients should be warned about possible damage to these two nerves.

Anatomically, the mandibular nerve crosses the facial artery at the lower border of the mandible. In 81% of cases the nerve lies at the level of the lower border posterior to the artery while in the remaining 19% lies anywhere up to 12mm below the mandible. For this reason the incision should be placed in a skin crease at least 2cm below the angle of the mandible. The nerve lies deep to platysma, enveloped in the deep fascia overlying the gland. Anteriorly it becomes more superficial at the angle of the mouth.

Indications for removal

- Chronic sialadenitis
- Stone in submandibular gland or posterior duct causing obstruction
- Benign tumour arising from gland
- Surgical management of intractable drooling in handicapped patients
- Removal as part of radical or selective neck dissection.

Equipment required

- Number 15 blade
- Bipolar diathermy
- Vacuum drain
- Vicryl ties and suture, 4/0 Prolene suture.

Position

Supine with head rotated to the opposite side supported by a head ring. Tilt the operating table into a head-up position.

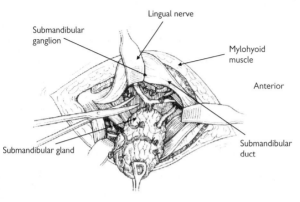

Fig. 15.5 Removal of the submandibular gland

Procedure

- Prepare the skin with Betadine or Chlorhexidine antiseptic. Infiltrate lignocaine subcutaneously with adrenaline to help haemostasis.
- Make a transverse incision placed in a skin crease at least 20mm below the angle of the mandible. Its posterior end should not extend beyond the posterior border of the mandible (Fig. 15.6).
- Divide skin, subcutaneous fat, and the platysma muscle. Continue dissection obliquely upwards through the deep fascia to the inferior aspect of the gland. Thereafter dissection is continued on the capsule of the gland (except for tumours where the surrounding fascia should also be removed). This avoids damage to the mandibular branch of the facial nerve. Mobilise the gland from the anterior, posterior and inferior aspect.
- Identify the facial vessels deep to the posterior part of the gland and divide them.
- Mobilise the superficial lobe of the gland anteriorly off the mylohyoid muscle and retract the muscle forwards. At this point the lingual nerve and submandibular duct can be identified on the deep surface of the mylohyoid muscle. The nerve is looped due to its attachment to the submandibular ganglion.
- Cauterise the attachments of the ganglion to the nerve and divide them. Continue mobilisation of the gland from the hyoglossus muscle leaves the gland pedicled on the duct. Divide the duct and ligate it as far forward into the mouth as possible.
- Carry out careful haemostasis, suture a vacuum drain in place. Close the platysma muscle with Vicryl sutures and the skin with 4/0 Prolene. Apply an Opsite dressing.

Postoperative care

Monitor blood loss in the drain. This can usually be removed the following morning and the patient should be discharged 3–4 hours later after checking that a haematoma has not developed.

Complications

Intraoperative

- Arterial haemorrhage if proximal end of facial artery not properly ligated
- Damage to mandibular branch of facial nerve, which is usually temporary, due to retraction injury or accidental diathermy
- Damage to lingual nerve if difficult to see, because of fibrosis following infection.

Postoperative complications

- Haematoma—this sometimes occurs after removal of drain
- Infection
- Nerve damage as previously mentioned
- Retained calculi in residual anterior submandibular duct.

Late complications

- Unsightly scar
- Infection caused by calculi in anterior duct—requires intraoral excision under general anaesthesia.

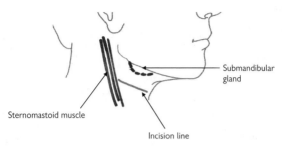

Fig. 15.6 Submandibular gland incision

Sublingual gland excision

Anatomy

The sublingual gland lies anteriorly in the floor of the mouth. It is bounded by the mucosa superiorly, the mylohyoid muscle inferiorly, body of the mandible laterally and the opposite sublingual gland anteriorly. The submandibular duct lies medial to the gland as does the lingual nerve which lies in close contact with the sublingual gland as it crosses under the submandibular duct. The gland drains mainly onto the mucous membrane via small excretory ducts and sometimes directly into the submandibular duct.

Adjacent structures encountered in surgery are the submandibular duct and lingual nerve, and the patient should be warned about the risk of a numb tongue or the (usually temporary) risk of submandibular gland enlargement related to duct obstruction.

Indications

- Ranula
- Tumours arising from the gland (rare).

Equipment required

- Number 15 surgical blade
- Bipolar diathermy
- Lacrimal duct dilator.

Position

Supine with the head up and supported on a head ring.

Procedure

With the exception of a plunging ranula, which is rare, this procedure can be achieved via an intra-oral approach. Infiltrate local anaesthetic (2% lignocaine with adrenaline 1 in 80 000) around the gland to reduce blood loss.

- Cannulate the nearby submandibular duct with a suitable lacrimal probe if technically possible. The probe will indicate the course of the duct and helps to locate the position of the lingual nerve.
- Make a mucosal incision running on the lingual side of the mandible lateral to the submandibular duct (Fig. 15.7).
- Expose the superior aspect of the sublingual gland. Raise medial and lateral mucosal flaps and mobilise the anterior border of the gland by blunt dissection and careful haemostasis.
- Use gauze pledgets and blunt dissection to mobilise the gland free of the duct from front to back.
- Carefully cautherise all vessels with bipolar diathermy. A branch of the lingual artery postero-medially may have to be tied off.
- Once the gland has been removed tack the mucosa lightly together with 3/0 Vicryl sutures.

Postoperative care

It is essential to monitor for postoperative haematoma in the floor of the mouth which may compromise the airway. This procedure can often be done as a day case.

Complications

Intraoperative
- Arterial haemorrhage
- Venous haemorrhage.

Postoperative
- Floor of mouth haematoma
- Lingual nerve damage
- Submandibular gland obstruction secondary to duct damage or oedema although in both cases this is usually temporary.

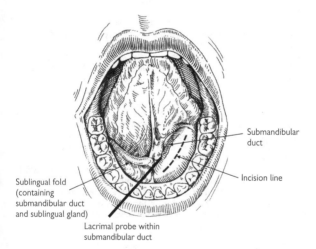

Submandibular duct

Incision line

Sublingual fold (containing submandibular duct and sublingual gland)

Lacrimal probe within submandibular duct

Fig. 15.7 Sublingual gland excision

Parotidectomy

The most common operation on the parotid is the *superficial parotidectomy*. Superficial parotidectomy is a technically demanding procedure that requires a thorough knowledge of facial nerve anatomy. There are a number of indications for this operation (listed below). As a general rule, surgery for removal of a benign tumour, e.g. pleomorphic adenoma, is easier than for chronic infection where fibrosis and inflammation may make the dissection difficult.

Anatomy

The parotid gland lies in the hollow between the sternomastoid muscle and the ramus of mandible. The anterior border is adherent to the masseter muscle. Posteriorly it is attached to the tragal cartilage and the external auditory meatus. Inferiorly it is attached to the sternomastoid muscle. The upper border of the parotid gland extends to the level of the zygomatic arch.

The parotid is enveloped within a dense capsule and Stenson's duct emerges from the anterior aspect to cross the superficial surface of the masseter muscle before passing through the buccinator muscle to open into the mouth opposite the crown of the upper second molar tooth.

Several important structures run through the gland. The most important structure is the *facial (VII) nerve* which divides the parotid gland into the superficial and deep lobes. The nerve emerges from the skull base at the stylomastoid foramen, pierces the postero-medial part of the gland and runs forward in the substance of the gland where usually it divides into two main trunks. The two main trunks then divide into the five main branches known as the temporal, zygomatic buccal, mandibular, and cervical branches (Fig. 15.8). There is considerable variation in the pattern of the trunks and branches of this nerve.

Other important structures include the *external carotid artery* which enters the deep part of the gland postero-medially and divides into its two terminal branches. The superficial temporal artery exits from the superior surface while the maxillary artery emerges from the antero-medial surface deep to the condylar neck of the mandible. The retro-mandibular vein lies deep to the plane of the facial nerve.

Indications

- Chronic sialadenitis
- Benign or some small malignant tumours arising within the gland (90% of tumours are benign)
- Sialosis
- Infection and pain related to Sjogren's syndrome.

Specific aspects of consent

- **Facial nerve paralysis** Emphasise the risk of temporary (33%) or permanent facial weakness (<2%) after superficial parotidectomy. Inform the patient that it is common for the nerve to be functioning well immediately after surgery, but to develop temporary paralysis on the first postoperative day as a result of oedema but that full recovery is expected.

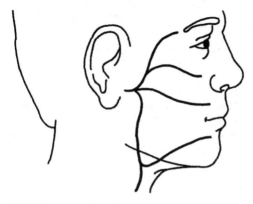

Fig. 15.8 Anatomy of the right facial nerve—typical pattern

- **Numbness of the ear** This is due to division of the great auricular nerve during surgery. This may be reduced by preserving the posterior branch of the nerve. There is often long term partial or complete recovery of ear sensation.
- **Frey's syndrome** Incidence varies according to the type of parotidectomy (8% for inflammatory disease, 20% for malignant lesions). A total parotidectomy increases the risk of Frey's syndrome. The syndrome usually develops several months after surgery and can be treated by Botulinum toxin.
- **Cosmetic problems** A retromandibular dent can be noticeable. The scar may heal badly, particularly the part in the neck.

Equipment required

- Number 10 and 15 surgical blades
- Bipolar diathermy
- Nerve stimulator
- A pair of magnifying loupes may help.

Position

Supine with head up with the neck extended and the head rotated to the opposite side supported by a head-ring. Clean the operative area with Betadine in aqueous solution and apply drapes. Keep the eye and the corner of the mouth visible during surgery. This can be done by applying an Opsite dressing. Place a Jelonet pack in the external auditory meatus to avoid postoperative deafness caused by blood. Infiltrate local anaesthetic (2% lignocaine with adrenaline 1:80 000) along the skin incision to assist haemostasis.

Incision

Make this in the preauricular area, extend under the ear and down into the neck as shown in Fig. 15.9. Raise a skin flap and extend it to the anterior part of the parotid gland. Use sutures to hold the flap forward.

Procedure

- Mobilise the gland from the sternomastoid muscle inferiorly. Identify the great auricular nerve and preserve its posterior branch while dividing the anterior branch. Separate the gland from the external auditory meatus posteriorly. Carry out dissection on a broad front to allow maximum exposure and facilitate the finding of the facial nerve.
- Be patient whilst identifying the nerve trunk. Two landmarks are helpful; the first is the pointed cartilaginous part of the external auditory meatus, the nerve lies approximately 1cm deep to this point. The second is McEwan's triangle which is the angle bisecting the anterior border of the posterior belly of the digastric muscle and the plane of the tympanic plate and mandibular ramus (Fig. 15.9).

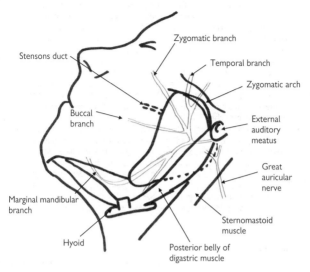

Fig. 15.9 Anatomy of the left parotid gland

- Identify the nerve and confirm it using a nerve stimulator, provided that the patient is not paralysed. Once located expose the main trunk by inserting fine artery forceps above the nerve along its course and divide the overlying tissue with a knife or scissors. The main trunk divides into two, approximately 1cm along. Thereafter, follow each individual branch through to the front of the gland. In the case of a tumour, carefully dissect it free even if a small branch of the nerve has to be sacrificed. Attempts have been made to classify the intraglandular course of the facial nerve, the pattern of branching is highly variable and necessitates cautious dissection to avoid inadvertent injury to anastomotic branches.
- It is not always necessary to remove the entire superficial lobe. For small benign tumours located within the lower pole of the gland a partial superficial parotidectomy is recommended. The technique is essentially the same as that for superficial parotidectomy but only the branches of the VII nerve related to the tumour are dissected out. This allows half of the superficial parotid gland to be retained and reduces the risk of damage to the nerve and the development of Frey's syndrome. Meticulous haemostasis will help to avoid damage to the nerve.

Closure

Irritate the wound and close the skin in layers using 3/0 Vicryl and 6/0 Prolene for the incision in front of the ear and 3/0 Vicryl and 4/0 Prolene or skin staples on the neck skin. A small vacuum drain should be sutured into place. The drain should not be placed directly on top of the facial nerve trunk.

Postoperative care

It is essential to monitor for excessive blood loss or haematoma. The sutures are removed on day seven.

Complications

Intraoperative
- Arterial or venous haemorrhage
- Difficulty locating nerve trunk.

Postoperative
- Haematoma—the patient should be made normotensive before closing the skin wound otherwise bleeding may occur
- Seroma
- Facial nerve damage—it can be reassuring to check facial nerve function at the end with a nerve stimulator provided that the patient is not paralysed
- Salivary fistula
- Sensory loss over the lower half of the pinna.

Long-term
- Cosmetic problem with retromandibular dent—a superiorly based sternomastoid muscle flap can be swung into this defect which may help
- Frey's syndrome several months later
- A poor scar
- Recurrent disease—tumour may recur, a superficial parotidectomy only does not cure all patients with chronic sialadenitis.

Other types of parotid surgery
- **Total conservative parotidectomy** indicated for chronic sialadenitis and deep lobe tumours. Following removal of the superficial lobe the facial nerve is dissected free from the underlying parotid tissue and retracted with vascular slings. The deep lobe is usually easily mobilised although the external carotid artery and the retromandibular vein may have to be divided and tied. The deep lobe is delivered between or below the branches of the facial nerve.
- **Total radical parotidectomy**—indicated for extensive malignant tumours with facial nerve involvement. Attempts should be made to preserve non-involved branches. Requires ligation of the external carotid artery. This operation can be performed in continuity with a radical neck dissection if lymph node metastases are present.
- **Extracapsular dissection**—this is a specialist technique and is not the same as a lumpectomy. It does not require dissection of the facial nerve. The incidence of temporary facial paresis and Frey's syndrome are reduced. The evidence suggests that this technique may increase the risk of recurrent tumour. It is most useful for superficially placed benign tumours.

Neck lump biopsy

Diagnosis

Preliminary investigation should include a CT and/or MRI scan. A fine needle aspiration biopsy (FNAB) with a 21 gauge needle may also give useful information.

If squamous cell carcinoma is considered a likely or possible diagnosis, carry out an examination under anaesthesia and examine the aerodigestive tract. An EUA can often include an ipsilateral tonsillectomy for biopsy and a fine needle aspiration biopsy of the neck lump.

It is not unusual to find that a CT scan suggests a benign lesion, an FNAB does not reveal malignant cells, no primary tumour is found, and although the patient may have no symptoms the lesion can turn out to be metastatic disease.

Equipment needed for biopsy of a neck lump

- Number 10 and 15 surgical blades
- Bipolar and monopolar diathermy
- Small vacuum drain.

Position

Supine with head up and neck extended with the head rotated to the opposite side supported by a head ring.

Procedure

Before starting the procedure it is advisable to mark the neck carefully with a marking pen. Outline the neck lump and then the neck should be marked with the incision lines for a radical neck dissection. For most biopsies the upper incision line for a neck dissection can be used as the access incision for the neck lump. If the lump turns out to be malignant then it is easy to carry out a radical neck dissection with excision of a large area of skin around the biopsy site.

- Make a transverse incision within the marked incision line. Divide the platysma with blunt dissection directly down to the neck lump. If the lump is a mobile node then the node itself can be dissected out once the node has been exposed.
- Do not dissect out a larger mass but rather carry out an incisional biopsy. Maintain haemostasis and close the wound in layers with or without a vacuum drain. Remove the sutures at day seven.

Postoperative care

Monitor the patient for an expanding haematoma. If a surgical drain has been left in place, keep the patient in overnight. If not the patient can be discharged on the same day.

Complications

Intraoperative

- Arterial haemorrhage
- Venous haemorrhage
- Accidental damage to a nerve, e.g. mandibular branch of facial nerve, accessory nerve.

Postoperative

- Haematoma
- Infection
- Atypical facial pain.

Neck dissection

A neck dissection is an operation carried out for the purpose of removing the lymph nodes of the neck en bloc as part of the treatment of malignant disease in the head and neck region. Cervical lymph nodes are divided into a number of levels (Fig. 15.10).

- **Level I**   Submandibular triangle
- **Level II** Upper jugular nodes
- **Level III** Middle jugular nodes
- **Level IV** Lower jugular nodes
- **Level V** Posterior triangle nodes.

As a result of this classification there are now a number of different types of neck dissections which can broadly be divided into *radical* and *selective* neck dissections.

A *radical* neck dissection involves removal of all five levels of lymph nodes in the neck while a full radical neck dissection removes lymph nodes at all five levels together with the accessory nerve, the internal jugular vein and the sternomastoid muscle.

If the accessory nerve is preserved then the operation is classified as a type I modified radical neck dissection. Preservation of the accessory nerve and the internal jugular vein makes this a type II modified neck dissection and preservation of the accessory nerve, internal jugular vein, and sternomastoid muscle is a type III modified radical neck dissection.

Selective neck dissections are usually carried out for the purpose of sampling the cervical lymph nodes at certain levels of the neck. Usually this operation is carried out when a patient has a head and neck tumour when the lymph nodes of the neck are not clinically enlarged and when no enlarged lymph nodes can be seen on a CT or MRI scan.

A good example is a squamous cell carcinoma of the tongue with no clinically obvious enlarged lymph nodes. It is known that this tumour has a high risk of developing metastatic lymph nodes in the neck. In these circumstances a supraomohyoid neck dissection, which removes level I–III lymph nodes, allows examination for micro-metastases which are not clinically apparent. The procedure limits morbidity and if the lymph nodes have micro-metastases radiotherapy can be given as adjunctive treatment with increased five year survival.

Indications

- Intraoral malignant tumours. Approximately 90% are squamous cell carcinomas, 8% are malignant salivary tumours, and 2% include other lesions such as melanomas and sarcomas.
- Squamous cell carcinomas and melanomas of the skin in the head and neck region
- Other head and neck malignant tumours, e.g. thyroid.

Equipment required

All instruments for a major soft tissue dissection:
- Number 10, 15 and 20 size blades
- Unipolar and bipolar diathermy
- Capillary slings, tissue holders
- Vicryl ties of various sizes, Vicryl transfixion suture.

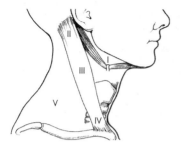

Fig. 15.10 Levels of the cervical lymph nodes

Incisions

- Two of the most commonly used are the Y-type incision (Fig. 15.11) and the McFee incision (Fig. 15.12).
- The anatomical limits of a radical neck dissection are from approximately 1cm above the clavicle inferiorly. An imaginary line drawn from the mastoid process to the angle of the mandible running along the lower border of the mandible to the midline is the upper limit. The anterior border of the trapezius muscle posteriorly, with an imaginary line running from the middle of the chin to the medial end of the clavicle is the anterior limit.
- If a McFee incision is used then the skin should be dissected off the underlying platysma muscle to the limits of the dissection described previously.

Procedure

- Carry out dissection from the lower end. Divide the platysma muscle, sternomastoid muscle and omohyoid muscle through the lower incision.
- Identify the lower end of the internal jugular vein under the omohyoid muscle and tie it off, passing an upper and lower transfixion suture through the vessel and divide it. Check that the thoracic duct has not been damaged. If there is a chyle leak, tie it off or clip it with a ligature. Identify and carefully dissect out the carotid artery and the vagus nerve, which are deep and slightly anterior to the internal jugular vein. Lift the fat of the posterior triangle off the prevertebral muscles and identify the phrenic nerve as it passes vertically across the scalenus anterior muscle.
- Once all of these structures have been identified, resect the posterior triangle contents, the sternomastoid muscle, the omohyoid muscle and the internal jugular vein which have been detached at their lower end upwards to the top of the neck preserving the phrenic nerve, the common carotid artery and the vagus nerve (Fig. 15.13). Divide branches of the internal jugular vein and the cervical nerve roots.
- Divide the sternomastoid muscle at the top end of the neck and amputate the lower part of the parotid gland. Tie and divide the

posterior facial vein just deep the parotid gland, carry out dissection anteriorly to include removal of the submandibular gland. Locate and divide branches of the external carotid artery such as the facial artery, preserving the hypoglossal nerve and the lingual nerve.

- Secure haemostasis once the dissection has been completed. Make a check for a chyle leak at the lower end of the internal jugular vein. Insert two small vacuum drains through the skin below the lower incision line. One drain should run along the anterior border of the trapezius muscle and the other should run up the anterior part of the neck to the submandibular region.
- Close the incision in layers with 3/0 Vicryl and the skin with clips and activate the vacuum drains.

Postoperative complications

Early

- *Bleeding.* The most common complication which usually necessitates a return to the operating theatre if severe. Carotid artery rupture is potentially lethal and occurs in over 2% of cases, usually at a later stage.
- *Infection.* Wound dehiscence, necrosis and infection can occur if there has been poor flap design or poor wound closure. It is more likely after previous radiotherapy. These problems are less common when the McFee incision is used.
- *Chyle leak.* This is uncommon. A small leak may resolve itself with pressure and intermittent suction. A severe leak requires total parenteral nutrition.
- *Cerebral or facial oedema.* This is due to poor venous drainage. It is rare with a unilateral neck dissection, but happens frequently with simultaneous bilateral neck dissections.
- *Stroke.* Manipulation of the internal carotid arteries in patients with known peripheral vascular disease can cause stroke.
- *Salivary fistulas.* This occurs in 6–30% of cases. Fistulas are usually small and resolve with regular dressings. Occasionally a fistula has to be excised.
- *Horner's syndrome.* This is caused by accidental damage to the sympathetic nerve trunk behind the carotid sheath. It causes an ipsilateral constricted pupil, ptosis and absence of sweating of the face and neck. This tends to improve spontaneously.
- *Death.* The operative mortality rate is 1%.

Late

- *Shoulder syndrome.* Sacrifice of the spinal accessory nerve usually results in a drooping shoulder, pain and reduced shoulder movement, particularly abduction. Physiotherapy may be helpful.
- *Painful dysaesthesia.* Patients may get severe discomfort when their neck is touched. This is thought to be caused by traumatic neuromas on surgically divided cervical nerves.

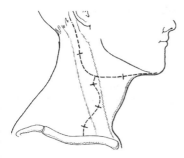

Fig. 15.11 Y-shaped neck incision

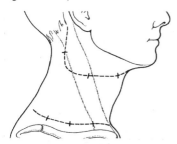

Fig. 15.12 McFee incision

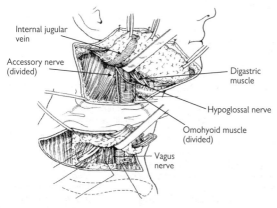

Fig. 15.13 Right, radical neck dissection with McFee incision

External carotid artery ligation

Anatomy

The common carotid artery bifurcates at the level of the upper border of the thyroid cartilage. After the bifurcation, the external carotid artery lies external to the carotid sheath. The artery runs deep to the posterior belly of the digastric muscle, crosses the styloglossus and stylopharyngeus muscles and pierces the parotid gland, where it terminates as the superficial temporal artery and the maxillary artery at the level of the neck of the condyle of the mandible.

Indications

Emergency

- Uncontrollable epistaxis
- Penetrating neck wounds

Elective

- Tumour resection
- Large arteriovenous malformation

Equipment required

- Number 10 and 15 blades surgical blades.
- Mono- and bi-polar diathermy.
- Vascular slings.

Position

Supine with the head turned to the opposite side and the neck extended.

Incision

Transverse lying within a neck crease about 2cm below the level of the mandible, at the level of the thyroid cartilage.

Procedure

- Divide the skin and the underlying platysma muscle with a number 10 blade and reflect the deep cervical fascia overlying the sternomastoid muscle to allow posterior retraction of the muscle.
- Identify the internal jugular and mobilise it and retract it posteriorly. Careful palpation of the artery will help the operator to bluntly dissect down to the vessel and expose it.
- Retract the hypoglossal nerve and posterior belly of digastric muscle superiorly (Fig. 15.14). Find the carotid bifurcation and identify the external and internal carotid arteries. The internal carotid artery can be identified by the vagus nerve which accompanies it. The external carotid artery should be identified by finding a branch such as the superior thyroid artery.
- Once the external carotid artery has been identified, dissect it out and pass a sling under the vessel. Place one or two ties around it with 1/0 Vicryl and at this point, check that the bleeding is controlled. If the vessel has been penetrated and cannot be repaired then tie the artery either side of the bleeding point. Clamp the vessel between the ties, divide it and then insert transfixion sutures at either end, again using a 1/0 Vicryl.

Closure

Close the incision in layers with a vacuum drain if necessary. Use skin clips to close the skin.

Postoperative care

The neck is inspected for haematoma. Skin clips can be removed at day seven.

Complications

Intraoperative

- Arterial haemorrhage
- Venous haemorrhage caused by injury to a large vein such as the common facial or internal jugular vein
- Accidental ligation of internal carotid artery. The incidence of permanent CVA is 30–35% and death approximately 20%.

Postoperative

- Haematoma
- Specific to the surgical site e.g.; damage to the mandibular branch of the facial nerve
- Infection.

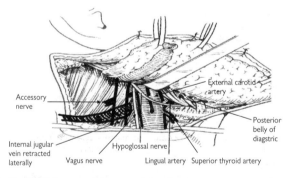

Fig. 15.14 Exposure of right external carotid artery

Excision of branchial cyst, sinus, or fistula

Anatomy

Branchial cysts are congenital second pharyngeal pouch abnormalities. They present as painless, fluctuant, slowly growing lateral neck swellings, anterior to the junction between the upper third and lower two-thirds of the sternomastoid. As they present in adolescence a congenital cause may be forgotten. It is equally important to ensure that the cyst is not a lower pole parotid tumour. A CT scan will usually distinguish where the cyst lies.

A *branchial fistula* is formed by the downgrowth of the 2nd branchial arch over the 2nd, 3rd and 4th branchial clefts. The fistula opening can be located in the lower third of the sternomastoid. As the fistula lies between 2nd and 3rd cleft structures, it passes between the internal and external carotid arteries.

Indications
- Recurrent infection
- Large cyst
- Persistent discharge from sinus.

Equipment required
- Number 10 and 15 surgical blades
- Monopolar and bipolar diathermy.

Branchial cyst
Mark the lesion preoperatively with surgical ink.

Position
Supine with the head-up tilt on the operating table. The neck extended and the head rotated, supported by a head ring.

Incision
Transverse directly over the swelling, but must be at least 20mm below the mandible to avoid the mandibular branch of the facial nerve.

Procedure
- Divide the platysma and incise the deep cervical fascia overlying the sternomastoid.
- Retract the sternomastoid posteriorly, allowing the cyst lining to be dissected free of adhesions. Carry out cautious mobilization on the deep surface of the cyst as it may extend between the internal and external carotid arteries. The accessory nerve lies close to the posteromedial surface and can be damaged by careless dissection or injudicious use of the diathermy.

Postoperative care
Monitor the patient for an expanding haematoma.

Complications
Intraoperative
- Arterial haemorrhage
- Venous haemorrhage
- Accessory nerve damage due to injudicious use of diathermy.

Postoperative
- Haematoma
- Seroma
- Infection.

Branchial sinus/fistula
Mark the lesion preoperatively with surgical ink and outline the ellipse of skin to be excised.

Position
Supine with a head-up tilt on the operating table with the neck is extended and head rotated, supported by a head ring.

Procedure
- Excise the skin sinus with an ellipse of adjacent skin (Fig. 15.15) and deepen to platysma. Divide the platysma and incise the deep cervical fascia overlying the sternomastoid.
- Retract the sternomastoid posteriorly, at the same time applying traction to the skin ellipse so that the tract can be identified and traced towards the carotid territory. Use a second transverse skin crease (step-ladder incision) to allow access to the carotid bifurcation. Locate the fistula between the arteries, passing over the hypoglossal nerve and alongside the glossophayngeal nerve until it terminates on the pharyngeal wall where it blends with the fibres of the middle constrictor muscle.
- Divide the fistula flush with the muscle, an intraoral approach is not required. Placing a finger in the mouth and manually displacing the pharyngeal wall can assist dissection.
- Place a closed suction drain along the length of the tract and close the tissues in layers.

Postoperative care
Monitor the patient for expanding haematoma.

Complications
Intraoperative
- Arterial haemorrhage
- Venous haemorrhage
- Hypoglossal and glossopharyngeal nerve damage due to careless dissection or injudicious use of diathermy.

Postoperative
- Haematoma
- Seroma
- Infection.

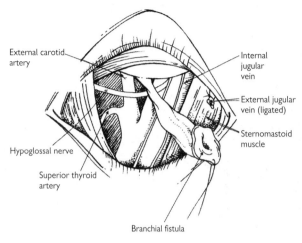

Fig. 15.15 Left branchial fistula

Pharyngeal pouch excision

Anatomy
A pharyngeal pouch is a posterior, midline, protrusion of the pharyngeal mucosa through a weakness (Killian's dehiscence) between thyro- and cricopharyngeus (Fig. 15.16).

Indications
- For relief of symptoms e.g.; dysphagia, halitosis, nocturnal cough
- Prevention of secondary complications e.g.; aspiration pneumonia.

Equipment required
- Number 11 and 15 surgical blades are needed
- Proflavin pack
- Monopolar and bipolar diathermy
- Nasogastric tube.

Position
Supine with head rotated to right, left arm by side, and a sandbag between the shoulders. Pack the pouch with proflavin on ribbon gauze, which assists in identifying the pouch. Insert a NG fine-bore feeding tube.

Incision
Make a transverse skin crease incision at the level of the cricoid cartilage.

Procedure
- Incise the platysma and deep cervical fascia and retract the sternomastoid, internal jugular vein and carotid arteries postero-laterally. Use blunt dissection to locate the sac, which is usually adherent to the oesophagus.
- Mobilise the sac and using gentle traction, identify the pedicle entering the inferior constrictor muscle. Withdraw the pack from the pouch. It is not essential to remove the sac, but simply to transfix the pedicle to prevent continued contamination.
- If the sac is excised, test the oesophageal patency with a 28–30 Fr gauge bougie before closing the wall defect.
- A cricopharyngeal myotomy is an essential adjunct to surgery and prevents postoperative fistula or late recurrence. Either insert a finger or curved artery forceps gently between cricopharyngeus and the oesophageal mucosa. Separate the two layers by opening the beaks of the forceps, followed by incising the cricopharyngeus with a No. 11 blade. This myotomy must be at least 40mm long and performed as far posteriorly as possible to avoid inadvertent damage to the recurrent laryngeal nerve.
- Close the mucosa with absorbable material (3/0 Vicryl) and the inferior constrictor muscles with 3/0 PDS. Close the wound over a suction drain.

Postoperative care
Keep the patient nil by mouth for 5 days. They can start clear fluids at 30ml/hr for the first 24 hours, before unrestricted free fluids.

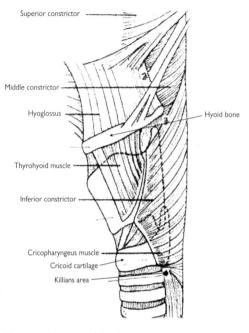

Fig. 15.16 Anatomy of the pharynx

Complications

Intraoperative
- Arterial haemorrhage
- Venous haemorrhage
- Recurrent laryngeal nerve damage
- Aspiration of pouch contents.

Postoperative
- Haematoma
- Seroma
- Chest infection
- Mediastinitis
- Fistula formation.

Alternative procedure

Dohlman's procedure. Requires specialist equipment and training. The oesophagus and pouch are cannulated and the adjoining wall is coagulated and incised.

Tonsillectomy

Anatomy

The tonsils are located on the lateral oropharyngeal walls. The main adjacent structures are:

- **Deep**   Superior constrictor muscle
- **Anterior**   Palatoglossus muscle
- **Posterior** Palatopharyngeus muscle
- **Superior**   Soft palate
- **Inferior**   Lingual tonsil

The arterial blood supply is through the external carotid artery and its branches. Of relevance are the ascending pharyngeal artery (tonsillar branches) and lesser palatine artery superiorly and the dorsal lingual and ascending palatine arteries and branches from the facial artery inferiorly.

The venous outflow drains into a venous plexus around the tonsillar capsule, the lingual vein, and the pharyngeal plexus. Lymphatic drainage is into the upper deep cervical and jugulodigastric nodes.

There is an extensive sensory supply from the glossopharyngeal nerve and the lesser palatine nerve.

Important structures deep to the inferior pole include the glosso-pharyngeal nerve, the lingual artery, and the internal carotid artery. These structures are at risk if the surgical plane in the tonsillar bed is not respected.

Indications

- Recurrent tonsillitis (>3 episodes requiring antibiotics in one year)
- Quinsy
- Lymphoma
- Malignant tumour
- To exclude primary squamous cell carcinoma in the tonsil when patient presents with an isolated neck node and no discernible primary lesion
- In conjunction with UVPPP for obstructive sleep apnoea.

Equipment required

- Monopolar and bipolar diathermy
- Boyle-Davis gag and attachment rods
- Tonsillar swabs
- Luc's forceps
- Pillar retractors
- Tonsillar guillotine
- Head light for surgeon.

Position

Supine with a sandbag between the shoulders to extend the neck, with the head supported by the table only.

Procedure

- Under direct vision, the field illuminated by a headlight, grasp the tonsil and elevate it out of the tonsillar fossa using Luc's forceps (Fig. 15.17).

The pillar retractor moves the anterior pharyngeal fold laterally and improves exposure.

- Incise the mucosa from the superior to inferior pole using either cutting diathermy or MacIndoe scissors. Either method can be used to mobilize the tonsil off its bed.
- Identify the peritonsillar plane, as this is a safe plane between the tonsillar capsule and superior constrictor muscle. Use careful dissection, sometimes using gauze swabs held in long handled forceps to sweep the tissues in a superior to inferior direction, mobilising the tonsil until it is held by the inferior pole. This contains the main blood supply. Clip it to excise the tonsil and carefully tie it. Haemostasis can be assisted by packing the tonsillar fossa with gauze and slowly checking the area for bleeding vessels in a superior to inferior direction. Pack gauze into the fossa while the contralateral tonsil is removed. At the end of the procedure haemostasis is rechecked and the pharynx careful aspirated to remove all clots that might compromise the airway on extubation.

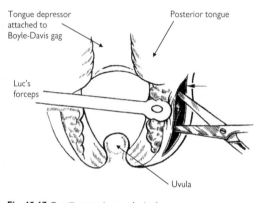

Tongue depressor attached to Boyle-Davis gag

Posterior tongue

Luc's forceps

Uvula

Fig. 15.17 Tonsillectomy (surgeon's view)

Postoperative care

Careful attention for postoperative haemorrhage, this may be hidden from the clinician as the patient the swallows blood.

Complications

Intraoperative

- Haemorrhage
- Dental trauma due to displacement of the mouth gag.

Immediate postoperative

- Haemorrhage; either primary or secondary. The overall bleeding rate is 2.3–3.4% of cases.
- Primary haemorrhage happens within the first 24hr, due to inadequate haemostasis at the time of surgery or the displacement of a tie from the inferior pedicle. Requires return to theatre in up to 1% of patients, although the majority of cases can be managed conservatively.
- Secondary, or reactive, haemorrhage occurs after discharge (1–10 days) and is due to separation of the slough in the tonsillar bed. The readmission rate is approximately 5%, of which less than 1% are returned to theatre.
- Pain. Discomfort at the operative site is to be expected, but can be referred (e.g. otalgia).
- Temporary dysphagia.

Late postoperative

- Temporomandibular joint pain.
- Oronasal fistula, producing hypernasal speech. This can happen due to overuse of the diathermy and failing to appreciate the relationship of the anterior tonsillar pillar to the soft palate.

Adenoidectomy

Anatomy

The posterior nasophayngeal wall contains a variable collection of subepithelial lymphoid tissue. If this tissue becomes infected, it hypertrophies to form masses that are commonly referred to as the adenoids (syn. pharyngeal tonsil). The adenoids are particularly prominent in children, and atrophy with age. When excessively enlarged, the adenoids can obstruct the posterior nasal aperture resulting in nasal congestion, mouth breathing and nocturnal snoring. The close anatomical relationship to the Eustachian tube can cause deafness and recurrent middle ear effusions (glue ear).

Blood supply is provided by the ascending palatine branch of the facial artery, ascending pharyngeal artery, pharyngeal branch of the internal maxillary artery, and the ascending cervical branch of the thyrocervical trunk. Venous drainage is into the pharyngeal plexus, pterygoid plexus and ultimately into the internal jugular and facial veins. Efferent lymphatic drainage flows from the retropharyngeal lymph nodes to the upper deep cervical lymph nodes, especially the posterior triangle nodes. Sensory innervation is derived from the nasopharyngeal branches of the glossopharyngeal and vagus nerves.

Indications

- Recurrent otitis media with effusion. Several studies report improvements in Eustachian tube function following adenoidectomy, regardless of the size of the adenoid
- Chronic mouth breathing
- Recurrent or chronic maxillary sinusitis
- Obstructive sleep apnoea.

Equipment

- Barnhill adenoid curette (Fig. 15.18)
- Boyle-Davis gag.

Position

Supine with the head extended.

Procedure

The transoral approach is commonly practiced and safer than transnasal adenoidectomy. The Boyle-Davis gag improves access to the posterior nasopharynx.

- Pass your index finger behind the soft palate and examine the postnasal space. This assists in determining the size, position, and consistency of the adenoid, the condition of the Eustachian tube orifices and the presence or absence of adhesions attached to the Eustachian tubes.
- Retract the soft palate by passing a vascular sling or paediatric urinary catheter through the nose and bringing it out through the mouth.
- If the patient also requires a tonsillectomy, always perform this after the adenoidectomy.

- Use an adenoid curette of appropriate size and place it against the posterior edge of the vomer. Using your thumb as a fulcrum, push the blade along the vault of the nasopharynx and over the odontoid process. This separates the adenoid free from its base and when it is withdrawn will shear the tonsil from the posterior nasopharyngeal wall. Avoid curettaging the Eustachian tube orifices.
- Observe for excessive haemorrhage, although packing is rarely required with the transoral approach.

Postoperative care

Most children recover rapidly. Short-term pain and discomfort is to be expected. Control it with simple analgesics. Encourage a normal diet.

Complications

Intraoperative

Bleeding (0.4%). Bleeding can be controlled by packing the site with a vasoconstrictor (e.g. oxymetazoline) on ribbon gauze. Rarely requires a return to the operating theatre.

Immediate postoperative

- Ear pain.
- Velopharyngeal insufficiency (0.05%). This occurs transiently in over 50% of all adenoidectomies as a result of removing the impingement to soft palate closure.
- Eustachian tube damage. This is rare and a result of uncontrolled use of surgical instruments.

Late postoperative

- Nasopharyngeal stenosis
- Chronic (persistent) otitis media with effusion
- Persistent symptoms, due to hypertrophy.

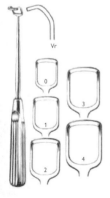

Fig. 15.18 Barnhill adenoid curettes of various sizes

Caldwell-Luc procedure

Although infrequently performed and to a greater extent superseded by endoscopic maxillary sinus surgery, the Caldwell-Luc procedure is still useful in gaining access to the maxillary sinus and pterygoid fossa.

Indications
- Chronic maxillary sinusitis
- Suspected neoplasm for biopsy
- Antrochoanal polyp
- Fungal sinusitis
- Drainage before radiation therapy
- Removal of displaced tooth roots
- Access for other procedures e.g. bone grafting prior to dental implants ('sinus lift').

Position
Supine. Use general anaesthetic and nasal intubation.

Incision
Make an intraoral incision through the free gingival tissues halfway between the gingival margin and the sulcus reflection. Avoid incision in the attached gingiva to allow the wound to be closed without tearing. Raise a mucoperiosteal flap to identify the intraorbital nerve and protect it.

Procedure
- Identify the canine fossa, distal to the root apex of the maxillary canine tooth.
- Create a window using a hammer and chisel and then enlarge with Hajek's forceps.

When performed for chronic sinus disease, the mucosa is radically debrided and an intranasal antrostomy is created below the inferior turbinate bone.

Complications
Immediate
- Pain
- Facial swelling and bruising
- Infraorbital nerve paraesthesia
- Damage to teeth apices.

Intermediate
Fistula.

Access incisions to the facial skeleton

Principles

Surgical exposure of the facial skeleton and access to the deeper structures of the oropharynx, nasopharynx and anterior cranial fossa fall within the armamentarium of the maxillofacial/head and neck surgeon. Adequate exposure is essential for the safe and efficient management of the surgical problem. Equally, any incision in the facial region must be designed to produce the minimum of visible scarring and avoid major neurovascular structures.

The main principles of incision design within the facial region are:

- **Allow adequate exposure** Incisions on the face should be as short as possible compatible with adequate exposure. Excessive traction on the soft tissues should be avoided.
- **Avoid neurovascular structures** The main neurovascular structures to be avoided are the sensory nerves of the face which include the supraorbital, infraorbital and mental nerves. Incision should avoid these areas and if necessary the nerves can be dissected out and carefully retracted.
- **Use relaxed skin tension lines** Incisions should be placed within lines of minimal tension, as the healed scar is imperceptible.
- **Incise perpendicular to the skin** This allows accurate reapproximation of wound edges. Oblique or tangential incisions are susceptible to over-riding and marginal necrosis.
- **In the scalp, place incision parallel to the hair to avoid damaging the follicle**

These criteria can be achieved through a number of approaches (Figs. 15.19–20).

- **Intraoral**
  - Maxilla: Le Fort 1 horseshoe degloving incision.
  - Mandible: Buccal sulcus degloving incision
- **Extraoral**
  - Coronal flap
  - Midface degloving approaches via the Weber-Ferguson incision (Fig. 15.19)
  - Periorbital
  - Rhytidectomy and preauricular.

Indications

Emergency

- Treatment of maxillofacial fractures.

Elective

- Tumour resection
- Assist neurosurgical approaches to the posterior orbit, anterior cranial fossa and pituitary gland
- Orthognathic surgery.

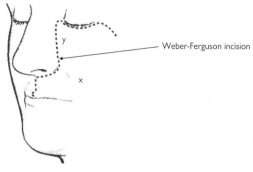

Weber-Ferguson incision

Fig. 15.19 Access incision to left maxilla

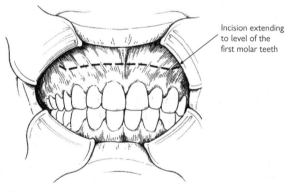

Incision extending
to level of the
first molar teeth

Fig. 15.20 Leforeone access incision

Equipment required
- Number 10 and 15 blades surgical blades.
- Mono- and bi-polar diathermy with access to Colorado needle if required.
- GOS (Great Ormond Street) solution (Table 15.1).

Position
Secure the head and support it with a head ring or neurosurgical craniotomy attachment. Place Jelonet in both ears and protect the eyes with simple eye ointment and tarsorraphy sutures.

Incision
Mark the incision line with surgical ink to avoiding areas of potential hair recession. The 'stealth' incision is commonly designed to avoid straight lines and sharp angles that might be subjected to tip necrosis. It also allows accurate repositioning.

Procedure: coronal flap
Advantage: wide exposure of cranial vault, medial and superior orbit, nasal bones and zygomatic arch.
- Make incision with a 10 blade or Colorado diathermy needle through skin, subcutaneous tissue and galea.
- Control bleeding from the scalp by using Rayney clips which are placed on the skin edge. Whether the dissection is carried out in the subpericranial or subgaleal plane depends on which part of the head or face needs to be exposed. If the cranial vault is to be excised then the dissection should proceed in the subpericranial plane leaving bare bone only.
- If the coronal incision is being used for access to the supraorbital ridge or orbit, then use a subgaleal dissection until within 20–30mm of the supraorbital ridge. At this point incise the pericranium and reflect it in continuity with the skin flap.
- If the zygomatic arch has to be exposed, incise the superficial layer of temporal fascia in continuity with the coronal flap. This offers satisfactory access to the zygomatic arch and at the same time protects the temporal branch of the facial nerve which lies superficial to the temporal fascia.
- Carry out meticulous closure to provide optimal healing. Use two small vacuum drains. Appose the galea and subcutaneous tissues with 2/0 Vicryl and use clips for skin.
- Insert closed suction drains to evacuate haematoma. Pressure dressings are optional.

Postoperative
Remove the drain at 24–48 hours.

Complications: immediate
- Subcutaneous haematoma
- Damage to the supraorbital nerves causing scalp numbness
- Later complications include facial ptosis and stretching of the scalp
- Incision leaving a broad visible scar within the hair.

Table 15.1 GOS solution

Hartman's solution	500ml
Adcortvl	50mg
Marcaine 0.25%	25ml
Lignocaine 0.5%	25ml
Hyalase 1500 IU	1amp
Adrenaline 1:1 000	0.5ml

Procedure: transoral approaches

Advantage: excellent exposure of entire maxilla and mandible.

- Infiltrate local anaesthetic widely. Design the incision so that it is placed 5mm away from the mucogingival junction (Fig. 15.20), this allows the unattached mucosa left on the alveolar segment to be reattached at the end of the procedure. Extend the incision as far posteriorly as necessary to facilitate tensionless exposure, although unnecessary lengthening may compromise mucosal vascularity.
- Deepen the incision through periosteum and raise the entire flap in a subperiosteal plane, with cautious dissection in the region of the mental or infraobital nerves.
- Then expose the maxilla or mandible.
- Close the mucosa with a tension-free continuous 3/0 Vicryl resorbable suture.
- Use an elasticated chin dressing after a mandibular degloving procedure to restrict haematoma and redrape the repositioned mentalis muscles.

Complications

Immediate

- Cutaneous paraesthesia due to traction neuropraxia
- Wound dehiscence

Late

- Gingival recession
- Facial ptosis
- Nasal alar flaring and shortening of the upper lip after
- Maxillary degloving procedure.

Acknowledgement

We wish to thank Mr Jerry Sharp FRCS, Consultant ENT surgeon, Derbyshire Royal Infirmary for his comments on the Thyroidectomy section.

Thoracic surgery

G. N. Morritt and A. N. Morritt

Bronchoscopy

This is performed using a rigid bronchoscope or a flexible fibreoptic bronchoscope.

The Negus rigid bronchoscope

- Different sizes e.g. adult, paediatric
- Halogen light source
- The three most commonly used telescopes are direct vision, 30° angled, and 90° angled.
- The telescopes are placed down the rigid barrel of the bronchoscope
- Instruments e.g. graspers, biopsy forceps, and suction devices
- Telescopes can be attached to a video camera for display on a monitor.

The flexible bronchoscope

- Fibreoptic bronchoscope
- Outer diameter—3–6mm
- Light transmitted via fibreoptic bundles
- Field of vision is usually 80°
- Can be attached to video camera for display on screen.

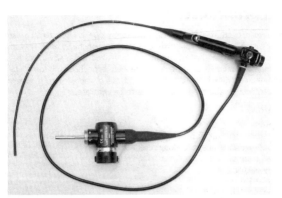

Fig. 16.1 The flexible bronchoscope

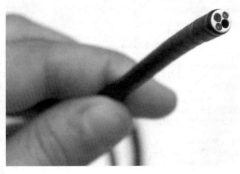

Fig. 16.2 The flexible bronchoscope. Light is transmitted via fibreoptic bundles

Rigid bronchoscopy

An invasive procedure where a rigid bronchoscope is used to visualise the oropharynx, larynx, vocal cords, and tracheobronchial tree. It may be combined with flexible bronchoscopy for improved distal airway visualisation and suctioning. It is preferred to flexible bronchoscopy for unstable patients, centrally located tumours, and cases where there is severe airway obstruction and the patient needs to be ventilated.

Indications
Diagnostic
- Biopsy (where flexible bronchoscope specimen is inadequate)
- Preoperative assessment for lung resection surgery
- Massive haemoptysis
- Airway obstruction
- Benign stricture
- Tracheobronchial toilet.

Therapeutic
- Removal of secretions
- Cauterisation of bleeding points
- Removal of foreign bodies
- Relief of airway obstruction
- Treatment of bronchopleural fistula
- Dilation of tracheal or bronchial strictures
- Laser therapy
- Insertion of airway stents.

Contraindications
Relative—uncontrolled coagulopathy.

Extra care should be taken with patients with active TB, HIV, and hepatitis to avoid the spread of infection.

Preprocedure preparation
- Bleeding time and PTT if a bleeding problem is suspected
- Atropine 0.6mg IM (to reduce secretions)
- Patient starved for six hours.

Position
Supine.

Anaesthesia
- General anaesthetic
- Ventilation is provided through a Sanders injector utilising a Venturi system to inject oxygen under pressure intermittently.

Procedure
- Aspirate pharyngeal secretions.
- Introduce the bronchoscope behind the tongue in the midline.
- Lift the epiglottis up using the beak of the bronchoscope to visualise the vocal cords.

- Turn the bronchoscope 90° and then pass through the vocal cords into the trachea (identified by the cartilage rings).
- Then rotate the bronchoscope back to its original position and note any tracheal narrowing, constriction, deviation or mucosal abnormality.
- Advance the bronchoscope to the carina. Significant enlargement of the subcarinal nodes will result in widening of the carina.
- If the pathology is unilateral, then do the examination of the contra-lateral side first ensuring a) a complete examination, and b) blood and cellular debris will not be carried to the other side.
- Biopsy any abnormal areas.
  - Control bleeding with a cotton pledget on a pledget holder.
  - If bleeding is uncontrolled pass a Thomson bronchial blocker (or Fogarty catheter) and occlude the lobar or segmental bronchus. If an Nd: YAG laser is available then this can be used to cauterise the bleeding area.
  - If bleeding remains uncontrolled, then turn the patient so the affected side is dependent to maintain the airway to the good side. Provisions should be made for immediate thoracotomy.
- When the preliminary examination is complete, address the indication for the procedure eg extraction of foreign body or biopsy.
- Collection of specimen and biopsy:
  - Collect aspirated material in a sputum trap and ensure the specimen bottle is labelled clearly before the specimen is sent for culture, sensitivity and cytology. Mark biopsies sent for histopathological examination.
  - If secretions are scanty, a lavage with 50ml of 0.9% saline solution will yield sufficient cells for study.
- Telescopes may be inserted into the bronchoscope to visualise the distal segments. The side viewing telescopes are used to visualise the upper lobe and segmental bronchi.
- For a more detailed examination a flexible bronchoscope can be used.

Complications

Are rare.
- Complications of general anaesthesia.
- Bleeding from biopsy site—control this by applying pressure at the bleeding point with a cotton pledget on a pledget holder soaked in 1:10 000 adrenaline solution. Repeat if necessary.
- Injury to the upper aero digestive tract e.g. teeth, gums.
- Tracheal or bronchial tears.
- Pneumothorax or subcutaneous emphysema.
- Arrhythmias.
- Death.

Flexible bronchoscopy

An invasive procedure where a flexible fibreoptic bronchoscope is used to visualise the nasal passages, pharynx, larynx, vocal cords and tracheo-bronchial tree.

Indications
Diagnostic
- Haemoptysis
- Abnormal finding on CXR e.g. undiagnosed pulmonary infiltrates, mediastinal lymphadenopathy
- Inhalation injury
- Bronchiectasis
- Cough
- Foreign body
- Intubation injury
- Lung abscess
- Sputum cytology suspicious for cancer
- Stridor or localised wheezing
- Thoracic trauma
- Vocal-cord paralysis.

Therapeutic
- Retained secretions or mucus plugs (bronchial toilet)
- Laser therapy
- Difficult endotracheal intubation
- Foreign body removal
- Lung abscess
- Brachytherapy
- Bronchopleural fistula.

Contraindications
Relative rather than absolute.
- Bleeding disorders
- Hypoxaemia and hypercapnia
- Cardiovascular instability—hypotension, uncontrolled angina, malignant arrhythmia, recent myocardial infarction
- Severe asthma.

Extra care should be taken with patients with active TB, HIV, hepatitis to avoid the spread of infection. Care should also be taken when there is tracheal obstruction, as there is the possibility of losing the airway.

Preprocedure preparation
- Bleeding time and PTT if suspected bleeding problem
- Atropine 0.6mg IM (to reduce oropharygeal secretions)
- Patient starved for 6 hours.

Anaesthesia
- Performed under sedation e.g. diazepam IV or midazolam (or under general anaesthesia if performed as an adjunct to rigid bronchoscopy to visualise segmental and lobar bronchi).

- Local anaesthetic spray (4% lignocaine).
- Two millilitres 4% lignocaine injected into the epiglottis and the entrance of the larynx while the patient takes a deep breath.

Position

Supine or lying at 45° facing the operator.

Procedure

- Pass the tip of the bronchoscope into the widest nostril and guid into the nasopharynx.
- From here, the procedure is as for rigid bronchoscopy however, the segmental bronchi can be visualised and biopsied with greater ease.

Complications

These are rare.
- Complications of general or local anaesthesia
- Respiratory depression
- Laryngospasm
- Bronchospasm
- Haemorrhage
- Pneumothorax
- Aspiration pneumonia
- Arrhythmias
- Cardiorespiratory arrest.

Cervical mediastinoscopy

Mediastinoscopy should be carried out in a thoracic operating theatre with full provision for immediate thoracotomy and appropriate staff available.

Indications
- Preoperative staging of lung carcinoma
- Diagnostic biopsy of mediastinal masses and lymph nodes e.g. tumours, sarcoidosis, lymphoma.

Preprocedure preparation
- Group & Save
- Benzodiazepine premedication.

Contraindications
Relative—superior vena cava obstruction.

Anaesthetic
General anaesthetic with endotracheal intubation.

Position
- Supine with neck fully extended
- A cushion is placed between the scapulae and the head is lowered to drop the patients shoulders and project the trachea forwards.

Incision
Transverse incision 3cm long, one fingerbreadth above sternal notch.

Procedure
- Divide the strap muscles in the midline.
- Enter the pretracheal fascia and tracheal rings visualised.
- Insert a finger anterior to the trachea and develop the pretracheal space into the mediastinum.
- Palpate the innominate artery anteriorly. Palpate also for any enlarged lymph nodes.
- Introduce the mediastinoscope into this space and visualise any abnormal lymph nodes.
- Perform biopsy of an enlarged lymph node with biopsy forceps after needle aspiration has confirmed that the structure is not vascular.
- Once biopsy has been performed, haemostasis is secured using diathermy cautery or pressure with gauze swab.
- Following haemostasis, withdraw the mediastinoscope.
- Close the wound in layers using absorbable sutures.

Postoperative management
Perform a chest radiograph.

Complications

- Control bleeding from biopsy site with a gauze pack.
- Severe bleeding is usually the result of damage to a large blood vessel e.g. superior vena cava, azygos vein, innominate artery, and arch of aorta or even right pulmonary artery. In this instance, pack the space with a gauze swab and proceed to immediate sternotomy. Identify the bleeding vessel and controlled by clamping and/or suture.
- Pneumothorax.

Anterior mediastinotomy

Used to sample lymph nodes in the subaortic and periaortic regions that are not easily accessible through cervical mediastinoscopy, and to assess operability of centrally located lung tumours. It is usually performed on the left side.

Mediastinotomy should be carried out in a thoracic operating theatre with full provision for immediate thoracotomy and appropriate staff available.

Indications
- Diagnostic investigation for staging lung cancer
- To assess operability of upper lobe and hilar lung tumours.

Anaesthetic
General anaesthesia with endotracheal intubation.

Position of patient
Supine.

Incision
Make a 4–6cm transverse incision in the left 3rd intercostal space just lateral to the sternal border.

Procedure
- Divide the subcutaneous tissues in the line of the skin incision.
- Divide the pectoralis major muscle fibres.
- Divide the intercostal muscles taking care to avoid the internal mammary artery. If the artery is seen or is in danger of damage it should be formally ligated.
- Enter the pleural space and carry out preliminary finger palpation of the following structures:
  - Pulmonary hilum.
  - Ascertain relationship of the tumour to the left atrium.
  - On the left side, the arch of aorta and subaortic lymph nodes.
- Introduce the mediastinoscope and tumour operability assessed.
- Signs of inoperability include:
  - Tumour invasion of the pericardium and left atrium.
  - Tumour invasion of the proximal pulmonary artery.
- Perform a biopsy of abnormal subaortic lymph nodes or of the tumour.
- Obtain haemostasis using diathermy cautery.
- Introduce an intercostal drain (size 24–28French, Silastic) through a separate stab incision in the left chest wall and connect to a bottle with an underwater seal.
- Close the wound in layers using absorbable sutures and apply a dressing.

Postoperative management
Perform a chest radiograph.

Complications

Complications are rare, but potentially life threatening.

- Control bleeding using diathermy or local pressure with a gauze swab (for bleeding following biopsy of the subaortic nodes, local pressure is preferred because of the risk of thermal injury and permanent damage to the recurrent laryngeal nerve from diathermy). If the bleeding is catastrophic then pack the mediastinum gauze while preparations are made for emergency thoracotomy or median sternotomy.
- Complications related to general anaesthesia.

Chest drain insertion: tube thoracostomy

Indications
- Pneumothorax
  - Spontaneous
  - Tension
- Haemothorax
- Pleural effusion
- Empyema.

Contraindications
- Relative
  - Coagulopathy
  - Pleural adhesions.

Equipment
- Sterile instrument pack
- Non-absorbable sutures
- Local anaesthetic e.g. lignocaine or bupivicaine
- Chest drain
- Bottle with underwater seal
- Dressing.

Chest drain tube
- Straight or right angled
- Silicone or plastic
- Most commonly use size 24 to 28Fr. gauge (a Bonnano suprapubic catheter can be used if the effusion is not viscous)
- Multiple drainage holes
- Radio opaque line for radiographic localization.

Preprocedure preparation
Premed e.g. benzodiazepine (if the patient is anxious).

Position
Patient sitting in a comfortable position on the edge of the bed resting on a pillow placed on the bedside table.

Procedure
- Chose the site depending on the location of collection. Usually 4th or 5th intercostal space in the anterior axillary line.
- Clean the skin with Betadine.
- Infiltrate local anaesthetic into the skin, subcutaneous tissues, muscle, and pleura at the chosen site.
- After 5–10 minutes, make a small incision (approximately 1.5cm) in the intercostal space.
- Deepen the incision using scissors or artery forceps to enter the pleura.
- Introduce a finger into the pleural cavity to ensure that the lung is free.

- Place a heavy non-absorbable suture on one side of the incision to secure the drain after insertion.
- Insert a second heavy non-absorbable vertical mattress suture in the centre of the wound in preparation for closure of the wound when then drain is removed. This method is preferable to a purse-string suture, which is commonly advocated, as the purse-string suture tends to convert the linear incision into a circle when it is tied. This may lead to the incision being held open resulting in poor wound healing.
- Introduce the drain through the opening, ensuring that all the drainage holes are within the pleural space.
- In the treatment of pneumothorax, direct the drain towards the apex of the chest whereas for the treatment of a pleural effusion the drain is directed basally.
- Secure the drain with the previously inserted suture.
- Connect the drain to a bottle with the underwater seal.
- Suction may or may not be applied depending on the surgeon's preference.
- In the event that the incision is too large for the tube, additional sutures are inserted.
- Apply a dressing.

Postprocedure management
- Perform a chest radiograph to confirm correct drain position and lung re-expansion
- Analgesia.

Complications
This is a potentially dangerous procedure.
- Bleeding—sometimes can be catastrophic e.g. from cannulation of large intrathoracic vessels (or even the heart). If recognised, the tube should be clamped and the patient resuscitated and transferred to theatre for emergency thoracotomy and control of bleeding.
- Pain from intercostal nerve damage.
- Pulmonary laceration.
- Air leak.

Chest drain management
Chest tube patency
Observe the underwater seal bottle for fluctuations of the fluid column with respiration (about 6cm). If no fluctuation occurs, then the tube is probably blocked and should be removed or replaced.

Air leak
- Bubbling in the underwater seal bottle generally indicates an ongoing air leak, which can be from the lung or a leak in the chest drain system. Place a Vaseline impregnated gauze around the tube at the skin exit site to prevent air from leaking into the chest through the tube tract when suction is being applied to the underwater sealed bottle.
- Repeat chest radiographs daily until the air leak stops. This may take several days.

- In the event that the air leak almost stops on normal respiration but some bubbles still appear when the patient is asked to cough, clamp the intercostal drain tube and take a chest radiograph after one hour. If there is no or minimal pneumothorax visible on the chest radiograph then the drain may be safely removed. If the patient experiences discomfort or the chest radiograph shows a significant pneumothorax release the clamp with a further period of suction instituted.

Fluid drainage

Note the quantity and character of the tube drainage regularly.

Chest tube removal

- Indications
  - When the drain has stopped draining air or fluid
  - The lung is fully expanded on chest radiograph
- Remove on breath holding (usually forced inspiration)
  - Drain should be pulled out rapidly and the suture tied before allowing the patient to breathe.

Posterolateral thoracotomy

Allows good access to all areas of the thoracic cavity.

Indications
- Unilateral lung resection
- Resection of chest wall neoplasms
- Unilateral lung volume reduction surgery
- Bullectomy
- Tumours of the posterior mediastinum
- Oesophageal surgery.

Contraindications
Inability to tolerate major surgery.

Anaesthetic
General anaesthesia with double lumen endobronchial intubation.

Position
- Left or right strict lateral position with break of table in the patient's chest area. Alternatively a pillow can be placed between the chest and operating table to elevate the chest and splay open the upper ribs to facilitate the incision.
- The upper arm is placed on an armrest elevating the scapula as far as possible to facilitate the incision.

Incision
Posterolateral incision in the line of the ribs 1–2cm below the angle of the scapula (5th or 6th intercostal space).

Procedure
- Divide the skin, subcutaneous fat, and latissimus dorsi muscle in line of the incision.
- Secure haemostasis using diathermy cautery or ligature.
- Retract the serratus anterior muscle anteriorly.
- Incise the fascia in the triangle of auscultation, just behind the angle of the scapula to expose the ribs and intercostal muscles.
- Divide the trapezius muscle (situated posteriorly) for approximately 2cm in the line of the incision.
- Retract the scapula superiorly using a scapula retractor.
- Then introduce your hand under the scapula and count the ribs from the top starting with the highest rib that can be felt, usually the 2nd rib. Mark the 5th or 6th rib with diathermy.
- Score the periosteum of the superior surface of the rib where entry into the chest is required with the diathermy cautery throughout its length.
- Elevate the periosteum along the length of the rib using a periosteal elevator.
- Divide the costo-transverse ligament posteriorly to facilitate movement of the rib.

- Cover the ribs with skin towels. Then introduce the rib spreader between the ribs and gradually open it to spread the ribs to gain adequate exposure.
- Deflate the lung.

Closure

- Insert two chest drains (24–28Fr., Silastic) through separate stab incisions one anterior and one posterior. Direct the anterior drain to the apex and the posterior drain to the base of the pleural space.
- Secure the drains to the skin with heavy non-absorbable sutures.
- Place three pericostal 'figure of eight' Vicryl sutures around the ribs on either side of the incision.
- Approximate the ribs with a rib approximator.
- Tie the pericostal sutures. Alternatively, suture the intercostal muscles in layers with a continuous absorbable suture (e.g. Vicryl).
- Suture the divided muscles individually in layers using absorbable continuous sutures e.g. Vicryl.
- Suture the subcutaneous fat in a similar way.
- Close the skin with an absorbable continuous subcuticular suture e.g. Monocryl.
- Apply a dry protective dressing.
- Connect the drains to bottles with underwater seals.

Postoperative management

- Transfer the patient to the HDU
- Connect the drains to suction (5KPa)
- Perform a baseline chest radiograph
- Provide analgesia with PCA, epidural or paravertebral block
- Monitor continuous ECG, O_2 saturations, and urine output.

Complications

- Complications of general anaesthesia
- Haemorrhage
- Pneumothorax
- Bronchopleural fistula
- Wound infection
- Post thoracotomy pain—due to damage to the intercostal nerve. 5% of patients have troublesome pain.

Anterolateral thoracotomy

Indications
- Open lung biopsy
- Closed mitral valvotomy
- Some anterior mediastinal masses
- Anterior mediastinal cysts
- Pericardial window for pericardial effusion that is resistant to drainage with a needle.

Anaesthetic
General anaesthesia with double lumen endobronchial intubation.

Position
Supine with the side to be operated upon tilted at 30°, by placing a pillow under the patients shoulder.

Incision
Anterior 5th intercostal space, from the midline to the angle of the scapula.

Procedure
- Incise the skin and the subcutaneous tissues in line of the incision.
- Divide the latissimus dorsi muscles in the line of the incision.
- Count the ribs downward on the surface of the chest from the angle of Louis (the level of the 2nd rib) and the 5th rib is scored with the diathermy.
- Enter the 5th intercostal space.
- Strip the periosteum from the inferior surface of the rib.
- Divide the pleura and enter the chest.
- Elevate the periosteum posteriorly to allow free movement of the rib.
- Cover with the skin towels. Introduce the rib spreader between the ribs and gradually open it to spread the ribs to gain adequate exposure.
- Deflate the lung.

Closure
- Insert two chest drains (24–28Fr. gauge, silastic) through separate stab incisions one anterior and one posterior. Direct the anterior drain to the apex and the posterior drain to the base of the pleural space.
- Secure the drains to the skin with heavy non-absorbable sutures.
- Place three pericostal 'figure of eight' Vicryl sutures around the ribs on either side of the incision.
- Approximate the ribs with a rib approximator.
- Tie the pericostal sutures. Alternatively, suture the intercostal muscles in layers with a continuous absorbable suture (e.g. Vicryl).
- Individually suture the divided muscles in layers using absorbable continuous sutures e.g. Vicryl.
- Suture the subcutaneous fat in a similar way.
- Close the skin with an absorbable continuous subcuticular suture e.g. Monocryl.

- Apply a dry protective dressing.
- Connect the drains to bottles with underwater seals.

Postoperative management
- Transfer the patient to the HDU
- Connect the drains to suction (5KPa)
- Perform a baseline chest radiograph
- Provide analgesia with PCA, epidural, or paravertebral
- Monitor continuous ECG, O_2 saturations, and urine output.

Complications
- Complications of general anaesthesia
- Haemorrhage
- Pneumothorax
- Bronchopleural fistula
- Wound infection
- Post thoracotomy pain—due to damage to the intercostal nerve. 5% of patients have troublesome pain.

Median sternotomy

The most frequently used approach for operations on the heart and mediastinum. In contrast to thoracotomy no muscles are divided so there is reduced postoperative pain.

Indications
- Mediastinal tumour resection (e.g. thymoma)
- Bilateral lung volume reduction surgery/bullectomy
- Transpericardial access to trachea/bronchus e.g. carinal tumours
- Resection of multiple pulmonary lesions e.g. metastectomy
- Trauma.

Position
Supine.

Anaesthetic
General anaesthesia with endotracheal intubation.

Incision
Vertical midline from the sternal notch to the xiphisternum.

Procedure
- Divide the skin and subcutaneous tissues in the line of the incision.
- Locate the middle of the sternum and score with diathermy cautery from top to bottom.
- Perform sternotomy using an oscillating electric sternotomy saw.
- Control bleeding from the periosteum with diathermy.
- Insert the skin towels on either side of the wound. Then insert the sternal spreader and open it to separate the two halves of the sternum. Avoid over distraction to prevent distraction injury to the lower cords of the brachial plexus.

Closure
- Insert two chest drains (24–28Fr., Silastic) into the mediastinum through separate stab incisions below the sternotomy.
- If the pleural space has been entered direct one of the mediastinal drains into the pleural space or use a third drain.
- Suture the drains in place with heavy non-absorbable sutures. Insert a closing stitch.
- Appose the sternal halves using six stainless steel wires, taking care to ensure that there is no bony step.
- Inspect the under surface of the sternum for bleeding at the wire entry and exit sites. Control this using diathermy or sutures.
- Twist the wires until the sternal edges are firmly approximated. Cut the wires using wire cutter and bend them so that the cut ends point into the sternum.
- Close the subcutaneous tissues using continuous absorbable sutures e.g. Vicryl.
- Close the skin using subcuticular continuous absorbable sutures e.g. Monocryl.

Postoperative management
- Transfer the patient to HDU (ICU in the event of cardiac surgery)
- Connect the drains to suction (5KPa)
- Perform a baseline chest radiograph
- Provide pain control with PCA, epidural, or paravertebral block
- Monitor continuous ECG, O_2 saturations, and urine output.

Complications
- Complications of general anaesthesia
- Bleeding—this can occur following damage to the internal mammary artery when the sternal wires are placed
- Instability of the sternum
- Wound infection
- Dehiscence of wound
- Osteomyelitis (rare).

Lobectomy

This is the removal of a single lobe of lung. Occasionally bilobectomy (e.g. middle and lower lobectomy) is performed.

Indications
- Lung carcinoma
- Benign tumours
- Chronic lung abscess
- Pulmonary tuberculosis
- Fungal infections
- Bronchiectasis
- Congenital abnormalities e.g. lung sequestration.

Preoperative preparation
- All patients should undergo bronchoscopy by the operating surgeon
- Results of lung function tests, chest radiograph, ECG, and CT scan must be available
- The patient should be warned about the possible conversion to pneumonectomy depending on intraoperative findings.

Position
Right or left lateral.

Incision
Posterolateral thoracotomy in the 5th intercostal space.

Anaesthetic
General anaesthesia with double lumen endotracheal intubation.

Postoperative management
- Nurse the patient on the HDU
- Monitor ECG, CVP, BP, oxygen saturation, respiratory rate, and urine output
- Perform a postoperative chest radiograph on arrival to the HDU
- Provide analgesia by PCA, epidural or paravertebral block
- DVT prophylaxis according to local protocols
- Use regular chest physiotherapy to help expectoration and deep breathing
- Carry out daily chest radiographs to assess expansion of the remaining lobe
- Remove the intercostal drains when there is no longer any drainage of fluid or air and chest radiograph appearances are satisfactory (this is usually 24–48 hours). Frequently after lobectomy the basal drain can be removed first and the apical one later. Confirm air leakage when bubbles appear in the underwater seal bottle when the patient is asked to cough.

Complications
- Complications related to general anaesthesia.
- Haemorrhage.

- Bronchopleural fistula.
  - Presents as an air leak lasting for more than one week.
  - Confirmed by the presence of bubbles in the underwater seal bottle during normal respiration or when the patient is asked to cough.
  - If the air leak is minimal the drain may be clamped for a period of one to two hours. A chest radiograph is taken. If the lung is still expanded or a very small pneumothorax is present the drain may be safely removed. A check radiograph is performed the following day to ensure the lung remains expanded.
  - As a last resort talc pleurodesis can be performed on the ward using a slurry of talc mixed with local anaesthetic introduced through the chest drain. This induces inflammation resulting in closure of the air leak.
- Cardiac arrhythmias (most frequently atrial fibrillation).
- Wound infection and empyema.
- Bronchopneumonia in the remaining lung.
- ARDS.
- Death (3–4% in the UK).

Right upper lobectomy

Indications
See p712.

Preoperative preparation
See p712.

Position
Right or left lateral position.

Incision
Posterolateral thoracotomy in the 5th intercostal space.

Anaesthetic
General anaesthesia with double lumen endobronchial intubation.

Procedure
- Carry out a posterolateral thoracotomy in the 5th intercostal space (see pp706–7).
- Divide any pleural adhesions to free the lung.
- Inspect the whole lung and palpate to ascertain location of the tumour and operability and to make sure that there are no other nodules in the other lobes of the right lung.
- Clean the pleural reflection at the top of the right lung.
- Identify the upper pulmonary vein and ligate it with two proximal non-absorbable ligatures and one distal ligature non-absorbable ligature and divide it between the proximal and distal ligatures. Alternatively, divide the vessel using an Endo GIA 30 vascular stapler (this places three rows of staples either side of the cut).
- Identify the upper pulmonary arterial branches and encircle them with right-angle forceps and a non-absorbable ligature. These can also be ligated with two proximal ligatures and one distal ligature and divided or secured using an Endo GIA 30 stapling device.
- Then pay attention to the posterior aspect of the lung where the pleural reflection onto the bronchus is cleared and identify the upper lobe bronchus.
- Isolate and staple with the TA 30 4.5mm stapler. Divide the bronchus just distal to the staple line and retract it to expose the recurrent branch of the right upper lobe. This branch is of varying size but is usually quite small; encircle it, ligate it, and divide it.
- Now separate the oblique fissure if not complete by dissection or by stapling it and dividing it.
- Deal with the horizontal fissure, which is invariably incomplete, in one of two ways, either by using the Endo GIA stapler or by applying traction on the right upper lobe bronchus to allow it to separate from the rest of the lung. This will inevitably leave a raw surface on the upper part of the middle lobe.
- Secure haemostasis on this raw surface with diathermy.

- Expand the remaining lung and test the bronchial staple line by covering it with 0.9% saline solution and increasing the intra airway pressure to 40mmHg. Seal any air leak using tissue glue e.g. Tisseal.
- Close the chest.
- Turn the patient into the supine position and reverse the anaesthetic.
- Transferred to the HDU for monitoring when the patient is breathing spontaneously.

Postoperative management
See p712.

Complications
See p713.

Right middle lobectomy

Indications
See p712.

Preoperative preparation
See p712.

Position
Right lateral.

Incision
Posterolateral thoracotomy in the 6th intercostal space.

Anaesthetic
General anaesthesia with double lumen endobronchial intubation.

Procedure
- Perform posterolateral thoracotomy in the 6th intercostal space (see pp706–7).
- Free the lung from the chest wall by dividing pleural adhesions.
- Identify the middle lobe between the horizontal and oblique fissures.
- Deepen the fissures at the point where the transverse fissure meets the oblique fissure if incomplete, and ligate the branches (usually two) to the middle lobe from the pulmonary artery and divide them between the ligatures.
- Then retract the lung backwards and clean the upper pulmonary vein. The middle lobe vein usually drains into the lower part of the right upper lobe vein. The middle lobe vein is the lowest tributary draining into the upper lobe vein. Identify it, ligate it with two ligatures and divided between the ligatures.
- Then identify the middle lobe bronchus by finger palpation. Clean it and visualise it and encircle it. Then staple the middle lobe bronchus using the TA 30 4.5mm stapler. Divide the middle lobe bronchus just distal to the staple line and the middle lobe specimen removed.
- Expand the remaining lung and test the bronchial staple line by covering it with 0.9% saline solution and increasing the intra airway pressure to 40mmHg. Seal any air leak using tissue glue e.g. Tisseal.
- Close the chest.
- Turn the patient into the supine position and reverse the anaesthetic.
- Transfer the patient to the HDU for monitoring when breathing.

Postoperative management
See p712.

Complications
See p713.

Right lower lobectomy

Indications
See p712.

Preoperative preparation
See p712.

Position
Right or left lateral position.

Incision
Posterolateral thoracotomy in the 6th intercostal space.

Anaesthetic
General anaesthesia with double lumen endobroncheal intubation.

Procedure
- Make a posterolateral thoracotomy in the 6th intercostal space (see pp706–7).
- Divide pleural adhesions to free the lung.
- Then inspect the lung and palpate to ascertain tumour operability and presence of any other lesions.
- Commence right lower lobectomy by separating the fissures at the point where the horizontal fissure meets the oblique fissure. If the fissures are incomplete, carry out dissection at this point inwards until the lower pulmonary artery branches become visible. Encircle them just below the middle lobe artery branch and ligate twice and divide them or staple with the Endo GIA 30 vascular stapler.
- Isolate the branch to the apical part of the lower lobe, which lies just above and ligate separately with two ligatures and then divide it. Then separate the rest of the oblique fissure.
- Isolate the lower pulmonary vein and divide it between ligatures, or with Endo GIA 30 vascular stapler.
- Then clean the lower lobe bronchus by removing lymphatic tissue and stapling it just below the middle lobe bronchus take off using the TA 30 4.5mm stapler. Resect the bronchus distal to the staple line and remove the lower lobe.
- Expand the remaining lung and test the bronchial staple line by covering it with 0.9% saline solution and increasing the intra airway pressure to 40mmHg. Seal any air leak using tissue glue e.g. Tisseal.
- Close the chest.
- Turn the patient into the supine position and reverse the anaesthetic.
- Transfer the patient to the HDU for monitoring when he/she is breathing spontaneously.

Postoperative management
See p712.

Complications
See p713.

Left upper lobectomy

Indications
See p712.

Preoperative preparation
See p712.

Position
Right or left lateral position.

Anaesthetic
General anaesthesia with double lumen endobronchial intubation.

Incision
Posterolateral thoracotomy in the 5th intercostal space.

Procedure
- Perform a posterolateral thoracotomy in the 5th intercostal space (see pp706–7).
- Divide any pleural adhesions.
- Inspect the lung (a puckered appearance on the surface of the lung suggests underlying tumour) and palpate it to assess operability of the lesion by lobectomy.
- Note any hilar or mediastinal lymphadenopathy.
- Proceed with lobectomy if the tumour is restricted to the lower lobe and there is no infiltration of the upper lobe or other adjacent structures.
- Clear the upper part of the pulmonary hilum to expose the large blood vessels clearly.
- Then enter the oblique fissure. If this is incomplete then dissect the fissure out to approach the branches of the left pulmonary artery in its depth. Identify the lower arterial branch. Then clear the lingular branch, isolate it and ligate it in continuity and divide it. There are two apical branches which can be quite large. Clear these isolate them and either ligate them between two non-absorbable ligatures or staple them using an Endo GIA 30 vascular stapler.
- If you encounter difficulty in isolating the apical arterial branches take the upper pulmonary vein first. If there is not sufficient length, open the pericardium, which will facilitate ligation or stapling of the vein.
- Clear the upper bronchus and its junction with the right main bronchus and demonstrate the right lower bronchus. Then staple the upper bronchus using the TA 30 4.5mm stapler and divide it distal to the staple line.
- Separate the remaining oblique fistula, staple it, and divide it and remove the upper lobe.
- Secure haemostasis using the diathermy cautery.
- Expand the left lower lobe and test the bronchial staple line by covering it with 0.9% saline solution and increasing the intra airway pressure to 40mmHg. Seal any air leak using tissue glue e.g. Tisseal.

- Close the chest.
- Turn the patient into the supine position and reverse the anaesthetic.
- Transfer the patient to the HDU for monitoring when he/she is breathing spontaneously.

Postoperative management
See p712.

Complications
See p713.

Left lower lobectomy

Indications
See p712.

Preoperative preparation
See p712.

Position
Right or left lateral position.

Incision
A left thoracotomy is performed in the bed of the 6th rib.

Procedure
- Perform a left thoracotomy in the bed of the 6th rib.
- Divide pleural adhesions if present to free the lung.
- Inspect the left lower lobe and palpate to assess tumour operability.
- Similarly inspect and palpate the upper lobe to make sure there are no other lesions present.
- Open the oblique fissure and the pulmonary arterial branches displayed deep within the fissure.
- Isolate the lower lobe arterial branches and ligate with two ligatures proximal and one distal, and divide between the proximal and distal ligatures. Alternatively, divide the branches using the Endo GIA 30 stapler. Isolate the apical branch of the lower lobe similarly, ligate it in continuity, and divide it.
- Divide the pulmonary ligament up to the lower pulmonary vein. Encircle this and either divided between two ligatures or stapled with the endo GIA 30 vascular stapler.
- Clean the lower bronchus through the bifurcation with the upper bronchus by removing lymphatic material surrounding it. Then staple the lower bronchus using a TA 30 4.5mm stapler. Resect the bronchus distal to the staple line flush with the stapler.
- Remove the lower lobe specimen.
- Ensure haemostasis using the diathermy cautery.
- Expand the left upper lobe and test the bronchial staple line by covering it with 0.9% saline solution or sterile water and increasing the intra airway pressure to 40mmHg. Seal any air leak using tissue glue e.g. Tisseal.
- Close the chest.
- Turn the patient into the supine position and reverse the anaesthetic.
- Transfer the patient to the HDU for monitoring when breathing is spontaneous.

Postoperative management
See p712.

Complications
See p713.

Pneumonectomy

Pneumonectomy is necessary for centrally placed tumours and can only be performed in fit patients.

Indications

* Lung carcinoma
* Chronic lung abscess.

Preoperative preparation

* All patients undergo bronchoscopic assessment by the operating surgeon
* Results of lung function tests, chest radiograph and CT scan must be available
* ECG.

Anaesthetic

General anaesthesia with double lumen endobronchial intubation.

Position

Lateral position.

Postoperative management

* The patient is nursed on the HDU.
* The drains are connected to a bottle with an underwater seal. A clamp is applied to the drain which is released for 5min every hour in order to keep the mediastinum central. *On no account should suction be applied to the drain.*
* Monitoring of continuous ECG, CVP, BP, oxygen saturation, respiratory rate, and urine output is performed.
* An immediate postoperative chest X-ray is performed on arrival to the HDU. This will be useful as a baseline in case there is any subsequent change in the patient's condition.
* Analgesia is provided by PCA, epidural, or paravertebral block.
* DVT prophylaxis is prescribed according to local protocols.
* Regular chest physiotherapy to help expectoration and deep breathing.
* A repeat chest X-ray is performed at 24 hours.
* The intercostal drain is removed after 24 hours providing there is no further blood leak and no air leak and the chest X-ray appearances are satisfactory.

Complications following pneumonectomy

* Complications related to general anaesthesia.
* Haemorrhage—blood loss over 200ml per hour for 4 consecutive hours, or more than 500ml per hour are indications for reopening the chest.
* Bronchopleural fistula—this may be suspected if the patient develops serosanguinous sputum or discharge from the thoracotomy wound. A drop in the fluid level on serial chest radiographs confirms the diagnosis. Immediate management:

- The patient is turned with affected side dependent so that there is no overspill of pneumonectomy space fluid into the good lung.
- An intercostal drain is inserted.
- Antibiotics are commenced.
- Suction bronchoscopy is carried out.
- Following stabilisation of the patient:
  - The patient is taken to the operating theatre and rigid broncho-scopy performed to suck out secretions or spill over into the good lung, and visualise the fistula.
  - If the fistula is small, treatment is with sodium hydroxide cauterisa-tion every 2 weeks. This is introduced on a cotton pledget through a rigid bronchoscope and neutralised with acetic acid. (This works by causing an inflammatory reaction followed by healing and fibrosis, which reduces and eventually closes the fistula).
  - If the fistula is large, the fistula is closed with a pedicled muscle flap.
  - If the bronchopleural fistula presents at a later date (weeks after surgery), diagnosis is made reduction in the fluid level within the pneumonectomy space on serial chest radiographs. The patient is treated as above.
  - Arrhythmias (most commonly atrial fibrillation).
- Wound infection and empyema of pneumonectomy space.
- Bronchopneumonia in the remaining lung.
- ARDS
- Death (mortality in the UK is between 5–8%).

Right pneumonectomy

Indications
- Lung carcinoma
- Chronic lung abscess.

Preoperative preparation
- All patients should undergo bronchoscopy by the operating surgeon
- Results of lung function tests, chest radiograph and CT scan must be available
- ECG.

Anaesthetic
General anaesthesia with double lumen endobronchial intubation.

Position
Lateral position.

Incision
Perform a posterolateral thoracotomy in the right 5th intercostal space.

Procedure
- Perform a posterolateral thoracotomy in the 5th intercostal space (see pp706–7).
- Divide pleural adhesions (if present) and free the lung.
- Palpate the lung to confirm the position and operability of the tumour and to assess whether any other lesions are present which have not been visualised on CT scan.
- Inspect the mediastinum for enlarged lymph nodes.
- Signs of inoperability: tumour invading adjacent structures e.g. pericardium, left atrium, aorta or oesophagus. (Diaphragmatic invasion is not a sign of inoperability as the affected part can be resected and the defect closed directly with non-absorbable sutures or a Dacron patch inserted to restore the diaphragm.)
- If the lesion is operable: clean the pleural reflection around the hilum, behind the phrenic nerve, below the azygos vein and in front of the oesophagus.
- Then free the superior pulmonary vein and encircle it with a stout non-absorbable suture using right angled forceps. This provides traction on the vein, which is either ligated in continuity with non-absorbable ligatures or stapled and simultaneously divided using an Endo GIA 30 vascular stapler.
- Isolate the lower pulmonary vein, encircle with a non-absorbable ligature and either ligate, divide, or staple it.
- Then clean the main right pulmonary artery and encircle with a stout non-absorbable ligature, which provides traction for application of the Endo GIA 30 vascular stapler, which staples on both sides and divides the vessel when it is fired.
- In the event that the pulmonary veins are too short for ligation or stapling then open the pericardium posterior to the phrenic nerve and divide the veins within the pericardium.

- Clean the right main bronchus by removing the subcarinal lymph nodes. The bronchus is then stapled as close to the main carina as possible using the TA 30 4.5mm stapler.
- Divide the bronchus distal to the staple line and remove the lung.
- Clip or ligate the bronchial arteries on the posterior aspect of the main bronchus.
- Remove and submit all visible lymph nodes for histological examination after clear labelling.
- Secure haemostasis using the diathermy cautery.
- If the pericardium has been opened, suture it with 4/0 Prolene. If the defect in the pericardium is too large for direct closure then suture a Dacron patch in place to close the defect in order to prevent herniation and strangulation of the heart.
- Cover the bronchial stump with adjacent pleura using interrupted 4/0 Prolene sutures.
- Then test the bronchial stump for air leaks by covering the hilum with 0.9% saline solution or sterile water and increasing the intratracheal pressure to 40mmHg. Suture any air leak with 4/0 Prolene.
- Insert a single intercostal drain (size 24–28French, Silastic) through a separate stab incision. Secure it with a heavy non-absorbable suture.
- Close the chest.
- Turn the patient into the supine position and reverse the anaesthetic.
- Transfer the patient to the HDU for monitoring when he/she is breathing spontaneously.

Postoperative management
See p712.

Complications
See p713.

Left pneumonectomy

Indications
- Lung carcinoma.
- Chronic lung abscess.

Preoperative preparation
- All patients should undergo bronchoscopy by the operating surgeon
- Results of lung function tests, chest radiograph and CT scan must be available
- ECG.

Anaesthetic
General anaesthesia with double lumen endobronchial intubation.

Position
Lateral position.

Procedure
- Perform a left posterolateral thoracotomy in the 5th intercostal space (see pp706–7).
- Divide any pleural adhesions and free the lung.
- Palpate the lung to confirm the position and operability of the tumour and to assess whether any other lesions are present which have not been seen on CT.
- Signs of inoperability: tumour invading adjacent structures e.g. pericardium, left atrium, aorta or oesophagus. (Diaphragmatic invasion is not a sign of inoperability as the affected part can be resected and the defect closed directly with non-absorbable sutures or a Dacron patch inserted to restore the diaphragm.)
- If the lesion is inoperable then take biopsies of the lung tumour and/or the mediastinal lymph nodes, insert an intercostal drain, and close the chest wall in layers.
- If the lesion is found to be operable then carry out the pneumonectomy as follows.
- Clean the pleural reflection around the hilum starting below the arch of the aorta, posteriorly in front of the oesophagus, and anteriorly behind the left phrenic nerve.
- Release the pulmonary ligament.
- Free the lower left pulmonary vein using sharp and blunt dissection and encircle with a stout non-absorbable ligature.
- Isolate the upper left pulmonary vein.
- Once it is clear that the lung can be removed without any problems, staple these two veins using an Endo GIA 30 vascular stapler.
- Clean the left main pulmonary artery, isolate it and retract it with a stout non-absorbable ligature. This facilitates the introduction of the Endo GIA 30 vascular stapler, fire it after ensuring the artery lies between the marks on the anvil of the stapler.

- Clear the left main bronchus by removing any subcarinal lymph nodes and staple it using the TA 30 4.5mm cartridge, and divide it as close to the main carina as possible.
- Remove the lung specimen.
- Remove any additional lymph nodes either in the subaortic area or mediastinum. Exercise great care in removing the subaortic lymph nodes because of the course of the left recurrent laryngeal nerve. Use diathermy with extreme caution.
- Secure haemostasis.
- Ligate or clip bronchial arteries with Liga clips.
- If the pericardium has been opened then suture this either sutured directly or patched using a Dacron patch, in order to prevent herniation and strangulation of the heart in the postoperative phase.
- Cover the bronchial stump with adjacent pleura using interrupted 4/0 Prolene sutures.
- Then test the bronchial stump for air leaks by covering the hilum with 0.9% saline solution or sterile water and increasing the intratracheal pressure to 5–6KPa. Suture any air leak with 4/0 Prolene.
- Insert a single intercostal drain (size 24–28Fr., Silastic) through a separate stab incision. Secure this with a heavy non-absorbable suture.
- Close the chest.
- Turn the patient into the supine position and reverse the anaesthetic.
- Transfer the patient to the HDU for monitoring when he/she is breathing spontaneously.

Postoperative management
See p712.

Complications
See p713.

Right intrapericardial pneumonectomy

Indication
Lung cancers situated at the hilum encroaching upon the pulmonary artery or pulmonary veins near the left atrium.

Anaesthetic
General anaesthesia with double lumen endobronchial intubation.

Position
Lateral position.

Incision
Perform a posterolateral thoracotomy in the 5th intercostal space.

Procedure
- Open the pericardium vertically behind the phrenic nerve to expose the junction of the pulmonary veins with the left atrium. Encircle the veins and staple or ligate as previously described.
- Encircle the right pulmonary artery in the recess between the ascending aorta and the superior vena cava and ligate or staple it.
- Staple the bronchus flush with the tracheobronchial junction as previously described.
- Close the defect in the pericardium by direct suture or insert a Dacron patch in order to prevent herniation of the heart.
- Subsequent steps of the operation are as for right pneumonectomy.

Postoperative care
See p712.

Complications
See p713.

Left intrapericardial pneumonectomy

Indication

Lung cancer at the hilum that has encroached upon the pulmonary artery or pulmonary veins.

Anaesthetic

General anaesthesia with double lumen endobronchial intubation.

Position

Lateral position.

Incision

Perform left posterolateral thoracotomy in the 5th intercostal space.

Procedure

- Clear the pulmonary artery and obtain further length by dividing the ligamentum arteriosum. Take *extreme care* during this manoeuvre to spare the recurrent laryngeal nerve, which is in close proximity. Do not use diathermy cautery.
- Make a vertical incision in the pericardium posterior to the phrenic nerve to expose the junction of the pulmonary veins with the left atrium.
- Isolate the pulmonary veins and staple them flush with the left atrium and divide them.
- Isolate the left pulmonary artery, staple it and divide it.
- Clean the bronchus to its junction with the trachea and staple it.
- Close the defect in the pericardium using a Dacron patch.
- Subsequent steps of the procedure are as for left pneumonectomy.

Postoperative care

See p712.

Complications

See p713.

Open parietal pleurectomy and bullectomy

Indications
- Non-resolving spontaneous pneumothorax
- Repeated spontaneous pneumothorax (more than two episodes)
- First spontaneous pneumothorax in airline pilots.

Anaesthetic
General anaesthesia with double lumen endobronchial intubation.

Position
Lateral position.

Preoperative preparation
Results of lung function tests, chest radiograph, ECG, and CT scan must be available.

Incision
Posterolateral thoracotomy through the 5th intercostal space.

Procedure
- After the chest is entered, retract the lung downwards to expose the apex where one or two thin walled cysts may be present. Sometimes only a scarred area may be visible.
- Remove the cysts using a stapling device endo GIA 30 (blue).
- Perform parietal pleurectomy by raising and excising the pleura starting at the pleural edge at the upper part of the incision and moving towards the apex of the pleural space. *Excise with great care* while the pleura is being stripped off the sympathetic nervous trunk.
- Control any bleeding points with diathermy.
- Close the chest.
- Turn the patient into the supine position and reverse the anaesthetic.
- Transfer the patient to the HDU for monitoring when is breathing spontaneously.

Postoperative management
- Suction is applied to the drainage bottles (5KPa) for 48 hours to encourage the lungs to expand and adhere to the raw surface of the chest wall created by the pleurectomy.
- Daily chest radiographs.
- Regular chest physiotherapy.
- Analgesia is provided with PCA, epidural or paravertebral block.
- The drains are removed when the drainage of air and fluid stops and the chest radiograph confirms the lung is fully expanded.

Complications
- Bleeding
- Prolonged air leak
- Permanent air space (lung not fully expanded)
- Wound infection
- Empyema.

Open lung wedge biopsy

Indications
Diagnostic for interstitial lung disease.

Anaesthetic
General anaesthetic with single lumen endotracheal intubation.

Preoperative preparation
Results of lung function tests, chest radiograph, ECG, and CT scan must be available.

Position
- Supine
- A pillow is placed under the shoulder on the side of the operation.

Incision
- Make a small anterolateral thoracotomy (10cm) in the 5th intercostal space.

Procedure
- After the chest has been opened, divide any pleural adhesions.
- Hold the edge of the lung with a Duval forceps and resect a wedge of lung using several applications of the Endo GIA 30 stapling device.
- Remove the specimen.
- Inspect the staple line for any air or blood leak. If present, suture these with 4/0 Prolene.
- Introduce an intercostal drain through a separate incision.
- Close the chest wall.
- Connect the intercostal drain to an underwater seal.
- Send the specimens for histopathology and microbiological examination.

Postoperative management
- Return the patient to HDU for monitoring and pain control.
- Attach the intercostal drain to suction (5KPa).
- Perform a chest radiograph as a baseline and at 24 hours.
- Provide analgesia through PCA, epidural or paravertebral block.
- Regular chest physiotherapy.
- Remove the drain after 24 hours, if the chest radiograph shows the lung is fully expanded.

Complications
- Pneumothorax
- Wound infection.

Open excision of pulmonary nodule

Indication
Solitary lung nodule on CXR and CT scan.

Preoperative preparation
Results of lung function tests, chest radiograph, ECG, and CT scan must be available.

Anaesthetic
General anaesthesia with double lumen endobronchial intubation.

Position
Lateral position.

Incision
Posterolateral thoracotomy in the 5th or 6th intercostal space.

Procedure
- Once the chest is opened, divide any pleural adhesions.
- Inspect the lung and palpate for the nodule.
- Grasp the nodule with tissue holding Duval forceps.
- Excise the nodule and surrounding lung as a wedge by applying the stapler (endo GIA 30) several times.
- Observe the staple line for air and blood leaks. If present suture these with a 4/0 Prolene.
- Insert two intercostal drains (24–28Fr., Silastic) through separate stab incisions. Direct the anterior drain to the apex of the pleural space and the posterior one to the base of the pleural space.
- Close the chest in layers as previously described.

Postoperative care
- Return the patient to HDU for monitoring and pain control.
- Attach the intercostal drain to suction (5KPa).
- Perform a chest radiograph as a baseline and at 24 hours.
- Regular chest physiotherapy.
- Provide analgesia by PCA, epidural or paravertebral block.
- Remove the drain after 24 hours, if the chest radiograph shows the lung fully expanded.

Complications
- Pneumothorax
- Wound infection.

Excision of mediastinal mass

Indications
Any anterior mediastinal mass e.g. thymoma, retrosternal thyroid, pericardial cyst, and germ cell tumours.

Position
Supine.

Anaesthetic
General anaesthesia with endotracheal intubation.

Incision
Vertical midline from the sternal notch to the xiphisternum.

Procedure
- Perform median sternotomy (see p710).
- Visualise and palpate the tumour or lesion and excise with care. Cauterise any arteries or veins supplying the tumour with diathermy or ligate them. Seek, identify, and ligate the thymic vein.
- In cases suffering from myasthenia gravis the whole thymic gland needs to be removed. This is an 'H' shaped structure and extends upwards into the neck as well as downwards to the phrenic nerves on either side of the pericardium. *Take great care* when the lower part of the thymus is being removed to avoid damage to the phrenic nerves.
- Secure haemostasis and introduce a single drain (24–28Fr, Silastic) into the mediastinum through a separate stab incision below the sternotomy.
- If the pleural space has been entered, direct either one of the mediastinal drains into the pleural space or insert a third drain.
- Suture the drain in place with a heavy non-absorbable suture. Insert a closing stitch.
- Appose the sternal halves using 6 stainless steel wires, taking care to ensure that there is no bony step.
- Twist the wires until the sternal edges are firmly approximated. Then cut the wires using wire cutters and bend so that the cut ends point into the sternum.
- Close the subcutaneous tissues using continuous absorbable sutures e.g. Vicryl.
- Close the skin using subcuticular continuous absorbable sutures e.g. Monocryl.
- Connect the drain to a bottle with an underwater and suction commenced (5KPa).
- Reverse the anaesthetic and once the patient is breathing spontaneously, transfer to the HDU.

Postoperative care
- Perform a baseline chest radiograph and repeated at 24 hours
- Provide analgesia through PCA, epidural or paravertebral block
- Regular chest physiotherapy

- Remove the chest drain at 24 hours if the chest radiograph appearances are satisfactory and drainage of blood and air has ceased.

Complications

- Complications of general anaesthesia
- Bleeding—this can occur following damage to the internal mammary artery when the sternal wires are placed
- Instability of the sternum
- Wound infection
- Dehiscence of wound
- Osteomyelitis (rare).

Thoracic neurogenic tumours

These usually lie in the paravertebral region at any level in the chest and are usually incidental radiological findings. They should be removed because:

1. They can grow into the intraveterbral foramen and cause spinal cord compression.
2. Sometimes they develop sarcomatous changes.

Preoperative preparation

- A CT scan or MRI scan study is essential to visualise any intra spinal extension.
- Neurosurgical input is essential if the tumour encroaches the spinal canal.
- The patient should be warned of the risk of damage to the sympathetic trunk which may result in postoperative Horner's Syndrome.

Position

Lateral.

Anaesthetic

General anaesthesia with double lumen endobronchial intubation.

Incision

Posterolateral thoracotomy in the 4th intercostal space.

Procedure

- Open the chest and deflate the lung and retract it. Incise the parietal pleural around the margins of the tumour using diathermy.
- Mobilize the tumour gradually placing traction sutures in the tumour tissue to assist the process.
- Cauterise and divide numerous blood vessels supplying the tumour.
- If the tumour rises from the sympathetic chain, the chain may be damaged during mobilisation.
- Carry out the resection all the way round until the tumour is on a stalk attached to the intravertebral foramen from which it is eased away with care. Ligate any veins.
- Use a pack to control any bleeding. Do not use diathermy because of proximity of the spinal cord.
- Close the chest as previously described.

Postoperative management

As for thoracotomy (see p712).

Complications

- Horner's syndrome
- Bleeding
- Complications related to general anaesthesia.

Pectus excavatum repair

Characterised by a deep depression of the lower half of the sternum.

Indication

Surgical treatment in most cases is for cosmetic reasons.

Preoperative preparation

The patient should be warned that one defect (pectus excavatum) will be replaced by another (a scar).

Anaesthetic

General anaesthetic with endotracheal intubation.

Position

Supine.

Incision

Make a vertical midline incision from the manubriosternal junction to 5cm below the xiphoid process.

Procedure

- Divide the skin and subcutaneous tissues in line of the incision.
- Raise a full thickness flap of skin subcutaneous tissue and pectoral muscles on either side to expose the relevant costal cartilages and ribs.
- Remove the deformed costal cartilages on both sides, preserving the perichondrium using a periosteal elevator.
- Then perform two parallel transverse sternal osteotomies using a powered saw. This is V-shaped in cross section with the broad part placed anteriorly so that elevation of the sternum results in correction of the deformity.
- Secure the sternum in its new position using two stainless steel wires passed through the two bits of sternum, which are twisted and tightened.
- Elevation of the lower sternum is made possible by inserting an Abrams bar of stainless steel under the lower sternum, which is attached on either end to the anterior end of the 4th or 5th ribs.
- Insert 2 Redivac vacuum drains.
- Close the muscle flaps using absorbable sutures.
- Close the subcutaneous tissues and skin using absorbable sutures.

Postoperative management

- Nurse the patient on HDU.
- Obtain a baseline chest radiograph.
- Provide analgesia through PCA epidural or paravertebral block.
- Regular chest physiotherapy.
- Repeat the chest radiograph at 24 hours, and if appearances are satisfactory and there is no further drainage of air or fluid, remove the drains.
- Remove the Abram's bar after six months under local anaesthesia via a 1cm skin incision.

Complications
- Bleeding—from intercostal or internal mammary artery
- Pneumothorax
- Wound infection
- Scar (hypertrophic or keloid).

Pectus carinatum repair

This deformity is characterised by prominence of the lower sternum or costal cartilages.

Indication
Cosmetic.

Anaesthestic
General anaesthesia with endotracheal intubation.

Position
Supine.

Incision
Make a vertical midline incision from the manubriosternal junction to 5cm below the xiphoid process.

Procedure
- Divide the skin and subcutaneous tissues in the line of the incision.
- Reflect the skin, subcutaneous tissues and pectoral muscles off the costal cartilages as a full thickness flap.
- Resect all the affected costal cartilages on both sides of the sternum leaving behind the perichondrium (from where new cartilage develops).
- Perform two parallel transverse sternal osteotomies close together using a power saw so that a wedge of sternum which is V-shaped on cross section is removed. The apex of the V lies anteriorly, so that the sternum moves inwards when the two edges are approximated.
- Fix the two parts of the sternum together with two stainless steel wires. These are tightened with the sternum in its new position.
- Secure haemostasis using diathermy.
- Insert two Redivac vacuum drains.
- Close the muscles, subcutaneous tissue and skin layers using absorbable sutures.

Postoperative management
As for pectus excavatum (p744).

Complications
As for pectus excavatum (p745).

Rib resection for empyema

Indications
- When decortication is contraindicated by a patient's age or debilitated state
- The presence of bronchopleural fistula or oesophagopleural fistula.

Anaesthetic
General anaesthesia with double lumen endobronchial intubation.

Position
Lateral position.

Procedure
- Look for the rib level at the most dependent part of the empyema cavity. This is identified on a PA and lateral chest X-ray after contrast material has been injected into the empyema cavity.
- Make a transverse incision (approx. 10cm) over the chosen rib. Divide the subcutaneous tissues and muscles along the incision and expose the rib. Elevate the periosteum using a periosteal elevator and excise a segment of rib (approx. 8cm).
- Aspirate through the periosteal bed to confirm the presence of pus.
- Send a pus specimen to microbiology for microscopy, culture and sensitivity.
- Enter the empyema cavity and remove the outer wall using diathermy. Ligate the intercostal vessels on either side in order to prevent later damage and haemorrhage by erosion from the intercostal drainage tube.
- Clean and wash out the empyema cavity.
- Insert a large bore Silastic drainage tube through the incision about 5cm into the pleural cavity. Then cut the tube short so that approximately 2cm project from the skin edge, and pierce its outer end with a large safety pin and secure it to the skin with adhesive strips.
- Leave the wound open, as it heals rapidly.
- Apply a dry dressing over the wound and drain. This can later be converted to a stoma bag.

Postoperative management
- Transfer the patient to the HDU.
- Obtain a PA and lateral chest radiographs to ensure that the chest drain is correctly sited.
- Change the drain dressings/stoma bag daily. When the drainage of pus ceases the drain is gradually shortened and eventually removed. This may take a few months.

Complications
- Complications of general anaesthesia
- Haemorrhage.

Decortication for empyema

Indication
- Chronic empyema
- Organised and unresolved haemothorax.

Contraindications
- In very elderly and debilitated patients.
- In the presence of severe systemic sepsis.

Preoperative investigations
- Chest radiograph—PA and lateral
- CT scan
- Needle aspiration of fluid for microscopy, culture, and sensitivity
- Rigid bronchoscopy.

Anaesthetic
General anaesthesia with double lumen endobronchial intubation.

Position
Lateral.

Incision
Perform a posterolateral thoracotomy in the 5th intercostal space when the empyema is near the apex, or in the 6th or 7th intercostal space when the empyema extends to the diaphragm.

Procedure
- Enter the chest and spread the ribs. In chronic empyema if the ribs are crowded it may be necessary to resect the rib to obtain access.
- Separate the outer wall of the empyema cavity from the chest wall as far as possible, using blunt and sharp dissection.
- Incise the outer cortex and enter the empyema cavity.
- Aspirate the pus and fibrin residue within the cavity and following this wash out the sac with sterile water.
- Dissect the outer wall of the abscess cavity further and remove by sharp dissection.
- Incise the cortex on the collapsed lung through the layers of the sac using a scalpel with great care.
- Develop a plane between the lung tissue and the cortex of the empyema sac.
- Then 'peel' the cortex off the collapsed lung tissue taking care to preserve the integrity of the visceral pleural surface of the lung as far as possible. Inevitably the superficial layers of the lung will be damaged in this process.
- Remove as much of the empyema sac cortex as possible.
- Score the bits of cortex, which are very adherent to the lung with a scalpel in a crosshatch pattern. The lung is simultaneously forcibly expanded by the anaesthetist so that the lung tissue expands through the incision.

- When maximum expansion of the lung is obtained there will be both air and blood leakage present.
- Obtain haemostasis with diathermy cautery. Use a dental mirror to visualise bleeding points on the lateral chest wall.
- Insert two intercostal drains (24–28Fr., Silastic), one anteriorly and one posteriorly. The anterior drains to the apex of the chest and the posterior drains to the base of the chest. Secure these to the skin with stout non-absorbable sutures. The air and blood leakage should settle over the next day or two.
- Connect the drains to suction (7–13KPa) in order to maintain lung expansion.
- Close the chest in layers as previously described.
- Send specimens of the contents of the empyema cavity and the wall of the empyema cavity to microbiology for microscopy, culture and sensitivity, and to histopathology.

Postoperative management

- Transfer the patient to the HDU.
- Daily chest radiographs.
- Continue suction on the drains until the lung is fully expanded and all air leaks have ceased, at which stage the chest drains are removed. This may take several days.
- Regular chest physiotherapy.
- Provide analgesia through PCA, epidural or paravertebral block.
- Remove the intercostal drains when there is no longer any drainage of fluid or air and chest radiograph appearances are satisfactory.

Complications

- Complications of general anaesthesia
- Bleeding
- Haemothorax
  - If severe, patient may need to be returned to theatre for evacuation of blood clots.

Airway stents

Indications
- Extrinsic airway compression e.g. tumours or other structures within the chest
- Intrinsic airway obstruction from benign or malignant diseases
- Sealing of airway fistulas
- Some cases of tracheobronchomalacia.

Contraindications
In addition to the contraindications for rigid or flexible bronchoscopy (see pp694, 696), stent insertion should be avoided if nonviable lung is present beyond the obstruction.

Types of stent
- Numerous types
- Silicone, metal or hybrid
- Insertion devices are specific to the stent.

Procedure
Insert with either flexible or rigid bronchoscope depending on the design of the stent. Radiological screening is sometimes necessary.

Postoperative management
- Humidified oxygen
- Regular chest physiotherapy.

Complications
In addition to the risks of flexible or rigid bronchoscopy (see pp695, 697)
- Migration of stent
- Infection
- Granuloma formation
- Breakage
- Haemoptysis
- Airway obstruction e.g. due to impaction or granulomas
- Pain
- Death.

Video assisted thoracic surgery (VATS)

Key points

- Patient placed in a lateral position.
- Position the patient to open the intercostal spaces as much as possible. This can be achieved by breaking the table at the chest level or placing a pillow between the patient's chest and the operating table.
- Use a triangular port arrangement.
- Avoid instrument 'fencing' (crossing the instruments).
- Create the ports under direct vision and ensure adequate haemostasis as bleeding will obscure the view.
- Using double lumen endobronchial intubation allows deflation of the lung and provides a larger space to work in.
- Divide all intrapleural adhesions before proceeding.
- Monitors should be positioned in front of the operating surgeon.
- Staples and cartridges must be selected according to the type and thickness of tissue to be divided.

Safety points

- Use bipolar diathermy near the heart, oesophagus, and spine.
- Always make sure the cutting instrument or stapler is positioned properly and in full view before dividing tissue.
- Ensure a full thoracotomy set is available in the operating room for immediate conversion to open thoracotomy in the event of severe intraoperative haemorrhage.

Location of ports

First port: 2cm incision in the 6th intercostal space below the tip of the scapula—insert the thoracoscopic camera via flexible port.
Second port: stab incision in the 4th intercostal space anterior to the latissimus dorsi muscle.
Third port: stab incision in the 5th intercostal space at the posterior border of the latissimus dorsi muscle.

Complications

- Bleeding. If uncontrolled, may require conversion to an open procedure.
- Infection of port sites.
- Complications of general anaesthesia.

VAT parietal pleurectomy and bullectomy

Indications
- Non-resolving spontaneous pneumothorax
- Repeated spontaneous pneumothorax on more than two episodes
- First spontaneous pneumothorax in airline pilots.

Anaesthetic
General anaesthesia with double lumen endobronchial intubation.

Position of patient
Lateral.

Procedure
- Insert ports (see p776).
- Deflate the lung.
- Divide pleural adhesions using endoscopic diathermy scissors.
- Examine the apex of the lung and identify bullae. Grasp these with an endoscopic grasper via the second port and stapled across the base using an Endo GIA 30 stapling device inserted through the third port.
- More than one staple application may be necessary.
- Carry out parietal pleurectomy by elevating the pleura with long Roberts forceps, starting at the anterior incision. A sheet of pleura is first rolled onto the forceps and then removed by gentle tracking on the video control.
- Alternatively the pleura may be abraded using a piece of mesh rolled on Roberts forceps.
- Aspirate blood in the pleural cavity. Secure haemostasis using diathermy.
- Insert two chest drains (one apical and one basal) under video vision. Connect the drains to underwater seal bottles, and commence suction (5KPa).
- Inflate the lung.
- Close the chest in layers with absorbable sutures.
- Transfer the patient to the HDU once the anaesthetic has been reversed and breathing spontaneously.

Postoperative care
- Obtain a baseline postoperative chest radiograph to ensure full expansion of the lung
- Perform daily chest radiographs
- Regular chest physiotherapy
- Remove the drains when they stop bubbling (no air leak) and the lung has expanded fully on chest radiograph.

VAT lung wedge biopsy

Indication

This is a diagnostic procedure for interstitial lung disease.

Preoperative preparation

- Chest radiograph
- CT scan
- Respiratory function tests.

Anaesthetic

General anaesthesia with double lumen endobronchial intubation.

Procedures

- Insert ports in a triangular configuration.
- Deflate the lung.
- Introduce the thoracoscope into the middle port (first port).
- Divide all pleural adhesions using the endoscopic diathermy scissors.
- Grasp the portion of lung containing the lung nodule with an endoscopic grasper via the second port.
- Introduce a stapler via the third port and fire several times around the lesion to remove a wedge of lung.
- Inspect the staple lines to make sure they are air and blood tight. If there is a leak, this is sutured with 4/0 Prolene.
- Aspirate blood in the pleural cavity.
- Place two chest drains (one apical and one basal) under video vision. Connect the drains to underwater seal bottles, which are connected to suction (5KPa).
- Inflate the lung.
- Close the chest in layers with absorbable sutures.
- Transfer the patient to the HDU once the anaesthetic has been reversed and breathing spontaneously.

Postoperative care

- Ensure adequate analgesia either by PCA, epidural or intercostal block
- Obtain a baseline postoperative chest radiograph to ensure full expansion of the lung
- Perform daily chest radiographs
- Regular chest physiotherapy
- Remove the drains when they stop bubbling (no air leak) and the lung has expanded fully on chest radiograph.

Principles of plastic surgery

P. Baguley

Introduction

Many branches of surgery have a well-defined anatomical area that they specialise in, whereas plastic surgery is generally a technique based speciality. This means that there are basic principles that can be used to help innumerable operative situations encountered.

The term 'plastique' was first used in 1798 and is derived from the Greek word plastikos, meaning 'fit for moulding'. Until the turn of the twentieth century most procedures were for reconstruction and there is a perceived distinction between aesthetic and reconstructive surgery. Sir Harold Gillies even defined the two: reconstructive surgery is an attempt to restore the individual to normal and aesthetic surgery attempts to surpass the normal. However, it is rare for any procedure not to need at least some degree of aesthetic consideration, so a sense of form and function as well as aesthetic judgement and an ability to conceptualise the final result are all essential to the application of plastic surgery.

As much of the surgery is technique-based then an appreciation of the underlying anatomy, particularly of skin, as well as factors such as healing and what may have caused the problem initially are vital. Following this an understanding of some of the basic principles of surgery must be appreciated. It is only when all factors are considered can a plan of treatment be formulated and a successful result be expected.

Plastic surgery covers an enormous range of procedures in all aspects of the body. However, in this chapter those aspects of plastic surgery, which are mainly applicable to general surgery are presented.

Anatomy of the integument

The integument consists of skin, subcutaneous fat and fascia.

Blood supply (Fig. 17.1)

The blood supply to the integument is divided into a number of transversely arranged plexuses.

- **Subpapillary plexus** At the junction of the papillary and reticular layers of the dermis; loops up to epidermis—papillary loops.
- **Subdermal plexus** At the lower border of the dermis; gives off branches to the subpapillary plexus and down to fat. The blood vessels that pass to the subdermal plexus come from the deep fascia.
- **Subcutaneous plexus** Within the adipose tissue.
- **Fascial plexuses** There are 2 fascial plexuses: *superficial fascial plexus* which is minor and cannot sustain flap and the *deep fascial plexus* which is dominant.

Relaxed skin tension lines

There is natural elasticity to the skin because of the elastin fibres that lie within the dermis. The skin is naturally under tension, as demonstrated by the gaping of an incised wound or the stretching of a healing wound. The degree of tension is greatest in one direction and this is termed the *relaxed skin tension line* (RSTL). An incision placed parallel to these lines is therefore subject to minimal tension and usually results in a better quality scar. Conversely an incision that transgresses these lines will gape widely and when healing is subject to tension that may cause the scar to gape or even develop a hypertrophic scar.

Wrinkle lines may be caused by either the pull of underlying muscles (around the eyes or mouth) or from movements around a joint (neck or wrist). In general these are similar to the RSTL, though may be different such as in the glabellar or the lateral palpebral fissure (crow's feet).

The RSTL can be found easily by pinching the skin between the thumb and index finger. A series of ridges and furrows develops which are made with greater ease and are more extensive when they are parallel to the RSTL.

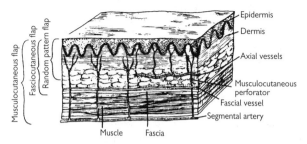

Fig. 17.1 Blood supply to the integument

Normal wound healing

There are 4 distinct but overlapping phases in wound healing (Fig. 17.2):

Haemostasis

- Occurs immediately after an injury
- Following vasoconstriction, platelets adhere to the vessels of the microcirculation leading to the release of cytokines
- The clotting cascade is initiated which leads to the deposition of a fibrin network.

Inflammation

- Polymorphs enter the wound, cleaning it of debris
- Monocytes follow which orchestrate the ingrowth of blood vessels and fibroblasts.

Proliferation

Four main events happen in this phase
- Fibroplasia
- Matrix deposition
- Angiogenesis
- Epithelialisation.

Remodelling

- Collagen is degraded and deposited in a more ordered fashion
- Myofibroblasts cause wound contraction
- Maximal tensile strength occurs by 12 weeks
- Ultimately the scar only has 80% of normal skin strength.

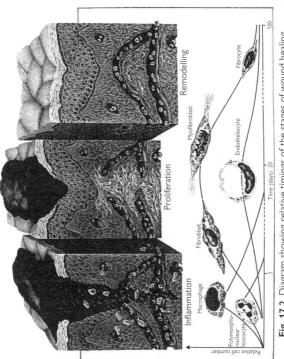

Fig. 17.2 Diagram showing relative timings of the stages of wound healing

Abnormal wound healing

Delayed wound healing develops when there is interference of one of the steps of wound healing. Factors that may be responsible are:

Local factors
- Foreign bodies
- Infection
- Ischaemia
- Arterial or venous insufficiency
- Smoking
- Neoplasia.

Systemic factors
- Nutritional deficiency
- Diabetes
- Ageing
- Liver disease
- Alcoholism
- Medications, particularly steroids and immunosuppessoats
- Immobility
- Cancer
- Anticancer therapy (X-rays).

Techniques to assess wounds
- Inspection
- Bacteriology swab
- Histological biopsy
- Radiological imaging
- Biopsy.

Types of abnormal healing
- Delayed
- Dehiscence
- Stretched scar
- Keloid
- Hypertrophic scar.

Keloids and hypertrophic scars

- Keloids and hypertrophic scars are characterised by excessive accumulation of collagen within the wound. There are abnormalities of cell migration and proliferation, inflammation, and the synthesis and secretion of matrix proteins and cytokines.
- Keloids grow beyond the borders of the original wound, can form some time after a tissue injury and generally do not resolve spontaneously. Hypertrophic scars stay within the limit of the original wound, usually develop soon after the tissue injury and tend to regress spontaneously.
- Histologically they differ from normal skin by having a rich blood supply, high cell density and a thick epidermal layer. Hypertrophic scars have collagen fibres arranged in a loose, wavy pattern. Keloids have irregularly shaped collagen fibres in a disorganized pattern.

Predisposing factors

That certain patients and conditions may predispose to hypertrophic scar formation is well known. Both hypertrophic scars and keloids occur more commonly in dark-skinned individuals. Wounds that cross skin tension lines or wounds that are located on the ear lobes or presternal and deltoid areas are common sites for these forms of abnormal healing. Conservative management includes pharmacologic therapy, pressure, laser, and radiotherapy. Each method has varying degrees of reported success.

- Black, Asian, and Celtic (red hair and freckles) skin.
- Wounds on the anterior chest, shoulders and anterior neck as well as wounds that cross skin tension lines.
- A wound that has healed by secondary intention, especially if the healing time is greater than 3 weeks.
- Wounds with prolonged inflammation (foreign body, infection, burn).

Treatment

No single, universally successful treatment for hypertrophic scars and keloids exists and the recurrence rate is high. Surgical treatment is reserved for cases that are unresponsive to conservative management.

- **Compression** dressings are custom-made for the patient and should be worn 24 hours a day.
- **Corticosteroids** injected directly into the lesion act by diminishing collagen synthesis and decreasing mucinous ground substance.
- **Excision** is most effective when combined with external radiation, steroid injection, ± pressure therapy. There is a high risk of recurrence.
- **Radiation** is most effective when used in the immediate postoperative period.
- **Cryosurgery** with liquid nitrogen is used to cause cell damage and to affect the microvasculature.
- **Laser therapy.**
- **Silicone sheets** sometimes in combination with compression applied over a scar are reported to reduce the bulk.
- **Massage** with aqueous cream may be effective.

Reconstructive ladder

When a plastic surgeon assesses a wound, or a situation in which a wound will result from resection, a basic set of rules guides the formulation of a treatment plan. The least complex methods, such as direct closure, are on the lower rungs whilst there is an increase in complexity to the top.

The size and nature of the injury as well as factors such as the patient's general condition will determine which treatment method is used. In general the least complex method of achieving the desired result is used.

Primary and secondary intention healing

Primary intention (primary closure)

This is where the edges of the wound are in direct contact. This is most appropriate for small and uninfected wounds. Methods of skin closure may be:

- Sutures
- Staples
- Glue (cyanoacrylate)
- Adhesive strips.

Secondary intention

This is where the wound edges are not in contact. Healing takes place by a combination of wound contracture and granulation/epithelisation. Whilst this generally leads to a wider and less attractive scar it may be appropriate in situations such as:

- Infection
- Wound breakdown
- Poorly vascularised areas
- Patient not fit for surgery.

Delayed primary and secondary closure

Can be used when an open wound is clean and free of infection or other underlying pathology.

Skin grafts

If a wound is too large for suturing, and healing by secondary intention or secondary closure is inappropriate, a skin graft may be suitable. A skin graft consists of the epidermis and a variable amount of the dermis. This is placed on the recipient site where it attains a new blood supply and integrates itself into the recipient site. The bed must be suitable for grafting and:

• Be free of friction.
• Have no contamination.
• Have no infection. *Pseudomonas aeruginosa* and group A β haemolytic streptococci are both particularly problematic.
• Have an adequate blood supply. Bare tendon or bone for example are not suitable.

Anatomy (Fig. 17.3)

In all skin grafts the epidermis is taken but the amount of dermis varies. If only part of the dermis is taken it is a *split thickness skin graft*; whereas in a *full thickness skin graft* the whole of the dermis is taken.

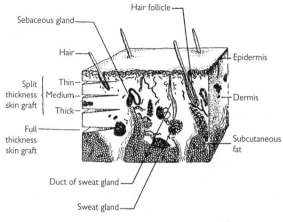

Fig. 17.3 Depth of skin grafts

Split thickness skin graft

This includes the epidermis and only part of the dermis.

Advantages
- Donor site heals by epithelisation from remaining dermal elements such as sweat glands and hair follicles
- Can be re-harvested
- Larger amounts can be harvested
- Can conform to defects as it is thin.

Disadvantages
- Less resilient to trauma
- Less aesthetically acceptable
- Can contract leading to secondary deformities.

Donor site
Virtually any part of the body can be used as a donor, including the scalp. Whilst the area does heal it leaves a scar and so a relatively hidden area is preferable. A variety of dressings have been used (alginate, semi-occlusive or occlusive) but they all aim to protect the healing donor site. It is not necessary to keep checking these sites unless specifically indicated such as the suspicion of infection. Healing takes from seven days to several weeks depending on the thickness.

Harvesting with hand knife
The commonest types of hand-held knife are the Watson or a modification of the Humby knife. There is a wide and sharp blade that has a depth guard running its length—this can be varied to cut to different depths. Holding the knife up to the light allows the depth to be seen and judged by experience; the depth is then locked.

Making the donor as taut as possible is essential, and an assistant to place traction on the skin is invaluable. The blade is then placed on the skin and an even reciprocating motion is used to harvest as it is advanced along the donor site. The angle and pressure used is a matter of preference as a correct balance is needed to harvest skin of the desired thickness.

Harvesting with dermatome (Fig. 17.4)
These may be either electric or air powered. The blade used is narrower than that in a hand knife and the power causes it to vibrate rapidly. There is a depth gauge that is graduated in thousandths of an inch.

Again having skin as taut as possible is helpful. The safety catch is released and the dermatome advanced along the donor site harvesting the skin.

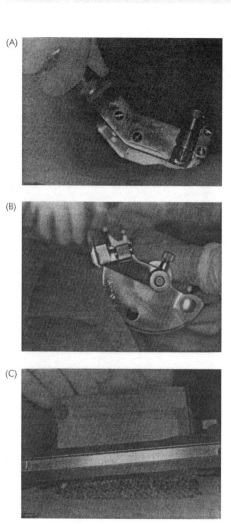

Fig. 17.4 (A–C) Sequence showing how to use a powered dermatome

Meshing

The skin is placed on a carrier board and passed through a hand powered device that cuts even fenestrations in it. The reasons for this are

- **Expansion** is usually 1.5:1 but can be up to 9:1
- **Conforming** allows the graft to fit irregular surfaces better
- **Fenestrations** help prevent collection of blood or serous fluid under
  graft.

Storage

It is possible to store a split thickness skin graft for a few weeks. This may
be useful if too much skin was harvested or the wound was not suitable
for immediate application. In the latter case the skin can be applied on
the ward with no need for further surgery.

Full thickness skin graft

This includes the epidermis and the whole of the dermis.

Advantages
- Better aesthetic appearance
- Less prone to contracture.

Disadvantages
- Less can be harvested
- Donor site has no dermal elements remaining and therefore usually needs suturing to close.

Technique
- A pattern of the defect is taken and then transposed onto the donor site. The graft is then harvested by incising around this pattern and dissecting the skin at the level of the subcutaneous fat. This is made easier by draping the graft over the surgeon's finger.
- If there is some fat remaining on the harvested graft this is then removed by trimming with scissors.
- The donor site is then closed by suturing, it is usually necessary to convert the defect into an ellipse.
- The graft is then sutured onto the recipient around the edges. Occasionally sutures may be placed across the surface attaching it to the bed; this is known as *quilting* and may help reduce shearing or haematoma development. The usual dressing is a *tie-over* which is formed by leaving the ends of the sutures longer than normal and then tied over a piece of gauze or cotton wool. The reason for this is to ensure there is maximal contact of the graft with the bed as well as reducing shearing, haematomas, and seromas. The sutures are then left in place for 5–7 days.

Flaps

Whereas a skin graft needs to acquire a new blood supply from the recipient site a flap takes its blood supply with it. The term flap originated in the sixteenth century from the Dutch word *flappe*, meaning something that hung broad and loose, fastened by one side. To help the understanding of flaps a number of classifications have been used based on the blood supply, contents, donor site, and geometry.

Blood supply

Flaps need an adequate blood supply to survive and the two types in this category are:
- **Random pattern** This is where the supply is only from the various plexuses discussed above and not derived from a recognised artery. Many skin flaps fall into this category. The relative dimensions of the flap are limited by the local blood flow; usually the base is the same length as the flap but in the face the length may be greater.
- **Axial pattern** Here the blood supply is from a recognised artery and as such can be relatively much larger. Some skin and most muscle flaps fall into this category.

Fasciocutaneous

Many skin flaps are random pattern and so a longer flap needs a wider base in order to supply adequate circulation. The ration of width to length may only be 1:1 in the lower limb but much greater, up to 8:1, in the head and neck because of the much greater inherent vascularity of this area. However, if fascia, as well as skin, is incorporated into a flap then the potential length of flap is greatly increased. The reason for this is the excellent blood supply to the fascia from the subfascial plexus. This type of flap is particularly useful in lower limb reconstruction.

Muscle

Because there is much variation in the blood supply to muscles a further classification of this has been formulated (see Table 17.1).

Contents

The following tissue or combinations of them can be used
- Skin   (cutaneous)
- Fascia   (fascio–)
- Muscle   (myo–)
- Bone   (osseo–)
- Visceral

Combinations include fasciocutaneous, myocutaneous, or osseocutaneous.

Donor site

- **Local** Tissue to be transferred is adjacent to the defect
- **Distant** Tissue to be transferred is from an incontiguous site to the defect
- **Pedicled** Transferred whilst the blood supply is still attached
- **Free** The flap is detached from its native blood supply and reattached to the recipient vessels.

Configuration
- Advancement
- Rotation
- Transposition
- Interpolation.

Table 17.1 Classification of muscle flaps

Flap type	Blood supply	Example
Type I	• One vascular pedicle	• Medial gastrocnemius • Lateral gastrocnemius • Tensor fascie lata
Type II	• Dominant vascular pedicles and minor vascular pedicle • Dominant pedicle is sufficient to sustain the flap	• Soleus • Gracilis • Trapezius
Type III	• Two dominant pedicles from separate sources • Muscle usually survives on one of the pedicles or can be split allowing the use of only part of the muscle	• Rectus abdominis • Gluteus maximus
Type IV	• Segmental vascular pedicle • Division of more than two or three of the pedicles usually results in necrosis of part of the muscle	• EHL • FHL • Tibialis anterior
Type V	• One large dominant and several segmental pedicles • Either is sufficient to sustain the muscle	• Latissimus dorsi • Pectoralis major

Types of local skin flap

Advancement flap (Fig. 17.5)

The tissue adjacent to the primary defect is mobilised and stretched to cover the defect. In its simplest form two parallel cuts are made along the sides of a defect and the intervening tissue undermined and advanced. Undermining around the defect minimises tension and promotes better scarring along the incisions. If there is wrinkling at the base of the flap it may be necessary to excise a small amount of tissue (Bürow's triangle).

A variation is the V-Y advancement flap where a triangular piece of skin is mobilised and then advanced to cover the defect. The donor area is then closed as a straight line.

Rotation flap (Fig. 17.6)

This rotates about a pivot point and is semicircular in shape. The steps to creating a flap are:

- Triangulation of defect
- Extend lower limb
- Draw semicircular line from the other edge of the defect to meet the above line
- Incision of the semicircular line
- Undermine the flap and advance it
- To reduce it is important to keep the arc of rotation as large as possible under tension; if this is too great a backcut or excision of Bürow's triangle may be necessary.

Transposition flap (Fig. 17.7)

In this type a flap is transferred laterally to cover the defect. For the basic transposition flap a defect is changed into a triangular shape. A rectangular flap is raised adjacent to the defect and transferred laterally. As the pivot point is at the base of the flap distal to the defect, then it is necessary to make the flap longer than the edge of the defect to allow adequate movement. The donor defect is usually covered with a skin graft.

Limberg flap (Fig. 17.8)

This is a form of transposition flap used to close a rhomboid defect, with no need to skin graft the donor as it can be closed. The markings are very precise and the steps are:

- Convert the defect into a rhomboid with angles of 60° and 120°
- Extend the short axis into an area of loose skin
- The length of this line is equal to the short axis of the defect
- The third limb of the flap is drawn parallel and equal in length to the edge of the defect.
- The flap is undermined and then transposed into the defect.

There are four possible flaps for each defect and which one is chosen depends on the orientation of the relaxed skin tension lines.

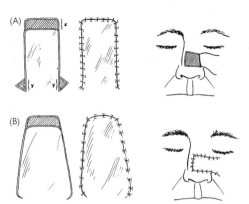

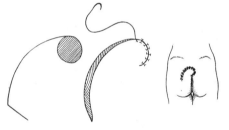

Fig. 17.7 Advancement flap

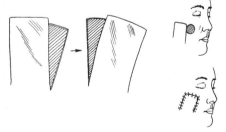

Fig. 17.8 Rotation flap

Fig. 17.9 Transposition flap

Z-plasty flaps (Fig. 17.9)

These are opposed transposition flaps that fill each other's defects. They are used to either lengthen a contracted scar or alter the orientation of a scar. The basic flap consists of central axis, along the line that needs lengthening, and two limbs orientated at 60° to it. All three parts of the flap are of the same length. The flaps are then undermined and transposed.

Whilst the classic Z-plasty has flaps of 60° they can vary from 30° to 90°. The theoretical gain in length of the tissue depends on the angle of the flap as outlined in Table 17.2.

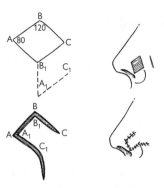

Fig. 17.10 Limberg flap

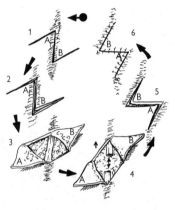

Fig. 17.11 Z-plasty flap

Table 17.2

Angles of Z-plasty	Theoretical gain in length (%)
30°	25
45°	50
60°	75
75°	100
90°	120

Free flaps and microsurgery

Microsurgery may used for both vessels and nerves; either in the trauma setting or for free flap surgery as part of reconstruction. It is time consuming, tiring and requires the utmost attention to detail and surgical technique.

Requirements

- **Magnification** using either a microscope or loupes
- **Microinstruments** consisting of forceps, scissors, needle holder, microvascular clamps, and vessel dilator
- **Microsutures** monofilament ranging from 8/0 to 11/0.

Vascular anastomosis

- **Support** of the arms so that the hand muscles allowed fine movement
- **Vascular clamp** is applied to allow accurate matching of the ends. Different types are available
- **Vessel ends** should be cleanly transected
- **Adventitia** is dissected free from the vessel
- **Intima** should be undamaged and free of clot or atheroma
- **Arterial flow** is checked by releasing the microvascular clamp
- **Anastomosis** may be end-to-end or end-to-side. If there is a discrepancy in diameters one vessel may be cut obliquely to give a better match
- **Suturing** is usually by single interrupted sutures taking care not to pass the needle through the back wall causing a stenosis
- **Patency** is checked after release of the clamps.

Vascular problems

- **No-reflow phenomena** is where there is reperfusion in the distal tissue despite an adequate anastomosis. This is due to capillary occlusion, with platelets and clot, resulting in shunting. The lack of perfusion leads to flap or replantation death.
- **Vasospasm** can be prevented by minimising the handling of vessels and keeping the patient warm and pain free (reduces circulating catecholamines). It can be temporarily reversed by mechanical dilatation with vessel dilators or pharmacological agents (papaverine, verapamil, lignocaine)
- **Thrombosis** at the anastomosis may develop if there has been damage to the intima.

Microneural surgery

This may be necessary to repair divided nerves, for an innervated free flap or if a nerve graft is used (cross facial re-animation of facial palsy). A nerve consists of 3 layers:

- **Endoneurium** is between the axons
- **Perineurium** surrounds fascicles
- **Epineurium** surrounds the nerve.

The types of nerve repair are:
- **Epineural** is the most commonly performed. It may be used for all types of nerve but particularly for smaller ones
- **Perineural (fascicular)** is more challenging and whilst theoretically advantageous this has not been proven
- **Grouped fascicular** is undertaken when specific branches can be identified such as in the median nerve.

Replantation

The decision to replant a severed body partly depends on a number of factors such as co-existing injury, time since injury, likelihood of future functional recovery, type of injury (guillotine better than avulsion) and body part.
- **Arm/digits** replantation is indicated if involving children, thumb, multiple digits, midpalm or more proximal.
- **Leg** replantation is rarely indicated because of the poor functional outcome.
- **Head/neck** scalp avulsions or amputated ears may be replanted as there is excellent vascularity and the late reconstructive options do not give a good aesthetic result.

Postoperative care

- **Access** should be easy to allow monitoring.
- **Dressings** should not compress the pedicle.
- **Visual observations** should be performed regularly noting colour, capillary refill, tissue turgor. A pale flap with poor turgor may indicate an arterial problem whereas a tense, cyanosed flap with brisk refill may indicate a venous problem.
- **Pain** should be minimal to reduce circulating catecholamine—may cause vasospasm and shunting leading to ischaemia and anastomotic problems.
- **Hydration** should be kept high to reduce blood viscosity and therefore the chances of thrombus formation.
- **Heat** either by keeping the room warm, or warming blankets maintains a hyperdynamic state and reduces circulating catecholamines.
- **Monitoring** with temperature probes or Doppler assessment of the anastomosis are useful adjuncts.

Ultimately there is no replacement for regular visual assessment by an experienced observer and senior advice should be sought if there is any doubt. If there are worries concerning the patency of the anastomosis then timely re-exploration in theatre is indicated.

Management plan

Risk factors

A number of factors may lead to an unfavourable result and may influence any plan of treatment.
- Unrealistic expectations
- Poor compliance
- Poor communication
- Child patients
- Surgeon's preconceptions
- Male aesthetic patients
- Psychiatric/psychological pathology.

Intrinsic factors

- **Endocrine disorders** particularly diabetes.
- **Nutrition** may lead to inadequate healing. Consider nutritional supplements or even nasogastric feeding (particularly in burns).
- **Mobility** may be poor and physiotherapy is vital to rehabilitation.
- **Cardiovascular compromise** can cause wounds in the lower leg to heal poorly.

Extrinsic factors

- **Infection** Chronic wounds should have a swab taken preoperatively and antimicrobial therapy (topical antiseptics ± IV/O antibiotics) given if appropriate.
- **Wheelchair etc.** Poorly fitted surgical appliances may be a cause of the problem and will need correcting.
- **Social** Burns in particular may be the first sign of inability to cope at home.
- **Surgical technique** This is a major cause of poor results.

Have a back-up plan

It is imperative that the pros and cons of each surgical option are considered. The reconstructive ladder is essential—formulate a plan and usually the simplest option is the safest. However, the simplest is not necessarily the one that will give the best result. Whatever plan is decided upon it is equally important to have an alternative should the original fail—Sir Harold Gillies described this as a 'lifeboat'.

Consider the donor

Steal from Peter to pay Paul only if Peter can afford it— i.e. tissue from one part of the body is used to reconstruct another only if the resultant donor is acceptable either cosmetically or functionally.

Body units

The body can be divided into units and each has still further subunits. It has been said that the most important aspects of a regional unit are its borders, which are demarcated by creases, margins, angles and hair liners'. It may be best to convert a partial defect of a unit to one that encompasses the whole unit.

Replace like with like

Skin from different parts of the body has different qualities—e.g. compare eyelid skin to palm skin. It is best to use as similar tissue for the reconstruction as was originally in the defect.

Postoperative care

Treatment does not finish with surgery and postoperative care may be more important. This may involve physiotherapy, occupational therapy, psychology and psychiatric help.

Plastic surgical technique

Factors
- **Body region** The sternal and shoulder region are particularly prone to poor quality scars.
- **Anatomical landmarks** Wounds close to landmarks such as the eyebrow or lips will produce a particularly noticeable scar if not sutured meticulously.
- **RSTL** The closer the line of a wound to these the better the cosmetic result.
- **Shape of incision** Curved or U-shaped incisions can cause unsightly scars called trapdoor deformity—the scar contracts causing a curved groove with the central area bulging.
- **Race** Black skin is more likely to develop keloids.
- **Age** Older skin is less elastic and so under less tension which can give a better quality scar.

Incision
The proposed incision is usually marked with ink prior to surgery. The skin is held taut and the incision itself should be perpendicular to the skin edge in the line of the RSTL.

Methods of skin closure
- Sutures
- Staples
- Glue
- Adhesive strips.

Suture material
There are so many types of suture—braided, monofilament, absorbable, non-absorbable that it is impossible to give definitive guidance. Indeed for most situations there are a number of equally acceptable alternatives that the choice is usually dictated by personal preference.

General suture technique
- Ensure that an elective incision runs along a RSTL
- Debride the wound, remove any foreign bodies, and irrigate it
- Ensure the wound edges are not under tension
- Ensure that the wound edges are well apposed (not inverted)
- Ensure that the forces acting on the wound only act in one direction, and minimise distracting forces
- Minimise tissue trauma when suturing
- Suture neatly with a gently everting wound edge
- Avoid materials that cause a bad tissue reaction e.g. silk on the face
- Make sure you immobilise the wound with Steri-strips, tapes, and even thermoplastic splints and plaster casts where necessary.

Simple interrupted suture

- A skin hook placed at either end of the wound can aid in suturing
- The thread should enter the skin at a distance from the wound border equal to the thickness of the skin
- It then passes through the skin slightly obliquely taking a larger bite more deeply (everts skin)
- The knot is tied with sufficient tension to evert the wound
- Enough sutures are used to satisfactorily approximate the wound edges

Mattress sutures

- **Horizontal** These complement the simple suture and help to achieve wound eversion
- **Vertical** Are used when there is extensive undermining or when the surgeon does not want to place deeper sutures. They should not be tied too tightly and may not actually coapt the wound edges in which case they will need to be alternated with simple sutures.

Continuous sutures

The continuous buried suture should leave no suture marks and gives good dermal approximation. However, there is little resistance to stretching, can be time consuming and is more difficult to achieve a satisfactory result.

Suture removal

An incised wound is epithelialised in 3–5 days and the strength of it for most of that time is due to the sutures. Sutures should be removed as soon as it is practicably safe to do so and the timing primarily depends on the anatomical site. In the face sutures should be left no longer than 5 days, in the hand this is usually 10–14 days and in the lower limb or back 14 days. If sutures are left too long and were tied too tight then stitch marks may remain.

Lower limb trauma

Lower limb trauma, particularly when high energy is involved, has a combination of bone and soft tissue injuries. Optimum treatment requires collaboration between plastic and orthopaedic surgeons from the start. The first crucial step is the recognition of a potential problem prior to surgery and to formulate a plan for the first few days after the injury. It is not adequate to realise a problem during or after bony fixation; the first call to a plastic surgeon should not be when the patient is on the way to theatre for bony fixation.

It is generally accepted that by the end of the 5th day all wounds should be covered; the success of microvascular free flaps is diminished after this time. Even if an operation for definitive soft tissue cover will be sometime after bony fixation then it may still be very useful for a plastic surgeon to be involved in the first procedure (or second look at 48 hours); either to advise on debridement or the placement of incisions/fixators so they do not compromise subsequent flap surgery.

History

There are some features that should alert a surgeon to the potential for problems

- Road traffic collisions
- Falls from a height
- Bullet/missile wounds
- Crushing mechanisms.

Examination

- ABC (airway, breathing, circulation)
- Coexisting injuries (cervical spine, pelvis)
- Skin (large wounds, degloving, crushing)
- Compartment syndrome
- Vascular compromise
- Nerve injury
- X-ray (comminution, segmental fractures, air in tissue).

Classification

The classification formulated by Gustillo is the most widely used and useful when discussing an injury.

- **Grade I**
  Low energy
  Skin opening of ≤1cm
  Quite clean
  Mostly from inside to outside
  Minimal muscle contusion
  Simple transverse or oblique fractures
- **Grade II**
  Moderate injury
  Laceration more than >1cm long
  Moderate crushing component
  Simple transverse or oblique fractures with minimal comminution
- **Grade III**
  High energy
  Extensive soft tissue damage including muscle, skin, neurovascular structures
  - IIIA
    Adequate bone coverage
  - IIIB
    Extensive soft tissue injury with periosteal stripping and bone exposure
  - IIIC
    Vascular injury requiring repair

Preoperative management

- **ABC**
- **Wound** Bacteriology swab, tetanus prophylaxis.
- **Antibiotics** Broad spectrum but consider adding penicillin (against clostridia).
- **Plan** An initial one should be made at this stage.

Initial surgical management

- **Skin** extension should be longitudinal (less likely to compromise subsequent flaps). All devitalised tissue must be removed but it may be possible to harvest skin grafts from degloved areas.
- **Muscle** can be difficult to accurately assess as it is very sensitive to trauma. Obviously dead muscle should be removed but a further inspection at 48 hours may be needed.
- **Fasciotomies** must be adequate and decompress all compartments (in lower limb; anterior, peroneal, posterior, and deep).
- **Closure** should not be attempted if there is any suggestion of skin tension—subsequent oedema will only worsen this.

Reconstruction (see Table 17.3)

Using the reconstructive ladder the 3 methods are

- Skin grafting
- Local flaps
- Free flaps.

Skin grafts

These must be applied only if there is a vascularised bed with no infection. If the bed is not vascularised then the next step up the reconstructive ladder is a local flap, either skin (fasciocutaneous) or muscle.

Fasciocutaneous flaps

These may be based on the medial or lateral aspects of the leg and either proximally or distally based.

Muscle flaps
- **Proximal third** Medial or lateral bellies of gastrocnemius.
- **Middle third** Anterior compartment muscles or soleus.

Free flaps

These are very flexible and can be applied to almost any situation. They may be either *muscle*—latissimus dorsi, rectus abdominis, gracilis or *skin*—antero-lateral thigh.

Table 17.3 Summary of treatment options for lower limb trauma

Region of defect	Flap
• Proximal third	• Gastrocnemius • Proximal fasciocutaneous • Free flap
• Middle third	• Soleus • Anterior compartment muscles • Proximal fasciocutaneous • Free flap
• Distal third	• Distally based fasciocutaneous • Free flap
• Ankle	• Distally based fasciocutaneous • Free flap

Neoplasia

Basal cell carcinoma
Basal cell carcinoma (BCC) is the most common skin tumour encountered in practice and is almost entirely, but not exclusively, confined to white caucasian individuals.

Aetiology
- Sun exposure
- Scars
- Irradiation
- Genetic syndromes—Gorlin's syndrome
  - Autosomal dominant (chromosome 9q)
  - Palmar pits
  - Jaw cysts
  - Parafalcine calcification.

Xeroderma pigmentosa
Presentation
- Nodulo-ulcerative
- Cystic
- Morphoeic
- Superficial
- Pigmented.

Treatment
- Curettage
- Cryotherapy
- Radiation
- Surgery
- Conventional
- Moh's microsurgery

Squamous cell cancer
Squamous cell cancer (SCC) is the second most common skin malignancy. Classified into:
- Well differentiated through to poorly differentiated.
- Kerato acanthoma—difficult to differentiate even pathologically and is considered a form of well differentiated SCC. It is self limiting.

Aetiology
- Sun exposure
- Human papilloma virus
- Exogenous carcinogens
  - Tobacco/pipe smoking
  - Petrochemical exposure
  - Radiation
- Genetic syndromes—xeroderma pigmentosa
- Marjolin's ulcer

Treatment
- Surgical excision with adequate margins is the treatment of choice
- Lymph node dissection should be considered in poorly differentiated or large cancers or if clinically enlarged lymph nodes
- Radiation therapy has been advocated in small cancers in anatomically important areas such as eyelids or in cases to control and palliate.

Melanoma

Melanoma is classified by description. Essentially all melanomas present pathologically as the same, but they are described by appearance
- Superficial spreading
- Nodular
- Lentigo maligna
- Acral lentiginous
- Amelanotic and unclassifiable.

Aetiology
- Sunlight
- Genetic
- Pre-existing naevus.

Staging
- Microstaging
  - Breslow—based on depth in millimeters
  - Clarke's level
    - I—within epidermis
    - II—within papillary dermis
    - III—within reticular dermis
    - IV—fills reticular dermis
    - V—into subcutaneous fat
  - AJCC classification 2002

Treatment
- Surgical
- Primary excision
- Margins
  - Less than 1mm Breslow depth—1cm margin
  - Greater than 1mm Breslow depth—2cm margin

Sentinel node

WHO recognise sentinel node as being the standard of care in melanoma greater than 1mm Breslow depth. In the UK it is still not accepted that sentinel node is the accepted standard of care.
Prognosis: lymph node status is the most important factor in assessing prognosis.
The AJCC Classification groups different aspects of melanoma, such as:
- Breslow depth
- Ulceration
- Mitoses per high power field
- Sentinel node positivity
- Number of nodes positive, and gives a prognostic figure.

The risk of recurrence may be stated approximately as:

Breslow 1mm	10% risk of recurrence
Breslow 2mm	20% risk of recurrence
Breslow 3mm	30% risk of recurrence
Breslow 4mm	40 % risk of recurrence
Breslow 5mm or greater	50% risk of recurrence.

Pressure sores

Pressure sores (bedsores and decubitus ulcers) are areas of tissue loss resulting from pressure. These areas are usually, but not exclusively, over bony prominences.

Aetiology
- Intrinsic factors
  - Paraplegia
  - Anaemia
  - Infection
  - Nutrition
  - General medical conditions such as diabetes etc.
- Extrinsic factors
  - Shear
  - Friction
  - Moisture
  - Pressure.

Classification
- Grade I—superficial redness and blistering
- Grade II—Partial thickness loss
- Grade III—Full thickness skin loss
- Grade IV—Deep to and including bone/periosteum.

Treatment
- Systemic
  - Nutrition
  - Correct anaemia
  - Treat infection
- Local
  - Conservative
  - Relief of pressure
  - Dressings
  - Catheterise
- Surgical treatment (Fig. 17.12)
  - Debridement
  - Resection of bony prominences
  - Resurfacing of defect
  - Design large flaps
  - Muscle flaps if necessary

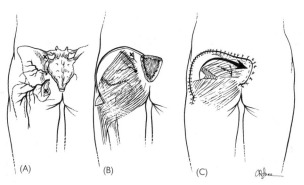

Fig. 17.12 Pressure sores Reproduced with permission from Mccarthy JG (1990) *Plastic surgery*, p3820.© Elsevier

The breasts

Breast cancer reconstruction

It is not in the remit of this chapter to discuss diagnosis and management of breast cancer, rather to focus on post cancer reconstruction. It is important, however, to comment on the approach of a clinician when confronted with a woman (or man) in the out patient setting immediately after diagnosis. The patient should have a frank and open discussion concerning reconstruction before definitive surgical treatment is performed. It should be in a no pressure situation with all the relevant personnel present—patient and partner/family (if she wishes), nurse specialist, surgeon, and oncologist.

It is the opinion of some clinicians that immediate reconstruction should not be offered. It is principally the decision of the patient after she has weighed all options. Immediate, even delayed, reconstruction is not for every woman, but it beholds us all to give as much information prior to surgery.

Reconstruction can be simply divided into expander based reconstruction and autologous tissue transfer. This latter may be divided into pedicled transfers and free tissue transfers.

Tissue expander reconstruction

Insertion of a tissue expander under the skin of the chest wall is a simple and 'one-stop' method of reconstruction. Not without complications, insertion of an expander partially filled with Silicone gel and partially with saline (Becker), this method allows a breast mound to be made with no additional scars elsewhere on the body.

After insertion of the Becker, expansion can be performed immediately on the operating table, or can be performed in out-patients after a period of one to two weeks post op. When the final volume is achieved further expansion should continue up to a point where 25–50% over expansion is achieved, this will allow for contraction post expansion (up to 25%) as well as allow a normal ptosis to develop. Insertion of an expander and then a second operation to insert a permanent silicone prosthesis is an acceptable option.

Contraindications for tissue expansion:

Absolute contraindications
- Do not place expander adjacent to obvious or suspected malignancy
- Do not place in an area of known infection

Relative contraindications
- Poorly vascularised tissue
- Chemotherapy
- Previously irradiated skin
- Psychological problems.

Autologous breast reconstruction

Use of the patient's own tissues, with or without a prosthesis or expander, is increasing in popularity.

Pedicled autologous transfers
- Latissimus dorsi
  - Based on the thoracodorsal artery or branches to serratus, the latissimus dorsi can be transferred with skin as a pedicled flap or a peforator flap with or without a prosthesis.
  - The 'extended' latissimus dorsi flap transfers a larger amount of skin and fat with the muscle thus obviating the need for a prosthesis.
- TRAM
  - Although not as reliable as a free TRAM, the pedicled TRAM is still a viable option for some cases of reconstruction.
  - Transfer should ideally be as a delayed flap when the deep inferior epigastric pedicle is ligated one week prior to the flap being raised and transferred on its superior epigastric pedicle.

Free tissue transfer
- TRAM—pedicle: deep inferior epigastric
- DIEP—deep inferior epigastric perforator
- SGAP—superior gluteal artery perforator flap
- TDAP—thoraco-dorsal artery perforator flap.

Aesthetic

Augmentation

Breast augmentation is the procedure where the breast is enlarged using autologous or alloplastic material. Prostheses may be saline filled or Silicone gel filled although the most common way is still using Silicone gel prostheses.

Incisions
- Inframammary
- Periareola
- Axillary.

Position of implant can be subglandular or subpectoral.

Complications (most common)
- Infection
- Bleeding
- Asymmetry
- Nipple sensory change
- Capsular contracture.

Reduction

Breast reduction is for women with gigantomastia. Essentially for women with cupsize DD or larger with associated symptoms of shoulder notching from the bra, painful neck, rashes under the breasts, and occasionally brachial plexus traction symptoms in the upper limb. It has been shown that if the BMI is >30, complications post operatively are higher.

There are a variety of techniques for reduction:
- Inferior pedicle
- Superolateral pedicle
- Superomedial pedicle.

There are an equal number of varieties of skin incisions:
- Inverted 'T'
- Single vertical scar
- Single horizontal scar
- Regnault 'B'

Complications (most common)
- Asymmetry
- Bleeding
- Infection
- Scarring
- Nipple sensory loss/hyperaesthesia
- Nipple necrosis.

Mastopexy

If the patient has ptosis of the breast but does not wish augmentation, or if skin tightening is required along with augmentation, the skin can be tightened around the breast volume. Common incisions use breast reduction techniques without removal of breast volume.

Burns

Children and persons over 75 years of age are more susceptible to burns of all kinds.

Burns can be classified into:
- Thermal
- Chemical
- Electrical
- Radiation.

Causes
- Flammable liquids
- Space heaters
- Electrical
- Outside fires
- House fires
- Self-inflicted.

Burn prevention
A strategy for burn prevention should include:
- Adequate and reliable data collection
- Recognition of a particular mechanism of injury on which preventative action can be focused
- Devising means of prevention
- Implementing these measures
- Assessing the effects
- Making improvements to the device or to its application as necessary.

Depth of burn injury
First aid
Remove the patient from the immediate vicinity and danger, but it is important to not endanger the rescuer.

Exposure
1. Stop burning process.
2. Cool area with water/wet dressings for 20min, but do not make patient hypothermic (patient may be in an external environment). It is important to realise that normal homeostatic mechanisms for temperature regulation are deranged by burns.
3. Remove clothing from affected area but *do not* peel off clothing stuck to the skin.
4. Cover wound 'Cling film' type of dressing is the best.
5. Antibiotics
   a. Antibiotics have no place in the management of burn injury unless there is microbiological proof of invasive infection.
   b. Scald injuries in children are susceptible to infection by streptococcus sp. There is a belief that children's scald injuries should be treated prophylactically with penicillin (or erythromycin for penicillin allergy).

Table 17.4 Classification and clinical appearance of thermal injury of different depth

Depth of burn		Usual history	Appearance	Blister formation	Sensation	Results
Superficial		Sunburn	Red, bloated	Absent	Painful	Heals in 7 days
Partial thickness	Superficial dermal	Scalds of limited duration	Red or pink with a capillary return	Present	Painful	Heals in 14 days
	Deep dermal	Scalds of long duration Contact with high temperature	Red without capillary return	Absent Wet or waxy surface	Painless	Heals in months
Full thickness		Contact with high temperatue Chemicals Electrical injury	Charred black-brown or white, dry, thrombosed vessels	Absent	Painless	Granulates

Assessment of area of burn and possible inhalation injury

1. History
   a. Explosion in confined space.
   b. Smoke inhalation.
   c. Consider electrical injury entry and exit wound as well as cardiac involvement.
   d. Chemical injury—acid/alkali.
   e. Burn may be secondary to:
      i. Stroke.
      ii. MI.
      iii. Seizure.
      iv. Non-accidental injury (child abuse).
2. Assess area of burn
   a. Wallace's rule of nines. (Fig. 17.13)
   b. Lund and Browder Chart for estimating the size of a burn as a percentage of body surface area (see Fig.17.14).

Airway and breathing

1. Smoke inhalation
   a. Confined space
   b. Confusion, agitation
   c. Burns to face
   d. Singeing of eyebrows or nasal hair
   e. Soot in the sputum
   f. Burning within the mouth
   g. Hoarseness or stridor.

Circulation

1. Burns involving >15% TBSA will require circulatory support—set up two large bore intravenous cannulas.
2. Choice of fluids—in the A&E department the choice of fluid is secondary to the need for urgent and adequate fluid replacement. Any fluid is adequate so long as it contains sodium in a concentration between 130 and 150mmol/l.
3. Fluid resuscitation
   a. Oral fluids
      i. <10% TBSA in children or <15% TBSA in adults
1. Dioralyte or Dextrolyte
2. Moyer's solution
   a. 4g NaCl/L and 1.5g NaHCO$_3$.
   b. intravenouis fluids
      i. Crystalloid
         a. 4ml/kg/% burn TBSA
         b. 50% in first 8 hours
         c. 25% in next 8 hours
         d. 25% in next 8 hours
         e. Routine daily maintenance fluids need to be added to the regime.
      ii. Colloid
         a. Muir and Barclay—First 36 hours divided into 4, 4, 4, 6, 6, 12 hour periods. Formula for replacement of fluid in each period. total % area of burn × weight (kg).

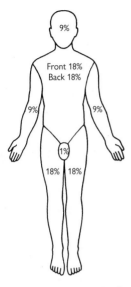

Fig. 17.13 Wallace's rule of nines

Burns surgery

Early surgery

1. Immediate—escharotomies.
2. Early excision and grafting.
   a. Tangential excision.
   b. Mesh grafts.
   c. Consider fascial excision.

Late surgery

1. Functional—scar excision and release.
   a. Skin grafting.
      i. split thickness.
      ii. full thickness.
   b. Z-plasties.
   c. Flaps.
      i. Local.
      ii. Free flaps.
2. Cosmetic.
   a. Facial surgery.
      i. nose.
      ii. eyelids.
      iii. lips.
   b. Trunk—breast reconstruction.

CHART FOR ESTIMATING SEVERITY OF BURN WOUND

NAME_____WARD_____NUMBER_____DATE____
AGE_____ADMISSION WEIGHT_____

LUND AND BROWDER CHARTS

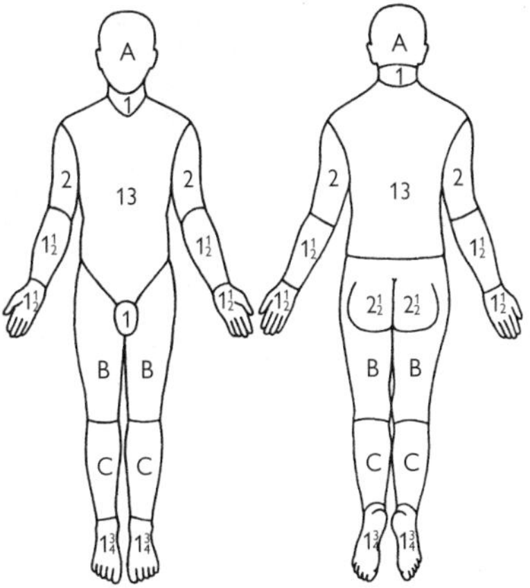

IGNORE
SIMPLE ERYTHEMA

Partial thickness loss (PTL)
Full thickness loss (FTL)

REGION	%	
	PTL	FTL
HEAD		
NECK		
ANT.TRUNK		
POST.TRUNK		
RIGHT ARM		
LEFT ARM		
BUTTOCKS		
GENITALIA		
RIGHT LEG		
LEFT LEG		
TOTAL BURN		

RELATIVE PERCENTAGE OF BODY SURFACE AREA
AFFECTED BY GROWTH

AREA	AGE 0	1	5	10	15	ADULT
A = ½ OF HEAD	9½	8½	6½	5½	4½	3½
B = ½ OF ONE THIGH	2¾	3¼	4	4½	4½	4¾
C = ½ OF ONE LEG	2½	2½	2¾	3	3¼	3½

Fig. 17.14 Lund and Browder chart

Trauma surgery

D. Southward and T. Friesem

Introduction

There are very few surgical procedures that are required in the acute resuscitative phase of trauma management. The priority in trauma management follows the ATLS© format of Airway, Breathing, Circulation. The procedures that may be required in trauma are outlined in that priority.

Surgical airway procedures
- Needle cricothyroidotomy
- Surgical cricothyroidotomy.

Procedures for breathing problems
- Needle thoracocentesis
- Intercostal drain insertion.

Circulatory procedures
- Venous cutdown
- Diagnostic peritoneal lavage.

Needle cricothyroidotomy

This technique is an emergency technique to oxygenate a patient. It does not provide 'ventilation' and is time-limited due to accumulation of carbon dioxide.

Indication

- Inability to intubate
- Airway burns
- Facial trauma
- Laryngeal fracture
- Emergency need for oxygenation, where non-surgical airway manoeuvres have failed or are not available.

Contraindications

Use with caution if complete airway obstruction is present. Reduce flow rates if there is complete obstruction.

Position

Supine. Neck maintained in neutral position with manual in-line immobilisation.

Equipment

- 14 gauge cannula (16–18 in children)
- 10ml syringe
- Oxygen tubing either connected to a three way tap or with a hole cut in the side of the tubing
- Oxygen supply with high pressure flow
- Cannula dressing.

Preparation

- Clean skin of neck with appropriate antiseptic
- Ensure all equipment available and connects together.

Anaesthetic

This is a procedure on a patient in extremis. Anaesthetic is not usually required.

Procedure

- Identify the cricothyroid membrane; find the thyroid cartilage and palpate in a caudal direction. The next rigid structure is the cricoid cartilage. The crico-thyroid membrane is between the two cartilages (Fig. 18.1).
- Stabilise the trachea with thumb and index finger of one hand.
- Attach a 14 gauge cannula to a 10ml syringe.
- Puncture skin with the cannula in a central position directly over the cricothyroid membrane.
- Direct the needle caudally at 45° while aspirating on the syringe.
- Puncture the crico-thyroid membrane, at this point air will be aspirated as the needle enters the trachea.

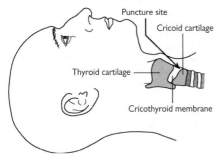

Fig. 18.1 Needle cricothyroidotomy

- While stabilising the needle, advance the catheter, then remove the needle. Respirate to ensure that the catheter has not been advanced against the posterior tracheal wall.
- Attach the oxygen tubing over the luer lock of the catheter.
- Occlude the aperture in the tubing (or three way tap) for one second and release for 4 seconds whilst observing for lung inflation. Exhalation occurs passively during the four seconds off.
- Secure the cannula in place with dressing or sutures.

Complications

- Inadequate ventilation leading to hypoxia
- Hypercarbia due to prolonged use of this technique
- Aspiration of blood
- Damage to posterior structures—posterior tracheal wall, oesophagus
- Subcutaneous emphysema
- Barotrauma to lung from high pressure insufflation. Be watchful to ensure the chest wall falls between inflations, if not you must reduce the flow rate to allow the chest to 'exhale' before the next insufflation.

Surgical cricothyroidotomy

This is an emergency technique to provide a definitive airway. It allows oxygenation, ventilation, and airway toilet to be performed. It is the surgical airway of choice in trauma because it is easier, quicker, and has less risks of bleeding than a tracheostomy. It is also more convenient in a patient immobilised in a semi-rigid collar. *Percutaneous tracheostomy* is not an acceptable alternative, as the neck needs to be hyperextended to perform this procedure.

Indication
- Inability to intubate and definitive airway required
- Airway burns
- Facial trauma
- Laryngeal fracture.

Contraindications
Children under the age of 12 years.

Position
Supine. Neck maintained in neutral with manual in-line immobilisation.

Equipment
- Scalpel with number 10 blade
- Skin cleansing fluid
- Working suction equipment
- Tracheal dilator (or artery forceps)
- 5.0, 6.0 tracheostomy tube
- 10ml syringe
- Endotracheal tube catheter mount
- Fittings to ventilate and deliver oxygen.

Preparation
- Clean skin of neck with appropriate antiseptic solution.
- Ensure all equipment available and connects together.
- Apply manual in-line immobilisation and remove collar, sandbags and tape.

Anaesthetic
If there is time and the patient is conscious local anaesthetic using lignocaine with adrenaline should be used. Local infiltration of the skin and subcutaneous tissues should be performed.

If the situation requires immediate action in an unconscious patient no anaesthetic should be used. Remember needle cricothyroidotomy may be used as an interim measure to buy time while preparing for this procedure.

Procedure
- Stabilise the thyroid cartilage with the left hand.
- Maintain stabilisation of the trachea until the airway is established.

- Make a 1cm skin incision transversely over the crico-thyroid membrane.
- Deepen your incision down through the membrane.
- Insert the scalpel handle into the incision and rotate 90° to open the cricothyroidotomy.
- Intubate the trachea with a cuffed tracheostomy tube (or endotracheal tube if no tracheostomy tube available).
- Inflate the cuff, attach the tube to oxygen and a ventilating device, and ventilate the patient.
- Check for correct placement; check chest movements are symmetrical, listen for breath sounds and verify using capnograph if available.
- Secure the tube with tapes.

You may now reapply the semi-rigid collar, sandbags and tape.

Complications
Immediate
- Aspiration of blood
- Malposition. Creation of a false passage into the tissues. Damage to posterior structures—posterior tracheal wall
- Laceration of trachea or oesophagus
- Haemorrhage or haematoma formation
- Subcutaneous emphysema
- Mediastinal emphysema.

Delayed
- Local infection
- Subglottic stenosis
- Laryngeal stenosis
- Vocal cord injury.

Needle thoracocentesis

Once the primary survey has been completed for Airway and interventions performed as required the primary survey continues with 'Breathing' and the management of respiratory disorders. Most patients can be managed without the need for surgical intervention. However in the primary survey needle thoracocentesis and/or intercostal drain insertion may be required for a patient in respiratory distress.

Following the primary survey most chest injuries are managed without the need for thoracotomy and can be managed conservatively or with the insertion of an intercostal drain.

Needle thoracocentesis, is an emergency technique to decompress a clinically suspected tension pneumothorax as a resuscitative procedure prior to chest drain insertion. High flow oxygen should be administered concurrently via an oxygen mask with reservoir bag.

Indication
Suspected tension pneumothorax.

Position
Supine. If not cleared the neck should be maintained in neutral with collar, sandbags and tape (or equivalent) or manual in-line immobilisation.

Equipment
- 14 gauge cannula
- 10ml syringe
- Cannula dressing.

Anaesthetic
Anaesthetic is not usually required.

Procedure
- Identify the appropriate side of the tension pneumothorax—side away from tracheal deviation, hyper-resonant, absent breath sounds.
- Identify the 2nd intercostal space in the mid-clavicular line.
- Clean skin with appropriate antiseptic (e.g. steret).
- Insert the needle at right angles to the chest wall through the chest wall. Pass the needle just superior to the upper border of the 3rd rib.
- Remove the hub from the cannula and listen for a hiss of air escaping under pressure from the tension pneumothorax.
- Remove the needle and advance the cannula to its hilt.
- Secure the cannula in place with dressing or sutures.
- Prepare for chest drain insertion.

Complications
- Local haematoma
- If there is no tension pneumothorax; creation of pneumothorax
- Direct lung injury.

Intercostal drain insertion

Indication

- As part of primary survey intervention in immediately life threatening chest conditions
- Tension pneumothorax
- Open pneumothorax
- Massive haemothorax
- Flail chest
- As part of ongoing treatment for other chest injury
- Haemothorax
- Pneumothorax
- Suspected severe lung injury and requiring transfer or general anaesthetic.

Position

- Supine. If not cleared the neck should be maintained in neutral with collar, sandbags and tape (or equivalent) or manual in-line immobilisation.
- Arm abducted with hand behind head.

Equipment

- Large intercostal drain with trocar removed
- Underwater seal and tubing or Heimlich valve
- Local anaesthetic
- Needles and syringe for administration of local anaesthetic
- Size 10 scalpel
- Large artery forceps
- Suture material—heavy guage non-absorbable suture (Nylon)
- Gauze dressing pads
- Adhesive dressing to secure drain and dressing
- Appropriate antiseptic solution for skin cleansing.

Preparation

- Clean skin of chest
- Ensure all equipment available and connects together
- Fill drain bottle to fill line.

Anaesthetic

Local infiltration of lignocaine in conscious patients. Anaesthetic to skin and subcutaneous tissue, including periosteum and pleura. Anaesthetised patients do not require local anaesthetics.

Procedure

- Position the patient.
- Identify the 5th intercostal space anterior to the mid-axillary line.
- Local infiltration with lignocaine, infiltrate the skin and deep to the 6th rib. Infiltrate around the rib and into the 5th space. Infiltrate the pleura.
- Clean area with appropriate skin prep.
- Make 2–3cm skin incision parallel to ribs in 5th intercostal space.

- Dissect down to pleura using blunt dissection with artery forceps.
- Puncture pleura with artery forceps and enlarge the opening by spreading forceps within wound.
- Explore the wound with finger and pass it through the pleura into the chest cavity. Check for any adhesions or abdominal contents within the cavity.
- Guide the drain using the artery forceps to avoid any structures within the thoracic cavity.
- Attach to underwater drain or Heimlich valve.
- Secure in place using horizontal mattress suture and drain sutures.
- Apply dressing and secure drainage tube.
- Check tube position with a chest X-ray.
- Reassess the patient.

Complications

- Malposition of tube—extra-thoracic, drain in thoracic cavity but drainage hole extra-thoracic
- Local infection
- Blockage of drain
- Subcutaneous emphysema
- Infection; wound, empyema
- Blockage of drain; kinking of tubing, clogging with solid debris, clotted blood, inappropriate clamping
- Damage to intra-thoracic or abdominal viscera
- Damage to neuro-vascular bundle under 5th rib.

Venous cutdown

This technique is a surgical emergency technique to establish venous access when peripheral access is unobtainable. Any superficial vein can be used; the most common choices are the long saphenous vein at the ankle and the basilic vein in the ante-cubital fossa. This section will describe the procedure for the long saphenous vein.

Indication
Venous access when peripheral route not available.

Contraindications
- Previous harvesting of long saphenous vein for arterial bypass procedure.
- Trauma to limb proximal to vein.

Position
Supine. If not cleared the neck should be maintained in neutral with collar, sandbags and tape (or equivalent) or manual in-line immobilisation. Leg rotated laterally.

Equipment
- Lignocaine
- Syringe and needles for administration of local anaesthetic
- 14 gauge cannula
- IV fluids with giving set
- Sutures.

Preparation
Clean skin with appropriate antiseptic.

Anaesthetic
Local infiltration with lignocaine.

Procedure
- Identify the anatomical landmarks for the long saphenous vein.
- 2cm proximal and posterior to medial malleolus
- Infiltrate with local anaesthetic
- 2cm transverse incision at identified site
- Blunt dissection with artery forceps down to vein and behind vein
- Pass two ties behind vein
- Tie one tie as distal as possible and use this to secure vein
- Pass second tie proximally
- Make a small transverse venotomy. Dilate the venotomy with the tip of the artery forceps and pass the cannula into the vein lumen
- Secure the cannula in place using the proximal tie
- Attach IV tubing, close the wound and dress the wound.

Complications
- Damage to vein and/or surrounding structures (especially nerve)
- Extravasation
- Local infection
- Cellulitis
- Thrombo-phlebitis
- Venous thrombosis.

Diagnostic peritoneal lavage

This procedure provides a rapid sensitive assessment for intraperitoneal blood. It should be performed by the surgeon responsible for managing the patient as it prevents accurate further assessment by clinical examination or ultrasound scanning.

Indication

In the haemodynamically abnormal patient:
- Change in level of consciousness (unreliable clinical examination)
- Change in normal sensation (spinal cord injury)
- Injury to neighbouring structures (rib, pelvis).

Patient away from regular clinical assessment for a long time (in theatre for limb/other non-abdominal procedure, or transfer to other provider including X-ray).

If a patient is not stable haemodynamically they should not be transferred to the imaging department.

Contraindications
- Patient requires laparotomy
- Relative contraindications include technical problems such as the possibility of adhesions or an obese patient
- Ultrasound may be considered and will be discussed later.

Position

Supine. If not cleared the neck should be maintained in neutral with collar, sandbags and tape (or equivalent) or manual in-line immobilisation.

Equipment
- Lignocaine with adrenaline
- Syringe and needles for administration of local anaesthetic
- Peritoneal dialysis catheter
- Minor procedures tray including small haemostats, small skin retractors.
- Antiseptic skin preparation fluid.
- 1 litre warmed Hartmann's solution
- IV giving set
- Urinary catheterisation equipment
- NG tube.

Preparation
- Decompress the stomach with oro-gastric tube
- Insert urinary catheter to ensure bladder is empty
- Clean skin. Include whole of abdomen.

Anaesthetic

Local infiltration with lignocaine in the midline over site of procedure.

Procedure

- Identify the operative area—1/3rd distance from umbilicus to symphysis pubis.
- Infiltrate the local anaesthetic.
- Vertical incision through the skin and subcutaneous tissue. This should be a bloodless field down to the linea alba.
- Lift the fascia with the haemostats and incise the peritoneum.
- Insert a peritoneal dialysis catheter into the peritoneum, and advance it down to the pelvis gently.
- Aspirate from the dialysis catheter with a syringe. **If gross blood is aspirated the test is positive.**
- If blood is not aspirated attach the catheter to 1 litre of warmed Hartmann's solution, and instil 10ml/kg into the abdominal cavity, via an IV giving set.
- Gently agitate the abdomen to distribute the fluid instilled.
- Allow the fluid to remain for 5–10min then drain by lowering the IV bag to the floor. Drainage by siphoning. The IV bag should be vented to allow easy flow.
- Analyse the fluid in the pathology laboratory—inform the haematology department that the sample is DPL fluid.
- A positive result is represented by RBC ≥100 000 per mm^3 or WBC ≥500 per mm^3.

Any food or faecal material is also indicative of the need for laparotomy.

NB A negative lavage does not rule out retroperitoneal injury.

Complications

- Haemorrhage from skin or subcutaneous tissues giving a false positive result
- Intestinal injury or other abdominal structures
- Bladder injury
- Wound infection.

A positive DPL is used as an indicator for the need for laparotomy.

If after blood is identified intra-abdominally the decision is made to treat conservatively, then subsequent observation is made more difficult due to the performance of the DPL. If non-operative treatment is to be considered then a senior clinician should consider the investigation to be performed. Abdominal ultrasound can be repeated and is non-invasive. It also allows for recurrent clinical examination to be performed.

DPL, ultrasound, CT, or laparotomy

Haemodynamically, trauma patients may be categorised into three classes:
1. Haemodynamically normal
2. Haemodynamically abnormal BUT stable
3. Haemodynamically abnormal AND unstable

In the first group it is unlikely that surgically significant blood loss has occurred, or that ongoing bleeding is present. This group may be investigated with less urgency and are safe to be transferred to a radiology department for departmental ultrasound or computed tomography.

The third group of patients require surgical intervention to identify the source of bleeding and to arrest further haemorrhage. If the site of bleeding is thought to be abdominal (other sites excluded—thoracic, pelvic, external, long bones) investigation is not indicated and the patient requires laparotomy.

In the second group the patient may have improved with resuscitation but not have normal parameters. If no further haemorrhage occurs they will remain abnormal but stable. These patients require further resuscitation to normalise their condition. It may be that they have a slow bleed and haemodynamic normality is not achievable. There is time to investigate these patients but they should not be transferred to a radiology department for CT. The option is DPL or ultrasound. These are summarised in the table opposite.

Table 18.1 Comparison of DPL and ultrasound in the assessment of abdominal trauma

	DPL	Ultrasound
Operator	• Surgeon	• Operator dependent
Gas shadowing	• Not affected by bowel gas or subcutaneous air	• Obscured by bowel gas and subcutaneous air
Limitations	• Only diagnoses haemoperitoneum or bowel contents from ruptured viscus	• Can pick up some retroperitoneal injuries • Will pick up peritoneal fluid (blood or faecal) but will miss some bowel injuries
Speed	• Readily available in resus	• Readily available in resus
Ongoing monitoring	• Not easily repeatable	• Easily repeatable
Sensitivity and accuracy	• High	• High but variable dependent upon operator

Transplantation

M. El-Sheikh and P. A. Lear

Organ donors

Specific organ criteria
- **Kidney** Age 4–70 years with acceptable renal function.
- **Liver** Age 1 month–55 years, with no known liver disease, viral hepatitis, or intravenous drug use.
- **Heart** Age 1 month–50 years, with no known cardiac disease.
- **Lung** No pulmonary disease or trauma. PaO_2, $PaCO_2$ acceptable on <50% FiO_2.

Living donors
- The number of patients waiting for transplantation increases by over 3% per year. Cadaveric donor numbers have declined over the past decade.
- In an attempt to reduce disparity, utilisation of living donor transplants has increased in recent years, particularly in kidney transplantation.
- Living donors comprise a first degree relative (parent, child, or sibling) or genetically unrelated (spouse or partner). Transplants between genetically unrelated individuals in the UK, are screened by ULTRA, the Unrelated Live Transplant Regulatory Authority.
- Donation requires meticulous work up. All donors must be fit and screened for any unrecognised disease which would prohibit safe donation.

Cadaveric donors
- Cadaveric donors comprise the majority of solid organ donors in the UK—770 (13 per million population) each year. Donor rates vary worldwide (e.g. Spain has 33.7 per million population).
- The UK adopts an 'opting in' policy whereby organ donation is only legally possible with consent from relatives and the Coroner.
- Suitability for donation is dependent upon the organ or tissue being considered and any pre morbid disease.
- All donors undergo blood grouping, tissue typing and assessment of viral status for hepatitis B, C, HIV, and cytomegalovirus. The presence of active extra cranial malignant disease precludes organ donation.
- Most commonly donors are heart beating (brain stem dead).
- Shortage of organ supply has resulted in re-extending the cadaveric donor pool to non-heart beating (NHB) donors.

Management of the heart beating (brain dead) cadaveric donor
- Causes of brain stem death: intra-cranial haemorrhage, trauma, viral/bacterial infection or primary intra-cerebral tumour.
- Diagnosis confirmed by CT and a series of clinical tests, performed by two senior doctors, establish brain stem death (Code of Practice 1983).
- Resuscitation of donors requires early recognition and assiduous support. Brain death causes a variety of scenarios which include hypothermia, coagulopathy, fall in T3 and T4, myocardial depression and diabetes insipidus.

Cardiovascular support

- Aim for mean arterial pressure of 60–70mmHg, central venous pressure ≥12cm H_2O, urine output ≥100ml/hour
- Inotropes are avoided if possible
- Adrenaline may be used for refractory hypotension
- Dopamine may exacerbate any polyuria and cause vaso-constriction; dobutamine may exacerbate hypotension.

Respiratory support

- Meticulous asepsis, especially if lung harvesting is envisaged.
- Oxygen delivery is optimised to achieve a normal $PaCO_2$; high PEEP should be avoided.

Hormone replacement therapy

Hormone replacement may be necessary.

- T3–bolus of 4mcg then infusion of 3mcg/hour.
- Diabetes insipidus–replace urine loss with 5% dextrose and water via a nasogastric tube. Vasopressin via an infusion may exacerbate the vasoconstriction. Desmopressin is a better anti diuretic. The aim is to achieve a 1.5–3ml urine/kg/hr output.

Haematological support

- Haematological support—coagulopathies are treated with blood products as guided by the local laboratory.

Management of the non-heart beating cadaveric donor

- NHB donors may be classified into 4 categories using the Maastricht criteria.

Category (1)	Patients dead on arrival to A&E
Category (2)	Unsuccessfully resuscitated patients
Category (3)	Patients awaiting cardiac arrest, where the treating clinicians have withdrawn treatment ('controlled' NHB donor)
Category (4)	Patients with cardiac arrest after being declared brain dead.

- Following cardiac arrest there is a stand off period (5–10min) to establish that an individual has changed from a dying patient to a donor.
- Minimising the time between death and administration of organ preservation fluid and cold storage, reduces detrimental effects on tissue viability and subsequent organ function.
- NHB donors have been mainly used for kidneys. The incidence of delayed graft function is higher in organs from NHB donors. There is no difference in long term outcome.
- Also now been used widely for livers; case reports of other organs.

Organ recipient preparation

Blood group compatible grafting is performed in heart and liver transplantation, tissue type-matched transplants are performed in all kidney and some pancreas transplants. Patients receiving a second graft must be screened for HLA antibodies whatever the organ. Investigation of patients for suitability for organ transplantation in all categories should include the following investigations:

- Full blood count and coagulation screen
- Blood group and antibody screen
- Urea and electrolytes
- Liver function tests
- Glucose and lipid profiles
- Hepatitis B, C, and HIV
- Cytomegalovirus (CMV), herpes simplex virus (HSV) and Epstein–Barr virus (EBV) status
- Chest X-ray
- Electrocardiogram
- MSU/sputum for culture and sensitivity
- Tissue typing—the recipient's lymphocytes are used to type the human leucocyte antigens (HLA) A, B, and DR.
- Detection of pre-formed anti-HLA antibodies in the serum. Performed against a panel of donors whilst on the waiting list, to detect sensitisation (panel reactivity) and immediately pre-transplant (crossmatch against the donor) in most cases. Sensitisation to foreign-HLA may occur by pregnancy, blood transfusion, or previous HLA mismatched transplantation.

Contra indications to organ transplantation
- Multi organ failure
- On-going sepsis
- 'Current' malignancy

Immunosuppression

- Drugs used in combination to provide optimal prophylaxis against rejection
- Ideally tailored to the specific requirements of both patient and organ graft.

Corticosteroids (e.g. prednisolone)

- Anti-inflammatory and immunosuppressive properties. Inhibit gene transcription of interleukin 1 (IL-1) and tumour necrosis factor (TNF). Non specific effects on immune response include lymphopenia and inhibition of monocyte migration. Induction dose (0.25mg/kg/day) then reducing dose (0–0.1mg/kg/day). Intravenous doses of methylprednisolone (500mg tds) used as first line treatment for acute rejection episodes.
- Side-effects: iatrogenic cushingoid syndrome, glucose intolerance, hypertension, osteoporosis, aseptic necrosis of femoral head.

Immunophillin binders: calcineurin inhibitors (e.g. cycoclosporin, tacrolimus)

- Cyclosporin binds to cyclophilin, and tacrolimus binds to FK-binding proteins. Leads to inhibition of the intracellular enzyme calcineurin, essential for the transcription of cytokines (IL-2, IL-4, interferon gamma and TNF-α). Inhibit T cell function. Induction dose (cyclosporin 12mg/kg/day; tacrolimus 0.15 mg/kg/day) then reduction to a maintenance level (ciclosporin 3–5mg/kg/day; tacrolimus 0.05–0.1mg/kg/day). Monitoring required (trough or levels 2 hours post dose).
- Side-effects: nephrotoxicity, neurotoxicity, impaired glucose metaboilism, hypertension, hypercholesterolaemia, gastrointestinal disturbance, hirsuitism, ginigival hyperplasia.

Immunophillin binders: non-calcineurin inhibitors (e.g. sirolimus)

- Binds FK-binding protein but does not inhibit calcineurin. Complex of drug and immunophilin acts on TOR (target of rapamycin) proteins and inhibits P7056 kinase which prevents the cell from moving G1 phase of the cell cycle. Prevents T cell proliferation in response to activation.
- Side-effects: thrombocytopaenia, hyperlipidaemia. Impaired wound healing. Possible increase incidence of lymphocoeles in renal transplantation.

Antimetabolites: (1) Azathioprine

- Metabolised in the liver to the active agent 6-mercaptopurine. Inhibits de novo purine synthesis, thus impair DNA synthesis and cellular proliferation. Dose 1–2mg/kg/day, monitor FBC.
- Side-effects: bone marrow suppression, hepatotoxicity, gastrointestinal disturbance, pancreatitis.

Antimetabolites: (2) Mycophenolate mofetil (MMF)

- Inhibits enzyme inosine monophosphate dehydrogenase (IMPDH), which is needed by activated lymphocytes to synthesise guanosine nucleotides and clonally expand. Most other cell types can bypass this pathway, so drug is selective for lymphocytes. Dose 1–2g/kg/day in divided doses, monitor FBC.
- Side-effects: Gastrointestinal side-effects (diarrhoea, gastritis, vomiting), bone marrow suppression.

Antibodies: polyclonal (e.g. ATG, ALG)

- Antibody binds to lymphocytes, which are cleared from the circulation, producing a profound drop in lymphocyte count. Used for induction therapy at transplantation or treatment of rejection. Monitor using absolute lymphocyte counts.
- Side-effects: Allergic reaction, thrombocytopaenia.

Antibodies: monoclonal (1) Anti CD3 (e.g. OKT3)

- OKT3 causes the T-cell receptor to be lost from the surface, and prevents T-cell activation. Used for induction therapy/treatment of rejection. Monitor using absolute lymphocyte counts.
- Side-effects: Non-cardiogenic pulmonary oedema, encephalopathy, aseptic meningitis, nephrotoxicity, high risk lymphoproliferative disease.

Antibodies: monoclonal (2) Anti-IL-2R (e.g. Basiliximab, Daclizumab)

Binds IL-2 receptor (CD25) and thus prevents the IL-2 driven proliferation of activated lymphocytes.

Important side effects of immunosuppression

Infection

Increased susceptibility to all infections.
- Opportunistic e.g. *Pneumocystis carinii* (*jiroveci*).
- Cytomegalovirus (CMV):
  - Transmitted within the graft. The latent virus may be activated and produce CMV disease particularly in CMV negative recipients.
  - Prophylaxis given using Acyclovir or Gancyclovir (6–12 weeks).
  - Patients treated with antibody therapy to combat rejection are most at risk of CMV disease.
  - Present with fever, respiratory symptoms, gastrointestinal disease and infection of the allograft with dysfunction. Renders the host more susceptible to opportunistic infection.
  - Treat with IV Ganciclovir and usually requires withdrawal of immunosuppression.
- Epstein–Barr Virus (EBV): active replication of virus predisposes to post-transplant lymphoproliferative disease (PTLD).

Malignancy
- Common neoplasms (e.g. breast, lung, colon) do not occur more frequently in transplant recipients. Neoplasms of the skin and lymphoid tissue are more common.
- Skin cancers are the most common malignant conditions in transplant recipients.
  - Basal cell carcinoma is seen 10 times more frequently than the general population.
  - Squamous cell carcinomas, which account for 90% of skin cancers in transplant patients, occur 65–250 times more in this population.
- PTLD
  - Occurs in around 2% of patients post-transplantation often within a year of transplantation. More common with more aggressive immunosuppressive regimens and in children.
  - The tumours are initially confined to the graft and are B-cell non-Hodgkin lymphomas. Often resistant to treatment with a high mortality.

Kidney transplantation

Indications

- Treatment of choice for end-stage renal failure. Recipients having a greater survival and improved quality of life. More cost effective than dialysis.
- Patients suitable for kidney transplantation are usually already established on dialysis. Transplantation pre-empting dialysis is becoming more common.
- Organs shared regionally and nationally, co-ordinated by UK Transplant. Selection of the most suitable recipient is primarily based on tissue matching of the HLA A, B, and DR antigens between the donor and recipient. Discrimination between equally matched pairs is performed using a scoring system based on age, matching, known sensitization of recipients to HLA antigens, and length of time on waiting list.
- Transplantation is only undertaken following a negative cytotoxic cross match between the donor cells and recipient serum.

Living donor kidney transplantation

- 361 (6.3 per million population) live donor kidney transplants performed in the UK in 2002, an increase of nearly 10% on the previous year.
- Long term outcomes in live donor kidney transplants are better than cadaveric.
- Immunosuppression now enables transplants to be safely performed in tissue-type mismatched individuals and an increase in unrelated living donors.

Organ retrieval—living donor: open donor nephrectomy

Incision

Flank incision at the level of the 12th rib. Preserve the lower rib as the incidence of wound pain is less.

Procedure

- Approach the kidney extra-peritoneally. Open Gerota's fascia and mobilise the kidney using blunt and sharp dissection to facilitate an extra-capsular dissection.
- Carefully dissect the hilum and identify the renal vessels. Preoperative imaging is helpful to determine both the number of renal arteries and to identify any extra-renal branches of vein or artery which may be encountered at this point.
- Dissect the ureter with preservation of the peri-ureteric fat and thus its blood supply. Divide the renal vessels to give adequate length for transplantation.

Complications

- The risks of death or major morbidity to the kidney donor have been estimated in the era of open surgery to be 0.03% and 0.23% respectively.
- Most common complications are respiratory (atelectasis, pneumonia and pneumothorax) and infective (wound and urinary tract).

Organ retrieval living donor: minimally invasive donor nephrectomy (MIDN)

MIDN may be performed by hand-assisted or total laparoscopic approach.

Position

In the transperitoneal laparoscopic technique, the patient is placed in a modified lateral decubitus position.

Procedure

- Establish four ports (iliac fossa, xiphoid, epigastric, and mid-axillary).
- Mobilise the colon and expose the kidney by a medial approach through Gerota's fascia. Dissect and divide the ureter.
- Expose the renal vein and artery and ligate tributaries by clips.
- Make a small 6–12cm lower umbilical incision to enable the kidney to be delivered.
- Divide the renal artery and vein using an endovascular stapling device and the kidney removed.

The hand assisted approach involves use of a hand-port device via the lower umbilical incision.

Advantages (cf. open): reduced recipient hospital stay; analgesia requirements and time off work.

Disadvantages (cf. open): longer graft warm ischaemia time and operating time.

Overall: donor and recipient outcomes appear to be similar.

Cadaveric organ retrieval

In multi-organ retrievals the kidneys are removed last. Both kidneys are removed en bloc and then separated on the bench.

- Divide the aorta in the posterior midline and the long left renal vein with a cuff of IVC.

The rest of the preparation is undertaken at the transplant centre. This involves the removal of the adrenal gland and perinephric tissue, and ligation of vessels not supplying the kidney. A Carrel patch of vena cava or aorta may be left around the renal vessels for anastomosis.

Ischaemic time, storage, and preservation

- Warm ischaemia is defined as the period from cessation of circulation until perfusion of the organ with cold perfusion fluid.
- The cold ischaemic time is defined as the time from cold perfusion to establishment of the new circulation within the transplant. The viability time of a kidney in simple cold storage is variable. 26 hours between explantation and implantation is recognised as being the maximum storage time if good immediate function is to be achieved.

Transplantation

- Antibiotic prophylaxis is important and immunosuppression is started perioperatively.
- The kidney is placed heterotopically into the iliac fossa using an extra peritoneal approach. The renal vessels are anastomosed to the external iliac vessels. The internal iliac artery end-to-end anastomosis has

been abandoned due to the significant incidence of postoperative erectile dysfunction. The ureter is anastomosed to the bladder which is close by. The ureter may be stented, depending on surgical preference.

- Preoperative native nephrectomy is rarely needed. It is considered for continued/recurrent urinary infection, tuberculosis of kidney, or massive polycystic kidney disease and uncontrolled hypertension.

Surgical complications

Vascular complications

- Graft thrombosis (renal vein thrombosis: 0.9–7.6%; renal artery thrombosis: 0.9–3.5%) results in pain, graft swelling and oliguria. Transplant nephrectomy is usually required.
- Stenosis (1.6–12%) of the renal artery presents initially with hypertension and progressing to graft dysfunction. Doppler ultrasound is the first line investigation. Treatment of arterial stenoses is by percutaneous transluminal angioplasty. Anastomotic stenoses are more safely treated by open surgery with a skip vein bypass graft.

Urological complications

- Urinary leaks (3%) may present with pain around the graft; a boggy swelling over the pubis; excessive wound drainage (high fluid creatinine to plasma creatinine ratio); reduced function or by ultrasound-detected perinephric collections. Small urinary leaks may be treated conservatively; larger leaks from ureteric necrosis, usually associated with damaged discrete lower pole vessels, require surgery (re-implantation, uretero-uretostomy, uretero-pyelostomy or Boari flap).
- Ureteric stenosis (6%) usually occurs distally and presents with oliguria and allograft dysfunction. Ultrasound shows hydronephrosis. ≥40% present more than 1 year following transplantation. Often associated with vessel occlusion concomitant with severe graft rejection episodes. Initial management of the obstructed kidney requires nephrostomy. Definitive management of the stenosis may be endoscopic or open.

Other complications

- Lymphocoele (0.6–18%). Result from damage to lymphatics surrounding the iliac vessels. Presents with pain, leg swelling, lower urinary tract symptoms, ureteric obstruction, or even vascular compression and thrombosis. Management options include percutaneous drainage ± sclerosant injection, or surgical marsupialization into the peritoneal cavity.

Rejection and function

- **Graft function** is monitored by daily urea and creatinine.
- **Delayed graft function** (DGF): the need for dialysis within the first week of transplantation. It should not be confused with primary non-function—defined as a graft which has never worked.
- **Causes for DGF:** acute tubular necrosis (secondary to the preservation injury), acute rejection, vascular thrombosis, and drug nephrotoxicity.

- **Investigations:** renal Doppler and ultrasound scanning. Flow is confirmed in transplanted vein and artery (usually intra-renal arcuate vessels) and overall graft resistive index (RI) calculated. RI is a non-specific measurement calculated as the difference in peak systolic and end-diastolic velocities, divided by the peak systolic velocity. The RI is normally less than 0.7. An RI >0.8 suggests rejection.
- **Management of DGF:** avoid use of nephrotoxic immunosuppressant drugs. Maintain adequate fluid balance.
- **Acute rejection** usually occurs in the first 3 months and affects up to 30% of kidney transplant recipients. The vast majority resolve with treatment.
- **Presentation:** asymptomatic, allograft dysfunction. Diagnosis is confirmed on biopsy. These are graded histologically using the Banff criteria.
- **Management:** parenteral steroid (IV methylprednisolone 500mg x 3 daily doses) and further immunosuppression, usually antibody therapy, if required.
- **Chronic allograft nephropathy** (CAN) is the result of both immune and non-immune factors. CAN is the major cause of long term declining graft function and eventual loss. 27–40% of all failed grafts between 1–3 years are due to CAN. Histological findings include tubular atrophy, interstitial fibrosis, intimal hyperplasia and glomerulo-sclerosis.

Graft and patient survival

- 1, 3 and 5 year allograft survival rates are approximately 90%, 80%, and 70% respectively.
- Graft survival is influenced by numerous factors including donor type (living versus cadaver) and HLA-mismatching. The 10 year graft survival is greater for kidneys from living donors (53–57%) compared to cadaveric organs (38%). 5 year patient survival is 90% and 80% for recipients of living donor and cadaveric kidneys respectively.

Pancreas transplantation

Solid organ pancreas transplantation

Indications

- Simultaneous pancreas–kidney transplantation (SPK) or pancreas after kidney transplantation (PAK) is indicated for diabetic patients in end-stage renal failure. Pancreas transplantation alone (PTA) is indicated in those patients who have hypoglycaemic unawareness, and/or aggressive non-renal complications of diabetes, e.g. neuropathy.
- The majority of transplants performed are SPK, with between 10% and 15% being either PAK or PTA.
- Most pancreases used for transplantation are cadaveric; a few centres worldwide have living donor programmes, using distal pancreatectomy.
- ≥14 000 transplants have been performed in the USA, with 1362 performed in 2001. Only 82 SPK transplants were performed in the UK in 2001.

Organ retrieval

- Harvest the pancreas as either a segment (tail and body) or whole organ with a cuff of duodenum.
- Carry out bench work at organ retrieval. Anastomose splenic and superior mesenteric arteries to a donor iliac artery bifurcated Y graft, which enables the arterial supply of the graft to be facilitated by a single anastomosis at transplantation.

Transplantation

- The technique associated with least complications involves transplantation into the opposite iliac fossa to the kidney (for SPK transplantation) using very similar extra-peritoneal techniques.
- The venous drainage of the pancreas is usually systemic (external iliac vein), and the drainage of exocrine function is to the bladder. Bladder drained exocrine secretions cause chemical cystitis or metabolic acidosis, and this requires changing the method of drainage. Portal venous drainage via a mesenteric vein is performed in less than 20% of transplants.
- Achieve enteric exocrine drainage via a Roux-en-Y loop of small intestine. Exocrine leakage of the enterically drained graft gives rise to peritonitis, intra-abdominal sepsis and the need for re-laparotomy in up to 70%.

Surgical complications

- Re-laparotomy within 3 months   15–35% in most large series
- Intra-abdominal sepsis   10–20%
- Pancreatitis   2–3%
- Exocrine leak rates   10%
- Vascular graft thrombosis   2–14%.

Rejection and function

- Rejection may cause graft loss due to difficulty in detection. Immunological damage to the pancreas is advanced before changes in blood sugar are recognised.

- Monitoring graft function in transplants drained by the bladder is performed by urinary amylase. C peptide/insulin levels also used as markers of function. In SPK transplants, kidney rejection is usually accompanied by rejection in the pancreas.

Graft and patient survival

- 1 year patient survival as 94–95% for SPK, 95–100% for PAK, and 97% for PTA. Graft survival at 1 year is 82–83% for SPK, 64–79% PAK, and 54–78% for PTA.
- 3 year graft/patient survival rates are approximately 83%/89% for SPK/PAK, and 60%/86% for PTA.

Pancreatic islet cell transplantation

In view of the surgical complications of solid organ transplantation the use of isolated pancreatic islets alone appears an attractive option.

Technique

- Islets comprise only 2% of solid pancreatic mass. These insulin-secreting cells must be isolated from the tissue. Cell isolation involves enzymatic digestion, mechanical disruption and purification using density gradients. Currently only a proportion of available islets are able to be isolated. This can provide 500 000 islet equivalent units, depending on the mass of the donor.
- Freshly isolated islets are infused via the radiologically cannulated portal vein (percutaneous transhepatic approach). This is done as a day case procedure.

Complications

Portal vein thrombosis (≤2%). Bleeding (requiring transfusion 5%).

Graft and patient survival

- Between 1989 and 1999, 267 adult patients received islet cell transplants; <10% were insulin-independent 1 year later.
- In 2000, the Edmonton group reported a series of islet cell transplants in 7 patients, all of whom were insulin independent at 1 year.
- Improvements were due to better islet cell isolation, steroid free immunosuppression and an increase in the total number of islets transplanted (average of 800 000 islets) by performing multiple transplants as necessary. By 2002, over 40 patients have received transplants (82% insulin independent at 1 year). A multi-centre trial is examining whether the results can be successfully replicated.
- The long term outcome of islet cell transplantation is unknown. The impact on secondary complications of diabetes is under review.

Liver transplantation

Indications

- Patients with acute or chronic end-stage liver disease may be considered.
- *Adults*: primary biliary cirrhosis; sclerosing cholangitis; alcoholic liver disease (active alcohol abuse is an absolute contraindication); cryptogenic cirrhosis; chronic active (autoimmune) hepatitis; chronic viral hepatitis (including hepatitis B and C); α-1-antitrypsin deficiency and drug induced hepatic failure. Liver transplantation may be considered as treatment for primary hepatocellular carcinoma.
- *Children*: biliary atresia, in-born errors of metabolism (Wilson's disease; α-1-antitrypsin deficiency; haemochromatosis), and idiopathic fulminant hepatic failure.
- Listing and timing patients in the UK is determined by the availability of organs. Timing of transplantation in chronic liver disease is ideally when there is <50% 2 year survival, without multisystem disease. Often patients are referred for transplantation late, once life threatening complications have developed (e.g. variceal haemorrhage, encephalopathy, spontaneous bacterial peritonitis), and quality of life has deteriorated considerably.
- The Child–Turcotte–Pugh score may be used as a prognostic tool, as shown below.

	1 point	2 points	3 points
Bilirubin (μmol/L)	<34	34–51	>51
Albumin (g/L)	>35	28–35	<28
Prothrombin time (seconds prolonged)	1–3	4–6	>6
Ascites	None	Slight	Moderate
Encephalopathy grade	None	I–II	III–IV

- The score is classified as A (5–6), B (7–9) or C (10–15). Patients with grade B have an 80% 5 year survival, whilst one third of patients with grade C die within 1 year.
- For patients with fulminant hepatic failure, King's College London has developed guidelines to determine when transplantation is indicated. Patients falling into these criteria have a high mortality without transplantation.

- Non-paracetamol   Prothrombin time (PT) >100 sec
  Or any 3 of the following:
  Age <10 or >40 years
  Aetiology: drug induced or nonA/nonB hepatitis
  PT >50 sec
  Bilirubin >300µmol/L
  >7 days of jaundice, prior to encephalopathy
- Paracetamol   Arterial pH <7.30
  Or all of the following:
  PT >100 sec
  Creatinine >300µmol/L
  Grade III/IV encephalopathy
- 698 cadaveric liver transplants were performed in UK (2002); 92 of these recipients being under 17 years of age.

Organ retrieval

- Cannulate both the aorta and the portal system via the superior mesenteric vein. Perfuse the portal system with cold University of Wisconsin solution and perfuse the arterial vasculature with Marshall's hypertonic citrate.
- Divide the common bile duct superior to the pancreas. Return the coeliac artery and an aortic patch with the common hepatic artery; ligate and divide all other branches.
- Divide the vena cava above the diaphragm, and above the right kidney.
- Divide the mesenteric and splenic veins at the portal vein confluence.
- Liver preservation is in cold storage in sterile bags. The liver is transplanted within 12 hours of retrieval.

Transplantation

The recipient undergoes hepatectomy.
- Divide the common bile duct at the level of the cystic duct, and ligate the hepatic artery beyond the gastrodudodenal artery.
- Prepare the portal vein to allow the placement of the patient on veno-venous bypass; cannulate the portal circulation and infra-hepatic systemic venous circulation (saphenofemoral vein) and blood returned to the heart by the axillary vein. Once bypass is established remove the liver and divide the caval attachments.
- Piggy-back transplantation involves preservation of the recipient vena cava, and division of the retro-hepatic veins.
- Anastomose the supra and infra hepatic vena cava followed by the portal vein. Following washout of air and preservation fluid the liver is reperfused by the portal system. Anastomose the hepatic artery end-to-end. Perform donor cholecystectomy and an end-to-end chole-docho-choledochostomy is performed over a T tube.

Split liver transplantation

First performed in 1988; allows a single donor liver to be divided for use in two recipients, and thus maximise the potential of donated organs.

- The segmental vascular and biliary anatomy of the liver allows the liver to be split typically into right (segments IV–VIII or V–VIII based on drainage by middle and right hepatic veins) and left lateral grafts (II–III or II–IV based on left hepatic vein drainage). The right graft is suitable for an adult, whilst the smaller left lateral graft is used for paediatric recipients.
- The liver may be split on the back table (ex-vivo) or in situ. Initial results showed increased incidence of primary non-function, biliary complications, and bleeding from cut surfaces. Increased experience and selective use of appropriate grafts have resulted in 1 year graft and patient survival of 88% and 90% respectively (Kings College Hospital, UK).

Surgical complications

Vascular: hepatic artery thrombosis is more common in paediatric than adult (1.6–10%) recipients. Presentation may vary from initial symptom. Early thrombosis demands surgical correction. Many adults require re-transplantation, particularly if presentation is late. The paediatric group may develop collaterals and not require re-transplantation. Venous thrombosis (1–2%) and haemorrhage may also occur.

Biliary: biliary obstruction 12–15% is generally dealt with non-operatively (ERCP and stenting, or PTC). Failure of initial treatment may require surgical reconstruction or re-transplantation. Bile leaks may present with non-specific symptoms of sepsis and abdominal pain, often in association with deranged LFTs. Bile leak may be secondary to ischaemic necrosis due to hepatic artery thrombosis and this must be excluded. Management is by percutaneous drainage ± re-laparotomy.

Rejection and function

- Monitoring is by liver function tests, coagulation tests and bile production. Function may be poor in the first week (IPF—initial poor function). Primary non-function (PNF) occurs in 2–10%, and requires immediate re-transplantation.
- Acute rejection occurs in up to 50% of patients and may lead to graft loss. Most episodes occur in the first month post transplantation. Presentation is non-specific and includes fever, graft tenderness/ enlargement and abnormal liver function tests. Biopsy is required for firm diagnosis. Treatment is by IV steroids. Chronic rejection is less common, presenting with progressive organ dysfunction often after repeated acute rejection episodes.

Graft and patient survival

1, 3 and 5 year graft survival for liver transplants performed in the U 80%, 73% and 64% respectively (1994–9 cohort). UNOS data gives 1 ar 3 year patient survival at 85% and 78%.

Cardiac transplantation

Indications

- Indications: cardiomyopathy, coronary artery disease, valvular disease, and congenital heart disease. Most patients have end-stage cardiac failure resulting from a dilated myopathy.
- Preoperative work up is extensive in both physical and psychological terms. All conventional treatment options for heart failure must be exhausted. Non cardiac co-morbidity must also be thoroughly assessed.
- Most candidates are New York Heart Association grade IV—equating to <50% 2 year life expectancy. Cardiac catheterisation provides confirmation of poor left ventricular ejection fraction (usually <20%) and a suitable pulmonary vascular resistance (<240–300 dynes/cm^5) for transplantation.
- Cardiac transplantation is contra-indicated in patients with pulmonary hypertension as this may lead to post operative right heart failure.
- Numbers of patients waiting and the number of heart-only transplants performed have declined gradually since 1992 (UK). In 2002, 157 heart-only transplants were performed, with 111 patients left on the waiting list.

Retrieval

- Donors are ideally ≤45 years of age with no previous cardiac history, requiring minimal inotropic support. Shortage of organs has meant donors of 45–65 years with acceptable echocardiography ± cardiac catheterisation are considered. Size matching of the graft is important for anatomical and physiological purposes.
- At the donor heart excision the heart is perfused with cold St. Thomas's cardioplegic solution and cardiac arrest occurs is diastole. The heart is stored in normal saline on ice and implantation performed as early as practicable. A cold ischaemic time of <4 hours is acceptable.
- A 'domino' heart transplant occurs when a viable heart from a patient receiving a heart/lungs transplant is then transplanted into another patient.

Transplantation

- The normal mode of transplantation is orthotopic. Heterotopic transplantation is rarely performed. There are two types of orthotopic transplantation commonly described: standard and bicaval. Most centres now the bicaval technique.
- The recipient is anaesthetised once the heart is in transit to the recipient hospital. Orthotopic transplantation involves full cardio-pulmonary bypass and explantation of the native heart. In the bicaval technique the right and left atrium are excised to leave only cuffs around the vena cava and pulmonary veins respectively. Transect the left and right pulmonary veins of the donor heart within the pericardial sac, but the left atrium left intact. Perform anastomosis between the cuffs of tissue around the right and left pulmonary veins in the recipient and the

- Infection is another major cause, particularly opportunistic respiratory pathogens such as CMV or pneumocystis. Prophylaxis against pneumocystis is given indefinitely.
- Airway complications occur in approximately 10–15%. Tracheal ischaemia may result in leak and mediastinitis.

Rejection and function
- Rejection episodes present similar to infection (fever/hypoxia/chest X-ray changes). Distinction is made by performing by transbronchial biopsy (bronchoscopic) and broncho alveolar lavage.
- Obliterative bronchiolitis occurs in 20–40% of lung recipients and is a major cause of morbidity. It presents with dyspnoea and a progressive obstructive airways disease. The mechanism is unknown, but rejection episodes increase the risk of disease.

Graft and patient survival
The patient survival rates in UK for lung-only transplants (performed between 1994 and 1999) are 67% at 1 year, 57% at 3 years, and 42% at 5 years. Heart/lung transplant results are similar.

Index